Current Topics in Pathology
80

Managing Editors

C.L. Berry E. Grundmann

Biological Characterization of Bone Tumors

Contributors

J. Althoff · D.B.v. Bassewitz · A. Bosse
V. Bouropoulou · J.J. Brooks · W. Dierschauer
G. Edel · E. Grundmann · A. Härle · W. Hiddemann
H.J. Höhling · N. Jiang · G. Jundt · M. Kolve
V.A. LiVolsi · W. Mellin · P. Quint · A. Roessner
A. Schulz · F. Sim · C. Sorg · T. Spelsberg
G.C. Steiner · J.Q. Trojanowski · E. Vollmer
L.E. Wold · P. Wuisman · G. Zwadlo

Editor

A. Roessner

Springer-Verlag Berlin Heidelberg NewYork
London Paris Tokyo Hong Kong

A. ROESSNER, Prof. Dr., Gerhard-Domagk-Institut für Pathologie der Universität, Domagkstraße 17, D-4400 Münster

C.L. BERRY, Prof. Dr., Department of Morbid Anatomy, The London Hospital Medical College, Whitechapel, London E1 1BB, Great Britain

E. GRUNDMANN, Prof. Dr., Gerhard-Domagk-Institut für Pathologie der Universität, Domagkstraße 17, D-4400 Münster

With 119 Figures, Some in Color

ISBN-13:978-3-642-74464-8 e-ISBN-13:978-3-642-74462-4
DOI: 10.1007/978-3-642-74462-4

Library of Congress Cataloging-in-Publication Data. Biological characterization of bone tumors/ contributors, J. Althoff ... [et al.]; editor, A. Roessner. p. cm. – (Current topics in pathology; 80) Includes index. ISBN-13:978-3-642-74464-8(U.S.:alk.paper) 1. Bones–Tumors–Histopathology. 2. Bones – Tumors – Diagnosis. 3. Diagnosis immunohistochemistry. I. Althoff, J. II. Roessner, Albert. III. Series: Current topics in pathology; v. 80. [DNLM: 1. Bone Neoplasms – pathology. W1 CU821H v. 80/WE 258 B615] RB1.E6 vol. 80 [RC280.B6] 616.07 s – dc20 [616.99'27107] DNLM/DLC for Library of Congress 89-11546 CIP

Softcover reprint of the hardcover 1st edition 1989

2122/3130-543210 – Printed on acid-free paper

List of Contributors

Althoff, J., Dr.	Institut für Medizinische Physik, Abt. Mikroanalytik, Schmeddingstraße 50, D-4400 Münster
Bassewitz, D.B.v., Prof. Dr.	Gerhard-Domagk-Institut für Pathologie der WWU, Domagkstraße 17, D-4400 Münster
Bosse, A., Dr.	Gerhard-Domagk-Institut für Pathologie der WWU, Domagkstraße 17, D-4400 Münster
Bouropoulou, V., MD	Department of Pathology, Apostle Paul Hospital, 4 Artemidos Street, Ag. Stefanos, GR-145 65, Greece
Brooks, J.J., MD	Surgical Pathology Section Hospital of the University of Pennsylvania, 3400 Spruce Street, Philadelphia, PA 19104, USA
Dierschauer, W.	Gerhard-Domagk-Institut für Pathologie der WWU, Domagkstraße 17, D-4400 Münster
Edel, G., Prof. Dr.	Gerhard-Domagk-Institut für Pathologie der WWU, Domagkstraße 17, D-4400 Münster
Grundmann, E., Prof. Dr.	Gerhard-Domagk-Institut für Pathologie der WWU, Domagkstraße 17, D-4400 Münster
Härle, A., Prof. Dr.	Orthopädische Klinik der WWU, Albert-Schweitzer-Straße 33, D-4400 Münster
Hiddemann, W., Prof. Dr.	Med. Klinik Abt. A der WWU, Albert-Schweitzer-Straße 33, D-4400 Münster
Höhling, H.J., Prof. Dr.	Institut für Medizinische Physik, Abt. Mikroanalytik, Schmeddingstraße 50, D-4400 Münster

JIANG, N., MD	Department of Pathology, Mayo Clinic and Mayo Foundation, Rochester, MN 55905, USA
JUNDT, G., Dr.	Zentrum für Pathologie, Klinikum der Universität, Langhansstraße 10, D-6300 Gießen
KOLVE, M., Dr.	Gerhard-Domagk-Institut für Pathologie der WWU, Domagkstraße 17, D-4400 Münster
LIVOLSI, V.A., MD	Surgical Pathology Section Hospital of the University of Pennsylvania, 3400 Spruce Street, Philadelphia, PA 19104, USA
MELLIN, W., Dr.	Gerhard-Domagk-Institut für Pathologie der WWU, Domagkstraße 17, D-4400 Münster
QUINT, P., Dr.	Institut für Medizinische Physik, Abt. Mikroanalytik, Schmeddingstraße 50, D-4400 Münster
ROESSNER, A., Prof. Dr.	Gerhard-Domagk-Institut für Pathologie der WWU, Domagkstraße 17, D-4400 Münster
SCHULZ, A., Prof. Dr.	Zentrum für Pathologie, Klinikum der Universität, Langhansstraße 10, D-6300 Gießen
SIM, F., MD	Department of Pathology, Mayo Clinic and Mayo Foundation, Rochester, MN 55905, USA
SORG, C., Prof. Dr.	Institut für Experimentelle Dermatologie der WWU, Von-Esmarch-Straße 56, D-4400 Münster
SPELSBERG, T., MD	Department of Pathology, Mayo Clinic and Mayo Foundation, Rochester, MN 55905, USA
STEINER, G.C., MD	Department of Pathology, Hospital for Joint Diseases, Orthopaedic Institute, 301 East 17th Street, New York, NY 10003, USA

Trojanowski, J.Q., MD	Surgical Pathology Section Hospital of the University of Pennsylvania, 3400 Spruce Street, Philadelphia, PA 19104, USA
Vollmer, E., Dr. Dr.	Gerhard-Domagk-Institut für Pathologie der WWU, Domagkstraße 17, D-4400 Münster
Wold, L.E., MD	Department of Pathology, Mayo Clinic and Mayo Foundation, Rochester, MN 55905, USA
Wuisman, P., Dr.	Orthopädische Klinik der WWU, Albert-Schweitzer-Straße 33, D-4400 Münster
Zwadlo, G., Dr.	Institut für Experimentelle Dermatologie der WWU, Von-Esmarch-Straße 56, D-4400 Münster

Preface

During the past few years, a considerable number of monographs on bone tumors have been published. They are mainly restricted to bone tumors as clinical-pathological entities, since their diagnosis, more than that of other tumors, requires the interdisciplinary cooperation between orthopedic specialist, radiologist, and pathologist. However, investigations concerning the histogenesis of bone tumors are rather limited, although they might be helpful in explaining the unique morphological heterogeneity of tumors of the skeletal system. Furthermore, the histogenetic approach in the study of bone tumors may facilitate the interpretation of the advanced cytobiological methods available for improving classification and diagnosis. Therefore, this volume presents recent pathological advances in the biological characterization of bone tumors. A major chapter deals with the differential diagnosis of Ewing's sarcoma as regards its demarcation from the so-called neuroectodermal tumor of bone.

The analysis of the ground substances in bone-forming tumors may be helpful for their classification. Therefore the volume includes a chapter on the biochemical and histochemical analysis of different osteosarcoma types. Recently it has become clear that in addition to different collagen types which are not specific for bone tissue, several bone-specific proteins occur, one of which is osteonectin. Its distribution is obviously important for the classification and diagnosis of osteoblastic tumors.

Proliferative behavior is of major importance for the diagnosis of malignant tumors. The present volume includes one contribution applying immunohistological methods and another using flow cytometry to study this problem. The results may facilitate the diagnosis of borderline malignant bone tumors.

The steroid receptors in giant cell tumor of bone have recently attracted clinical interest. This problem is discussed in an additional chapter. As is well known, the histogenesis of chordoma is peculiar and immunohistochemical methods have proved valuable for further characterizing this tumor and facilitating its differential diagnosis. Special interest is focused on the entity of chondroid chordoma.

Finally, the group of so-called fibrohistiocytic tumors has been under discussion in recent years. As several bone tumor entities belong to this group (malignant fibrous histiocytoma of bone, benign fibrous histiocytoma, giant cell tumor, nonossifying fibroma), a critical consideration of the group in the light of recent results with advanced morphological methods seems necessary.

We hope that the use of cytomorphological investigations for the biological characterization of bone tumors may improve the understanding of their morphological heterogeneity. For practical purposes, this volume offers new data on advanced morphological methods promoting the classification and diagnosis of bone tumors.

I would very much like to thank all contributors for their cooperation. Special appreciation is due to the staff of Springer-Verlag for their excellent cooperation in preparing this volume.

A. ROESSNER

Contents

Neuroectodermal Tumor Versus Ewing's Sarcoma – Immunohistochemical and Electron Microscopic Observations. With 20 Figures
G.C. STEINER 1

Immunohistological Demonstration of Osteonectin in Normal Bone Tissue and in Bone Tumors. With 12 Figures
A. SCHULZ and G. JUNDT 31

Tumor Bone Formation in Different Osteosarcomas: Topological, Biochemical, and Histochemical Analyses. With 17 Figures
J. ALTHOFF, P. QUINT, H.J. HÖHLING, A. ROESSNER, and E. GRUNDMANN 55

The Proliferation Behavior of Bone Tumors Investigated with the Monoclonal Antibody Ki-67. With 15 Figures
E. VOLLMER, A. ROESSNER, P. WUISMAN, A. HÄRLE, and E. GRUNDMANN 91

Flow Cytometric DNA Analysis of Bone Tumors. With 8 Figures
W. MELLIN, W. DIERSCHAUER, W. HIDDEMANN, A. ROESSNER, G. EDEL, P. WUISMAN, A. HÄRLE, and E. GRUNDMANN 115

Steroid Receptors and Giant Cell Tumor of Bone. With 6 Figures
L.E. WOLD, T. SPELSBERG, N. JIANG, and F. SIM 153

Chondroid Chordoma: A Low-Grade Chondrosarcoma and Its Differential Diagnosis. With 10 Figures
J.J. BROOKS, J.Q. TROJANOWSKI, and V.A. LIVOLSI 165

Immunohistochemical Investigation of Chordomas: Histogenetic and Differential Diagnostic Aspects. With 16 Figures
V. BOUROPOULOU, A. BOSSE, A. ROESSNER, E. VOLLMER, G. EDEL, P. WUISMAN, and A. HÄRLE 183

The Cytogenesis of Macrophages and Osteoclast-like Giant Cells in Bone Tumors with Special Emphasis on the So-Called Fibrohistiocytic Tumors. With 15 Figures
A. Roessner, E. Vollmer, G. Zwadlo, C. Sorg, M. Kolve, D.B. v. Bassewitz, P. Wuisman, A. Härle, and E. Grundmann 205

Subject Index 229

Indexed in ISR

Neuroectodermal Tumor Versus Ewing's Sarcoma – Immunohistochemical and Electron Microscopic Observations

G.C. STEINER

1	Introduction	1
2	Material and Methods	2
3	Ewing's Sarcoma of Bone	3
3.1	Histological Features	3
3.2	Immunohistochemistry	5
3.3	Electron Microscopy	7
4	Neuroectodermal Tumors	10
4.1	Concept and Terminology	10
4.2	Histological Features	12
4.3	Immunohistochemistry	13
4.4	Electron Microscopy	17
5	Other Small Round Cell Tumors	18
5.1	Metastatic Neuroblastoma	20
5.2	Embryonal Rhabdomyosarcoma	20
5.3	Non-Hodgkin's Lymphoma	23
6	Conclusions	24
References		26

1 Introduction

Malignant small round cell tumors of bone and soft tissue are relatively rare neoplasms of children and adolescents. Because of their similar morphological appearance, they have presented a diagnostic challenge to pathologists. The age of the patient, radiographic appearance, and site of the tumor may help in some cases to distinguish between the different categories of lesions. Ewing's sarcoma, for example, is a tumor more common in children and adolescents, producing an osteolytic destruction of bone often with soft tissue invasion (DAHLIN and UNNI 1986). Lymphoma of bone, which resembles Ewing's sarcoma radiologically, predilects adults. Embryonal rhabdomyosarcoma, which can mimic Ewing's sarcoma histologically, is a tumor of soft tissue origin.

Routine histological examination including hematoxylin and eosin, reticulin, trichrome, and glycogen stains sometimes may give adequate information to establish the correct diagnosis. However, because of their undifferentiated morphology, the study of small round cell tumors requires the application of modern techniques useful in diagnostic pathology such as immunohistochemistry and electron microscopy.

The diagnostic problems of small round cell tumors became more difficult in recent years with the description of Ewing's tumors occurring in extraosseous sites, that resemble their osseous counterparts (ANGERVAL and ENZINGER 1975; GILLESPIE et al. 1979; ENZINGER and WEISS 1983; HUNTRAKOON 1987). In addition, tumors that mimic Ewing's sarcoma in their clinical presentation and morphology were found to have neural features (SCHMIDT et al. 1982) and a presumptive neuroectodermal origin. Evidence of neural differentiation was established by the application of immunochemistry and electron microscopy, and tumors with such characteristics have been described in the soft tissue as well as in bone (VOSS et al. 1984; JAFFE et al. 1984; SCHMIDT et al. 1985). The development of these new categories of neoplasms has imposed a diagnostic challenge to the pathologist when confronted with a small round cell tumor arising in those sites. This diagnosis has clinical implications as new models of treatment using different protocols of chemotherapy are being applied to each category.

The purposes of this presentation are first, to review the current knowledge of the pathology of Ewing's sarcoma and the information obtained by the use of immunohistochemistry and electron microscopy; second, to discuss the concept of peripheral primitive neuroectodermal tumors (PNETs) in the light of new developments; third, to give a brief review of other small round cell tumors of bone and soft tissue; and finally, to offer general comments on the usefulness of immunohistochemistry and electron microscopy in the diagnosis and distinction between Ewing's sarcoma and peripheral PNET.

2 Material and Methods

All the small round cell tumors of bone from the pathology files of the Hospital for Joint Diseases Orthopaedic Institute were reviewed from 1979 to 1986. Cases were excluded in which the tissue from the biopsy or resection was inadequate for study due to small sampling or necrosis. Eighteen cases of Ewing's sarcoma, three PNETs, and one probable neuroectodermal tumor were selected for light microscopy including immunohistochemistry.

For immunohistochemistry, only paraffin blocks of tissue fixed in 10% buffered formalin were available and in some cases decalcified tissue was used for the study. The avidin-biotin-peroxidase technique was used (HSU et al. 1981).

Tissue sections were stained with polyclonal antibodies against neuron-specific enolase (NSE) and S100 protein (Dako Corp., St. Barbara, CA). In addition, monoclonal antibodies were used against leukocyte common antigen (LCA) (Dako Corp., St. Barbara, CA), vimentin (Biogenex, Dublin, CA), neurofilaments (Cambridge Res. Cambridge MA – 70 and 200 kD), cytokeratin (Becton Dickinson, Mountain View, CA – 39, 43, and 50 kD keratin), and chromogranin A (Boehringer Mannheim Bioch., Indianapolis, Ind). Pepsin digestion was used for cytokeratin and protease digestion for S100 protein to enhance the immunostaining.

For electron microscopy, well preserved tissue was available in seven Ewing's sarcomas, three PNETs, and one possible PNET. The tissue was double fixed in glutaraldehyde 3% and osmic acid 1%, both in cacodylate buffer, and then

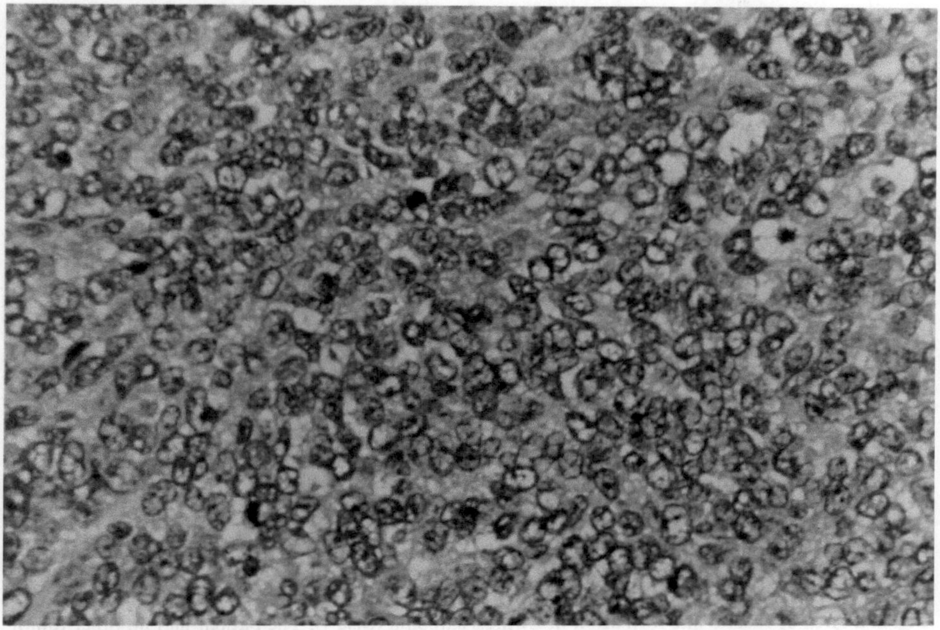

Fig. 1. Photomicrograph of Ewing's sarcoma. The tumor cells have uniform rounded nuceoli and the cell boundaries are ill-defined. There is a diffuse pattern of growth. (H&E, ×350)

it was processed in a routine fashion. The sections were stained with uranyl acetate and lead citrate and they were examined in a JEOL 100X electron microscope.

3 Ewing's Sarcoma of Bone

3.1 Histological Features

This tumor was first recognized as a clinical entity by Ewing in 1921 and 1924. Some authors in the past doubted the existence of this tumor, but there is general agreement nowadays that Ewing's sarcoma of bone is a true clinical pathological entity (JAFFE 1958; SCHAJOWICZ 1981; DAHLIN and UNNI 1986). It predilects children and adolescents and it is quite rare under the age of 5 years (DAHLIN and UNNI 1986). The most common sites in bone are femur, tibia, and humerus as well as the pelvis.

Histologically, the cells of Ewing's sarcoma are uniformly rounded with clear cytoplasm and indistinct cell boundaries (KISSANE et al. 1983). The nuclei are round with faint chromatin, inconspicuous nucleoli, and mild to moderate mitotic activity (Fig. 1) . Among the typical cells described above, small cells with denser nuclei (dark or secondary cells) are also noted (LLOMBART-BOSCH

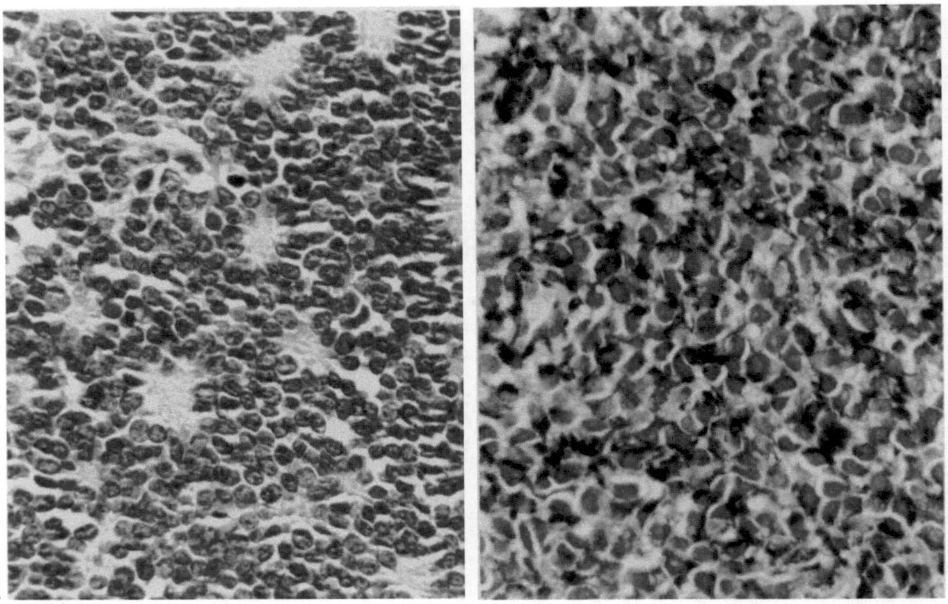

a b

Fig. 2. a Area of rosette-like formation in Ewing's sarcoma (case 4). The patient had no other tumor outside the bone. NSE was negative. (H&E, ×350). **b** Ewing's sarcoma cells showing positive reaction to vimentin in the cell cytoplasm. This reaction indicates a mesenchymal phenotype. (×400)

et al. 1982). Several microscopic patterns of growth have been described in Ewing's sarcoma such as diffuse, lobular, and organoid, the latter including the filigree pattern (Kissane et al. 1983). The diffuse growth pattern was the most common pattern observed in our material. Occasionally, the tumor cells are disposed circularly in a pseudorosette or rosette-like formation (Fig. 2a). The center of the rosette-like structures may contain degenerated and necrotic cells (Jaffe 1958) or immature connective tissue fibrils (Takahashi et al. 1976). These structure usually lack the fibrillary center that is associated with the Homer-Wright type of rosettes of neuroblastoma (Hashimoto et al. 1983). Sometimes it is histologically difficult to distinguish between the pseudorosettes of Ewing's sarcoma and those of neuroblastoma.

In addition to the classic Ewing's sarcoma described above, a small group of these lesions has been classified as atypical or large cell Ewing's sarcoma (Nascimento et al. 1980; Llombart-Bosch et al. 1982). They differ from the classic Ewing's tumor because the cells are larger, more irregular, and pleomorphic with often prominent nucleoli. The clinical presentation and behaviour are similar to the classic Ewing's sarcoma (Nascimento et al. 1980).

Reticulin fibers are seen only occasionally around some cells of Ewing's sarcoma and usually they are present around the vascular component or in the fibrous septae. Glycogen is present frequently in substantial amounts in at least 50% of cases fixed in formalin (Kissane et al. 1983). We found, like others, that tissue fixation in alcohol and particularly imprint preparations can demonstratet glycogen in a higher percentage of cases (SCHAJOWICZ 1981; YUNIS 1986). In our experience, the glycogen content is only partially affected by chemotherapy treatment of the tumor. Because a substantial number of Ewing's sarcomas lack glycogen, the absence of glycogen in a primary round cell tumor of bone does not preclude the diagnosis of Ewing's sarcoma.

Ewing's sarcoma lacks a specific enzyme pattern characteristic of this lesion (JEFFREE 1973; TAKAHASHI et al. 1976; POVYSIL and MATEJOWSKY 1977; LLOMBART-BOSCH et al. 1982; NAVAS-PALACIOS et al. 1984). This tumor is known to produce in tissue culture collagen types I, III and IV, and these collagen profiles led some authors to conclude that Ewing's sarcoma derives from multipotential primitive mesenchymal cells (DICKMAN et al. 1982). However, other authors found that collagen was restricted only to the stroma and they considered that collagen analysis is not useful to distinguish Ewing's sarcoma from other round cell tumors (HARVEY et al. 1982). Chromosomal studies have demonstrated translocations between chromosomes 11 and 22 and trisomy 8 (MALETZ et al. 1986). The former abnormality has been consistently described in Ewing's sarcoma, but it is also found in peripheral neuroepithelioma and it is probably not a diagnostic feature of Ewing's sarcoma (MALETZ et al. 1986).

3.2 Immunohistochemistry

Our experience and that of others has demonstrated that most Ewing's sarcoma cells lack the surface markers characteristic of hemopoietic cells such as LCA and immunoglobulins (NAVAS-PALACIOS et al. 1984; LONING et al. 1985; MIERAU et al. 1985). Only two of our cases (Table 1) showed LCA reaction in a small number of tumor cells. Similarly, immunomarkers that identified histiocytes (lysozyme, AIAT, and AIACT) and muscle (myosin, myoglobin, desmin) were all negative (MIETTINEN et al. 1982; NAVAS-PALACIOS et al. 1984; MIERAU et al. 1985). Recently, however, some macrophage markers were described as being present in Ewing's sarcoma (LONING et al. 1985; LLOMBART-BOSCH et al. 1986). While factor VIII–related antigen has been found to be negative (MIETTINEN et al. 1982; NAVAS-PALACIOS 1984), some authors found it to be positive in some Ewing's sarcoma cells (ROESSNER et al. 1982).

Neuron-specific enolase is negative in typical examples of Ewing's sarcoma (MIERAU et al. 1985; MOLL et al. 1987). With few exceptions, NSE was negative in our series (Table 1). Cases 2 and 5 showed a questionable focal positive reaction. The strong background staining made difficult the interpretation of the results. This problem has also been observed by others (THOMAS et al. 1987). A positive NSE reaction usually excludes a Ewing's sarcoma and categorizes the lesion most likely as a neuroectodermal tumor. One case in our files that clinically, histologically, and by electron microscopy had features of Ewing's sarcoma, showed a positive NSE reaction. This case is considered to be a probable PNET and is discussed later (see Fig. 17).

Vimentin, which is an intermediate filament associated with mesenchymal derivation, is present in Ewing's sarcoma (Fig. 2b). In our experience, staining

Table 1. Ewing's sarcoma of bone: clinical data and immunohistochemistry

Case	Sex/age	Site	Vimentin	Cytokeratin	LCA	NSE	Neuro-filaments
1	17M	Scapula	20%–30% positive cells	NEG.	NEG.	NEG.	NEG.
2	13F	Clavicle	NEG.	Rare positive cells	NEG.	±[a]	NEG.
3	11F	Rib	10%–20% positive cells	NEG.	NEG.	NEG.	NEG.
4	11M	Clavicle	NEG.	NEG.	NEG.	NEG.	NEG.
5	14M	Fibula	1%–5% positive cells	NEG.	NEG.	±[a]	NEG.
6	8F	Femur	10%–20% positive cells	NEG.	NEG.	NEG.	NEG.
7	11M	Clavicle	1%–5% positive cells	NEG.	NEG.	NEG.	NEG.
8	15M	Ilium	NEG.	NEG.	Rare positive cells	NEG.	NEG.
9	17F	Ilium	Rare positive cells	NEG.	NEG.	NEG.	NEG.
10	39F	Fibula	1%–5% positive cells	NEG.	NEG.	NEG.	NEG.
11	11F	Humerus	1%–5% positive cells	NEG.	NEG.	NEG.	NEG.
12[b]	13F	Femur	5%–10% positive cells	60%–70% positive cells	Rare positive cells	NEG.	NEG.
13	8M	Ilium	Rare positive cells	NEG.	NEG.	NEG.	NEG.
14	18F	Scapula	1%–5% positive cells	NEG.	NEG.	NEG.	NEG.
15	16M	Tibia	NEG.	NEG.	NEG.	NEG.	NEG.
16	17F	Scapula	10%–30% positive cells	NEG.	NEG.	NEG.	NEG.
17	12F	Femur	5%–10% positive cells	10%–20% positive cells	NEG.	NEG.	NEG.
18	16M	Humerus	NEG.	NEG.	NEG.	NEG.	NEG.

[a] In case 2 and 5, although several cells were NSE positive, the presence of strong background staining raised questions about the validity of the results
[b] This case has been previously reported (GRECO et al. 1988)

for vimentin varies in distribution and it was found in the tumor cells of 13 out of 18 cases (Table 1). The negative reaction of some tumors and weak reaction of others may be attributed to loss of vimentin antigenicity due to formalin fixation (AZUMI and BATTIFORA 1987). Vimentin was present in the nonneoplastic mesenchymal tissue of the sections, and this was used as a built-in control. MIETTINEN et al. (1982) and MOLL et al. (1987), using immunofluorescent techniques, found vimentin in all their cases of Ewing's sarcoma.

Cytokeratin was present in substantial amounts in cases 12 and 17 of our series (Fig. 3). In case 12 [previously reported – GRECO et al. (1988)] tonofilaments were identified by electron microscopy in the original tumor (Fig. 6) and in the liver metastasis. In case 17, electron microscopy revealed occasional intermediate-type filaments, but not tonofilaments. In a third case (case 2), rare

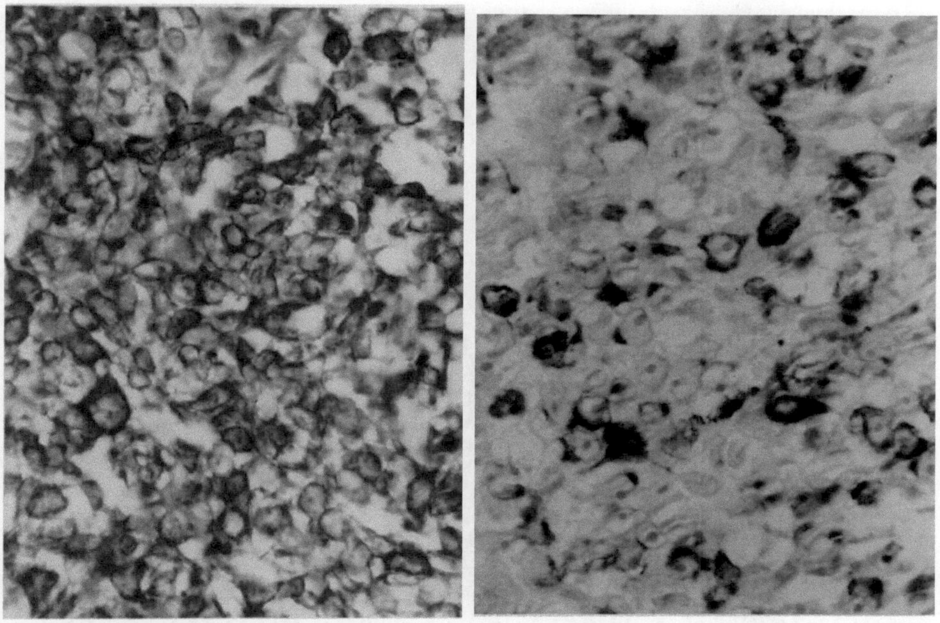

a b

Fig. 3. a Prominent reaction to cytokeratin in the tumor cell cytoplasm of case 12. This tissue was obtained from a recurrence in the femur following chemotherapy and radiotherapy. Tonofilaments were seen by electron microscopy (see Fig. 6). (×400). **b** Cytokeratin reaction from case 17. No tonofilaments were identified by electron microscopy. (×400)

cells were stained with cytokeratin. MOLL et al. (1987) have also demonstrated cytokeratin in Ewing's sarcoma cells. Neurofilaments were not demonstrated in our cases. They were observed by MOLL et al. (1987) in 3 out of 11 cases.

3.3 Electron Microscopy

The morphology of the seven cases selected for study was basically similar to that described in the literature (AYALA and MACKAY 1977; MAHONEY and ALEXANDER 1978; LLOMBART-BOSCH et al. 1982; NAVAS-PALACIOS et al. 1984).

The most common tumor cells of Ewing's sarcoma are rounded, polygonal, or ovoid and they are usually referred to as principal or primary tumor cells. They are often in close contact to each other, forming dense aggregates, and the cell membranes are in close proximity to each other. Nuclei are usually rounded with few indentations. The chromatin is finely dispersed and occasional clumping is seen along the nuclear membrane. Nucleoli are small and are inconspicuous in many cells (Fig. 4). Cytoplasm varies in amount but generally it is not abundant. The organelles are sparse in most cells and consist mainly of mitochondria, small numbers of ribosomes, rare rough endoplasmic reticulum, and occasional poorly developed Golgi apparatus (Fig. 5). Lipid droplets

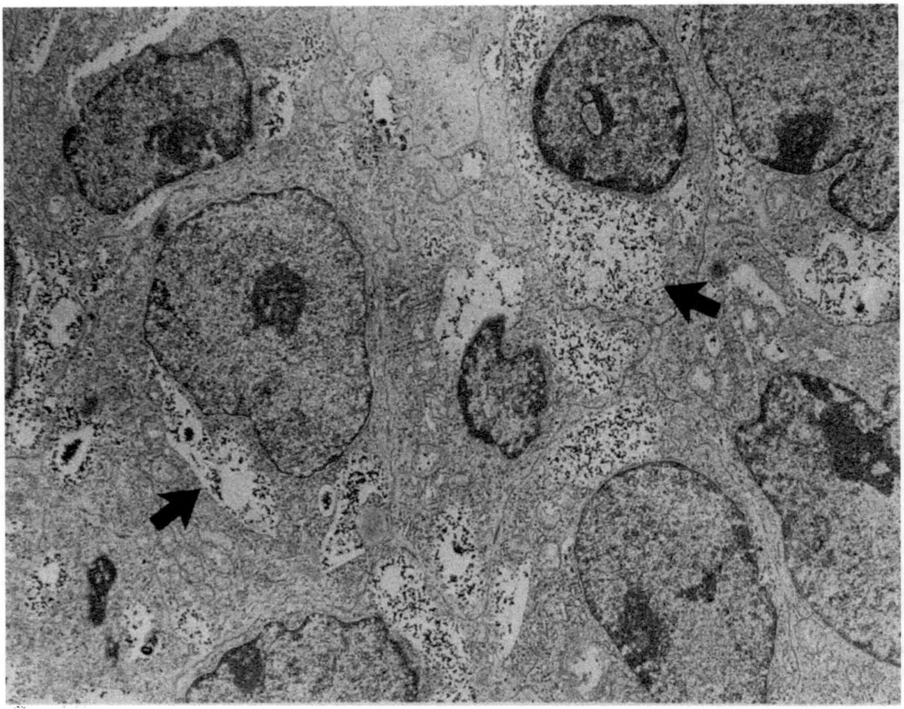

Fig. 4. Electron micrograph of Ewing's sarcoma. The cells have slightly indented nuclei. The cytoplasm contains abundant glycogen (*arrows*) and sparse organelles. Some of the glycogen has been extracted during the processing of the tissue. (×3800)

are also seen occasionally, as well as microtubules. There is a variable amount of glycogen in all of our cases, usually in the form of both monoparticulate beta and rosette alpha forms (NAVAS-PALACIOS et al. 1984) (Fig. 4).

Intermediate-type filaments were usually sparse in our cases. In case 12 (GRECO et al. 1988) intermediate filaments were seen in the form of tonofilaments (Fig. 6). Some authors have described the presence of occasional "rhabdoid cells" with acidophilic cytoplasm and eccentric nuclei, containing large amounts of cytoplasmic intermeditate-type filaments (ERLANDSON 1983). Cell junctions of different types are frequently seen but fully developed desmosomes are not usually identified (Fig. 7a). Recently authors have found by immunoelectron microscopy that most cell junctions are associated with vimentin intermediate filaments; there are other junctions that morphologically are "rudimentary" but they are positive for desmoplakin and therefore are considered to be true desmosomes (MOLL et al. 1987).

Ewing's sarcoma cells usually contain a few cytoplasmic processes or projections and usually can be recognized in greater detail when the cells are isolated. Most of these projections are short and blunt (Fig. 5), but some are elongated and they project away into the neighboring cells (TAKAHASHI et al. 1975; POVYSIL and MATEJOWSKY 1977; AKHTAR et al. 1985) (Fig. 7). Occasional microtubules

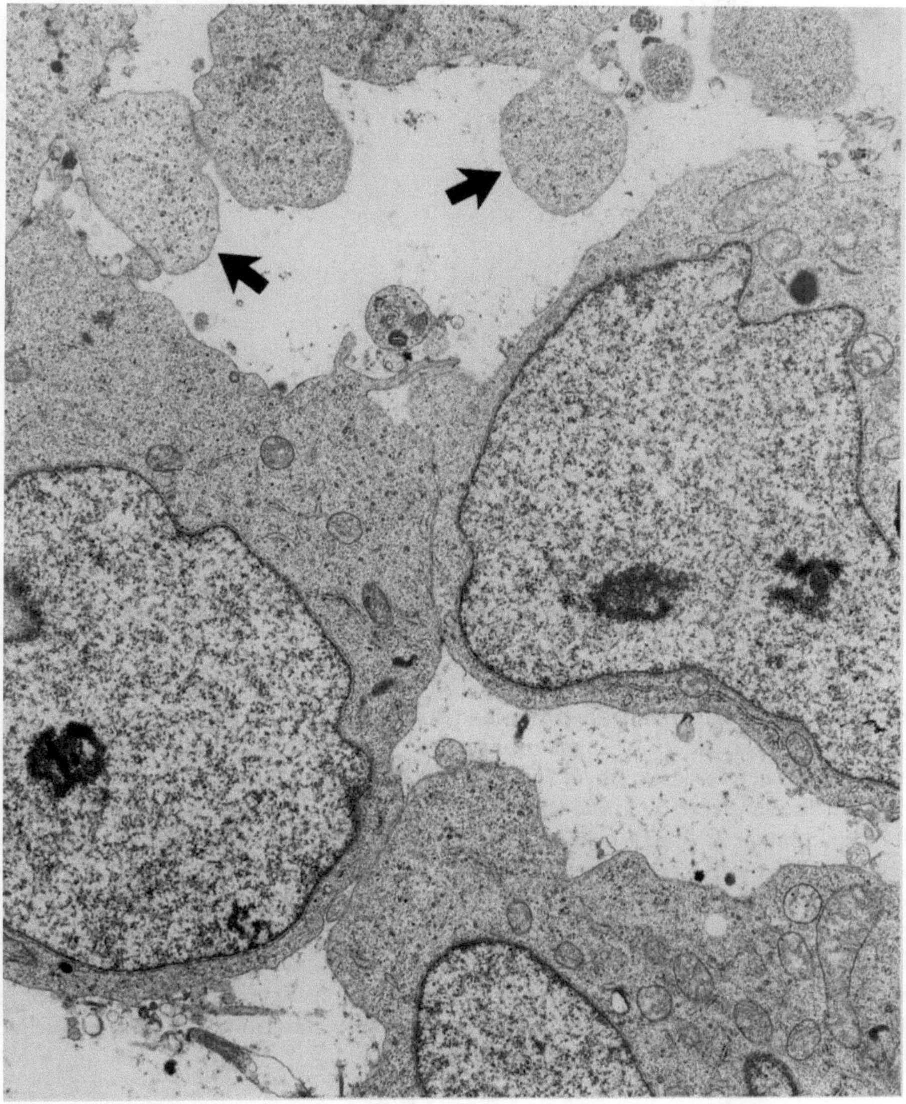

Fig. 5. Ewing's sarcoma cells. The cytoplasm contains a sparse number of mitochondria and ribosomes. There are short blunt processes arising from the cell periphery (*arrows*). (×8250)

and dense membrane-bound bodies have been described within the cell projections (NAVAS-PALACIOS et al. 1984) Pinocytotic vesicles are rarely found. No true basal lamina is found around the cells but dense amorphous material resembling basal lamina was seen on occasions in our cases. Some authors describe the presence of long-spacing collagen fibers around the blood vessels of the tumor (NAVAS-PALACIOS et al. 1984). Rosette-like formations have been studied by electron microscopy; these structures contain part of the cell processes or

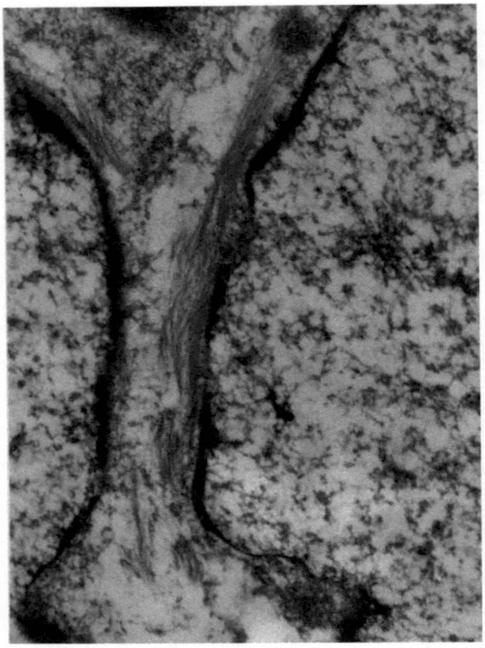

Fig. 6. Tonofilaments are seen around the cell nuclei of case 12. This material was originally embedded in paraffin; it was deparaffinized and then processed for electron microscopy (see Fig. 3a). (×20800)

cell bodies, which are centrally oriented (POVYSIL and MATEJOWSKY 1977). Other authors have found in the pseudorosettes that the tumor cells are disposed around connective tissue fibers (NAVAS-PALACIOS et al. 1984).

The above electron microscopic description of Ewing's sarcoma refers to the principal or primary cells of the tumor, which are those most commonly seen. We have observed in several typical examples of Ewing's sarcoma, tumor cells containing abundant organelles and indented nuclei, that have histiocytic features. Some authors refer to these cells as "secondary cells" of the tumor (MAHONEY and ALEXANDER 1978; LLOMBART-BOSCH et al. 1982). The group of cases that by electron microscopy are classified as atypical Ewing's sarcoma represents the large cell Ewing's sarcoma already mentioned in the histologic description (LLOMBART-BOSCH et al. 1982).

4 Neuroectodermal Tumors

4.1 Concept and Terminology

Peripheral PNETs include a group of small cell neoplasms that arise in the peripheral sites of the nervous system. They probably develop from embryonic migrating cells of the neural crest and show varying degrees of neural differentiation (SEEMAYER et al. 1975; DEHNER 1986). The prototype of the peripheral PNET is the classic neuroblastoma, which is a tumor of infants and young

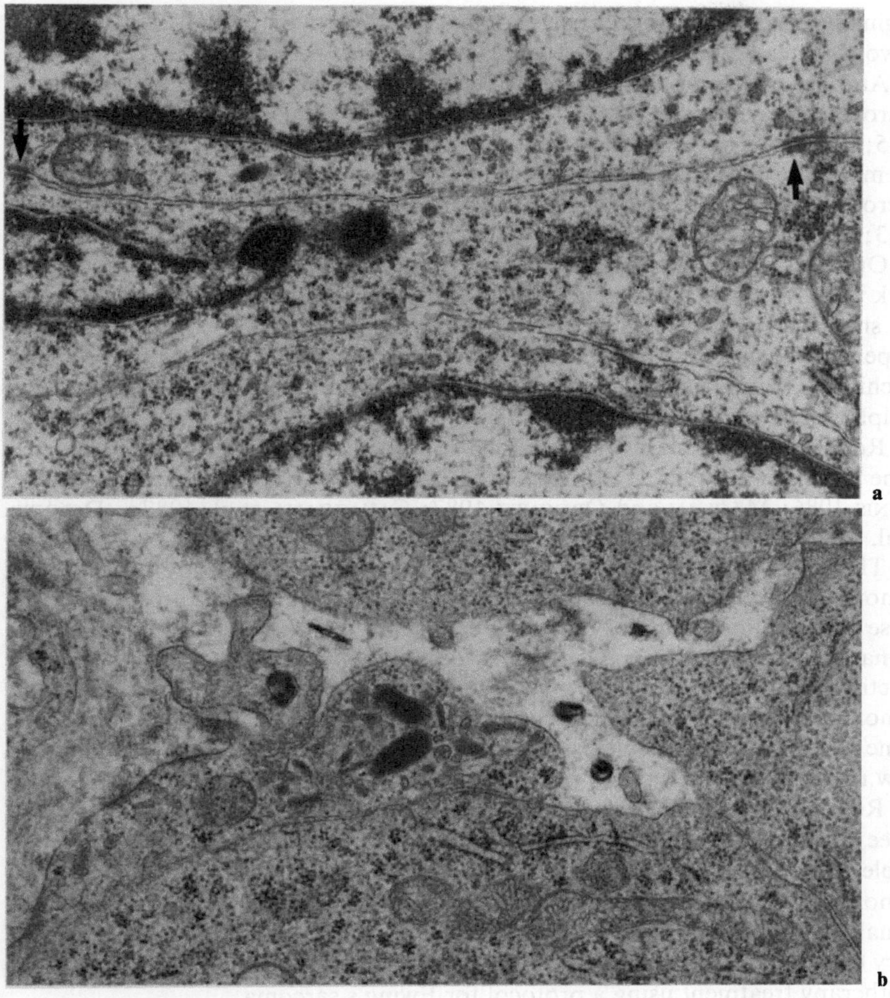

Fig. 7. a Elongated tumor cell at the *center* with cytoplasmic projection to the *right*. Primitive cell junctions are noted (*arrow*). (× 20800). **b** Cell process containing mitochondria, lysosome-like granules and ribosomes. (× 25000)

children arising from the adrenal medulla or other sites of the sympathetic nervous system, and which is usually associated with elevated catecholamine values (SEEMAYER et al. 1975; DEHNER 1986).

There is another group of peripheral PNETs different from the classic neuroblastoma; this group arises in the soft tissues or in the bone, sometimes at the site of a peripheral (nonautonomic) nerve. These lesions usually affect older children or adults and with rare exceptions they are not associated with elevated serum or urine catecholamine levels (ENZINGER and WEISS 1983; VOSS et al. 1984; DEHNER 1986). Many of the peripheral PNETs are reported in the literature under neuroepithelioma, which is a somewhat confusing term originally used to describe malignant neuroectodermal tumors of the central nervous system (BAILEY and CUSHING 1926).

Another confusing term used for peripheral PNETs is peripheral and adult neuroblastoma (MACKAY et al. 1976; HASHIMOTO et al. 1983; ALESHIRE et al. 1985; NESLAND et al. 1985; MACKAY and ORDONEZ 1987). Some of these tumors resemble morphologically the classic neuroblastoma in that rosette formation, microtubules, and dense core granules are often demonstrated (HASHIMOTO et al. 1983; MACKAY and ORDONEZ 1987).

One of the first descriptions of a peripheral neuroectodermal tumor dates back to 1918, when STOUT reported a tumor arising from the ulnar nerve showing small round cells with many rosettes. VOSS et al. (1984) collected 38 cases of peripheral neuroepithelioma from the literature, fifteen of which occurred in children, and some but not all the lesions were anatomically related to a peripheral nerve.

Recently, several cases of PNET have been reported as primary within the bone (JAFFE et al. 1984; USHIGOME et al. 1984; KAWAGUCHI and KOIKE 1986; YUNIS 1986; MACKAY and ORDONEZ 1987; CAVAZZANA et al. 1987a; DONNER et al. 1987).

The application of immunomarkers and electron microscopy to small cell tumors of uncertain histogenesis has recently clarified the nature of some of these lesions. For example, the malignant small cell tumor of the thoracopulmonary region in childhood, originally described by ASKIN et al. (1979), shows reactivity to NSE and it is now considered to be a peripheral neuroectodermal tumor probably arising in intercostal nerves (LINNOILA et al. 1986). Similarly, some cases of extraskeletal Ewing's sarcoma react positively to NSE and are now reclassified as peripheral neuroectodermal tumors (MIERAU 1985).

Review of our material of round cell tumors primary of bone demonstrated three cases that are classified as PNETs, and the clinical data are shown in Table 2. None of these patients had evidence on clinical workup of a primary tumor elsewhere. Cases 1 and 2 of the series were initially thought to be conventional Ewing's sarcoma. Case 3 was suspected to be a neuroblastoma, but urinary catecholamine levels were normal. All three patients initially received chemotherapy treatment using a protocol for Ewing's sarcoma.

4.2 Histological Features

The morphological appearance of our three cases of neuroectodermal tumors was similar to the description in the literature. The main cell type was a small, uniform cell with an often ill-defined cell membrane. The cytoplasm was pale pink, sometimes eosinophilic, and scanty, and the nuclei were rounded with indistinct nucleoli. Mitoses were not infrequent and mild cell pleomorphism was noted. The cells were disposed in diffuse, dense aggregates which were occasionally separated by thin fibrous septae. Rosette-like formation varied from being absent in one case, rare in another, to quite extensive in case 3 and resembling the Homer-Wright rosette of classic neuroblastoma (HASHIMOTO et al. 1983) (Figs. 8a, 9a, 10). Necrosis was particularly extensive in case 2,

Table 2. Neuroectodermal tumors of bone: clinical data and immunohistochemistry

Case	Age/sex	Site[a]	Symptoms	VMA	Treatment	Follow-up
Clinical data						
1	28M	Right ilium	1 month	Not done	Chemotherapy, surgical resection	Alive and free of tumor, 1 1/2 years
2	27F	Right ilium	4 years	Not done	Chemotherapy, surgical resection	Recurrence and metastases, died 1 1/2 years after diagnosis
3[b]	15F	Right ilium	7 months	Normal	Chemotherapy, surgical resection	Alive and free of tumor, 2 years

Case	NSE	Vimentin	S100 protein	LCA	Neuro-filaments	Cyto-keratin	Chromo-granin
Immunohistochemistry							
1	Focally +	10%–20% positive cells	NEG.	NEG.	NEG.	NEG.	NEG.
2	Focally +	60%–70% positive cells	NEG.	NEG.	NEG.	NEG.	NEG.
3	Focally +	90% positive cells	20%–30% positive cells	NEG.	NEG.	NEG.	NEG.

[a] The frequent localization in the ilium may be coincidental, because PNET has been described in other bones (JAFFE et al. 1984)

[b] This case has been reported previously (STEINER et al. 1988)

which required a second biopsy to establish a definitive diagnosis. Glycogen was present in the imprints as well as tissue sections of the three tumors, particularly case 3, where it was quite prominent. Glycogen was found in several PNETs reported in the literature (JAFFE et al. 1984; SCHMIDT et al. 1985). Reticulin fibers were scanty and almost absent between the tumor cells.

4.3 Immunohistochemistry

One important immunomarker found to be present in the neuroectodermal tumors is NSE. NSE, previously called 14-3-2-protein, is an isoenzyme (2 gamma subunits) of the glycolytic enzyme enolase; it is demonstrated in normal neurons and normal cells of the neuroendocrine system and has been considered to be a good marker for neuroectodermal tumors (VINORES et al. 1984; LLOYD and WARNER 1984). NSE was present in our three PNETs. The reaction was observed focally in small groups of cells scattered in the tumor. The intensity of the staining was not too strong, and it was difficult to reproduce in a black-and-white photomicrograph (Fig. 8b, 9b). NSE is positive in most peripheral PNETs (HASHIMOTO et al. 1983; JAFFE et al. 1984; TSOKOS et al. 1984; ALESHIRE

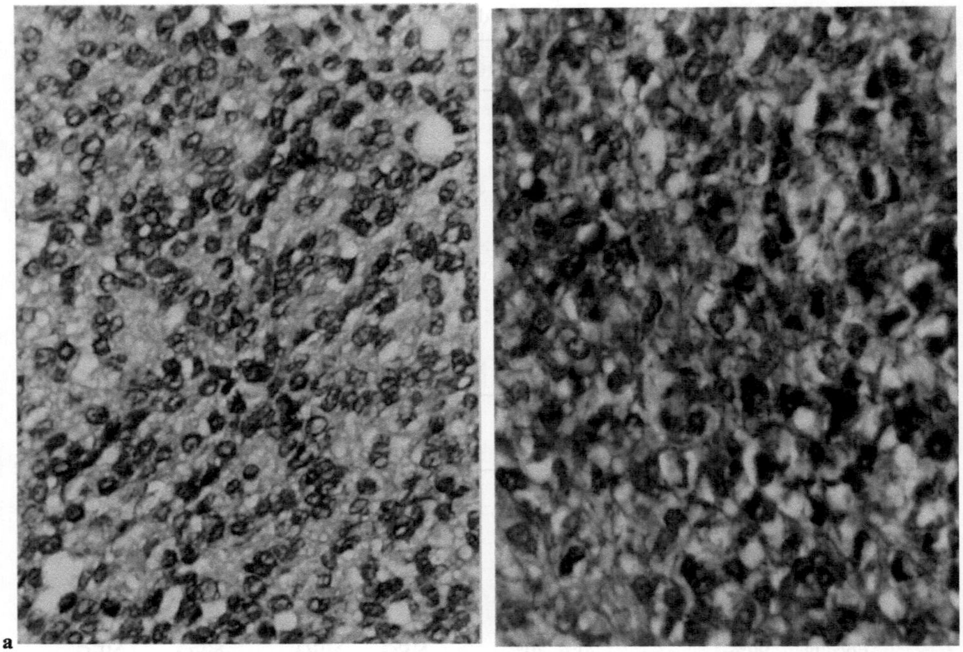

a b

Fig. 8. a Neuroectodermal tumor (case 1). Photomicrograph showing uniform round cells which are disposed around irregular spaces suggesting pseudorosettes. In most areas, the tumor shows a solid growth pattern. (H&E, ×350). **b** NSE reaction of case 1. The reactivity was focal throughout the tumor. (×400)

et al. 1985; MIERAU et al. 1985; SCHMIDT et al. 1985; LINNOILA et al. 1986; KAWAGUCHI and KOIKE 1986; MACKAY and ORDONEZ 1987). In our study of small cell round tumors, we found that NSE (Dako, St. Barbara, CA) cross-reacted with skeletal muscle and sometimes there was a nonspecific background staining that made interpretation of the results difficult. Another problem with NSE is that it has been found to be positive in a number of tumors that do not belong to the nervous system or APUD system, such as rhabdomyosarcomas, chordomas, and certain carcinomas (HASHIMOTO et al. 1983; TSOKOS et al. 1984; VINORES et al. 1984; MIERAU et al. 1985; TRICHE et al. 1985; OSBORN et al. 1986; PAHLMAN et al. 1986; THOMAS et al. 1987). These findings have raised questions about the specificity and usefulness of NSE as a marker for the diagnosis of PNET. A positive NSE reaction should be interpreted critically and in conjunction with other immunomarkers and electron microscopy.

A negative NSE reaction can occur in PNETs and this is probably due to the fixation, decalcification, or processing of the tissue (HASHIMOTO et al. 1983; JAFFE et al. 1984). It does not rule out a PNET if all the other morphological characteristics of neural differentiation are present (SCHMIDT et al. 1985), including those revealed by electron microscopy.

The positive reactivity of NSE in rhabdomyosarcoma is apparently due to the presence of some gamma isoenzyme in the nonneural enolase of the skeletal

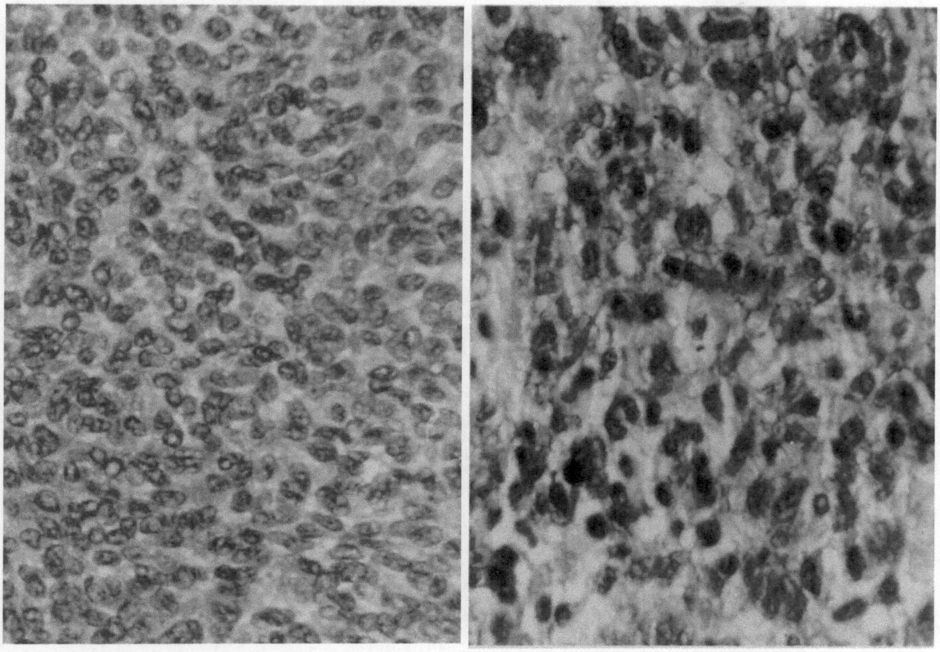

a b

Fig. 9. a Neuroectodermal tumor (case 2). Small round cells disposed in diffuse and dense aggregates. (H&E, ×350). **b** NSE reaction of case 2. The reactivity in this case was also focal in the tumor. (×400).

muscle (TRICHE et al. 1985). This diagnostic problem is avoided by using immunomarkers for skeletal muscle in combination with electron microscopy (MIERAU et al. 1985).

Recently, a new monoclonal antibody to human NSE was found to show less background staining and more specificity than a commercial polyclonal antibody (THOMAS et al. 1987). This or any other monoclonal antibody may prove to be more specific to neuroectodermal tumors than the presently available polyclonal antibodies.

Vimentin is an intermediate-type filament that was found to be present in our neuroectodermal tumors as well as in other reports in the literature (SCHMIDT et al. 1985; CAVAZZANA et al. 1987a). The presence of this marker indicates a mesenchymal phenotype. It is interesting to know that in classic neuroblastoma, vimentin is only occasionally present (OSBORN et al. 1986; MACKAY and ORDONEZ 1987; AZUMI and BATTIFORA 1987).

S100 protein is a highly acidic protein that is present in cells of both the central and peripheral nervous system and it is a useful marker to identify brain tumors, Schwann cell tumors, and other tumors of the peripheral nervous system (NAKAJIMA et al. 1982; WEISS et al. 1983). The presence of S100 protein in one of our PNETs and in other reports in the literature (SCHMIDT et al. 1985; TRICHE et al. 1985; CAVAZZANA et al. 1987a) probably indicates Schwann cell differentiation (NAKAJIMA et al. 1982; TRICHE et al. 1983). However, the

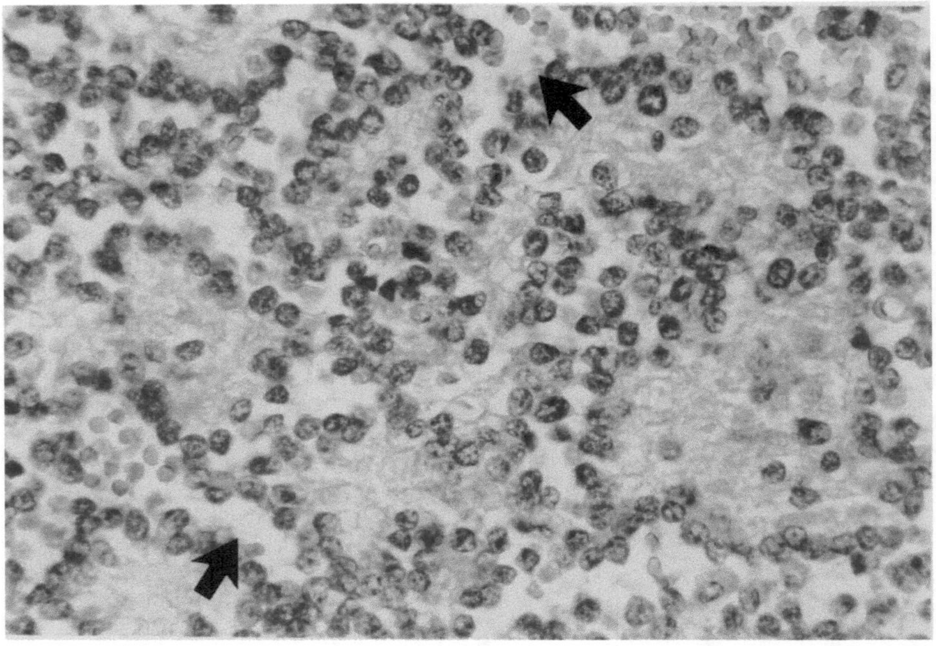

Fig. 10. Neuroectodermal tumor (case 3). The small round cells are disposed in a rosette pattern, at the center of which there are cell projections. In addition, there is also an alveolar or gland-like pattern (*arrows*) around spaces that are empty or contain hemorrhage. These latter areas are probably an artifact. Antimuscle antibody was negative. (×350)

S100 cells in our case (case 3) were round or polygonal rather than spindle shaped, as one would expect if they were Schwann cells (NAKAJIMA et al. 1982). S100 protein is usually negative in neuroblastoma (NAKAJIMA et al. 1982; WEISS et al. 1983). This marker is not a specific indicator of neuroectodermal tumors because it has been found in many nonneural neoplasms, including mesenchymal lesions (NAKAJIMA et al. 1982; WEISS et al. 1983).

Neurofilamentous proteins, which are another intermediate-type filament, were absent from our cases and other cases of PNET (MACKAY and ORDONEZ 1987; CAVAZZANA et al. 1987a), although this marker may occasionally be positive (SCHMIDT et al. 1985). In classic neuroblastoma on the other hand, neurofilaments have been present in all cases examined recently (OSBORN et al. 1986; MUKAI et al. 1986). Formaldehyde fixation reduces the antigenicity of neurofilaments (OSBORN et al. 1986), and this may account for the negative results in our cases. Glial fibrillary acid filament (GFAP) has been occasionally reported in PNETs (SCHMIDT et al. 1985).

Chromogranin is a constituent of secretory granules and is used as a marker for neuroendocrine tumors (WILSON and LLOYD 1984). Chromogranin was not detected in our cases of PNET, probably due to the sparsity of the granules (WILSON and LLOYD 1984). It was present in a PNET of bone recently reported (MACKAY and ORDONEZ 1987).

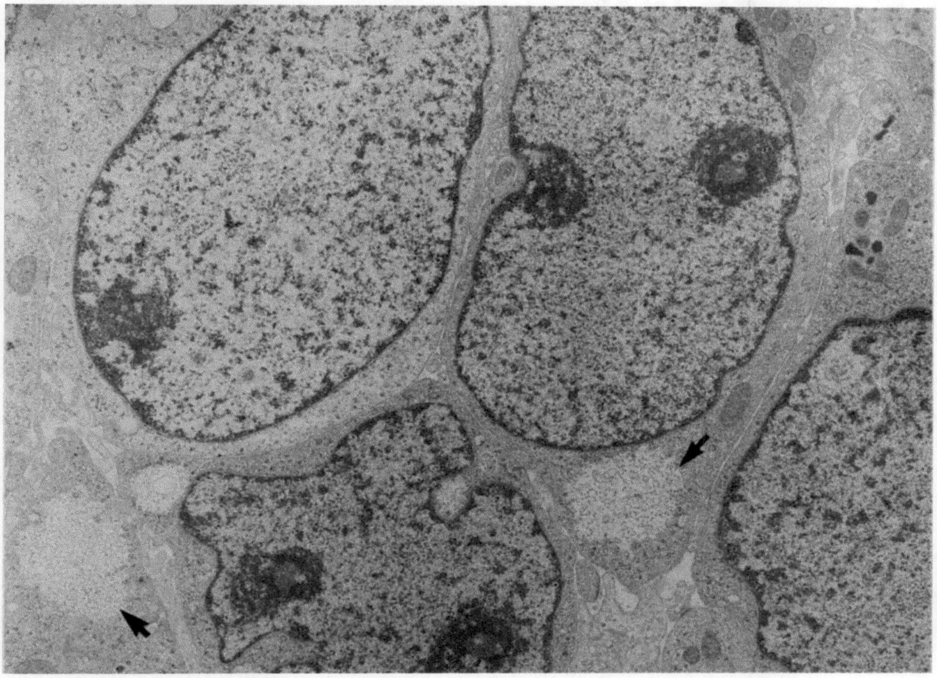

Fig. 11. Electron micrograph of neuroectodermal tumor (case 1). The cell nuclei are focally indented. Glycogen is seen focally in the cytoplasm (*arrows*). It was present in moderate amounts in the tumor. (× 7500)

4.4 Electron Microscopy

The tumor cells of our three cases were rounded to polygonal and contained round and ovoid nuclei with dispersed heterochromatin and occasional nucleoli. Cytoplasmic organelles in general were more abundant than in Ewing's sarcoma. Free ribosomes were numerous and intermediate-type filaments were inconspicuous. Occasional lysosomes were seen. Glycogen was present in the three cases, particularly in case 3, where it was so prominent that it distorted the cell contour (Figs. 11 and 13).

As mentioned in the literature (JAFFE et al. 1984; SCHMIDT et al. 1985; MACKAY and ORDONEZ 1987), numerous cell processes were noted in all three cases of PNET, particularly in case 2, where they were prominent and often demonstrated microtubules and some dense core granules (Figs. 14, 15). In case 3, showing rosette formation, the central area contained numerous cell projections (MACKAY and ORDONEZ 1987) (Fig. 13). Cell junctions usually of the primitive type were occasionally seen in all three cases and electron-dense material that resembled basal lamina was focally adherent to the cell membrane particularly in case 1 (Figs. 14, 15a).

Of particular interest was the demonstration of annulate lamellae in a few cells of case 1 (Fig. 16). The highly characterisitc parallel membrane arrays of

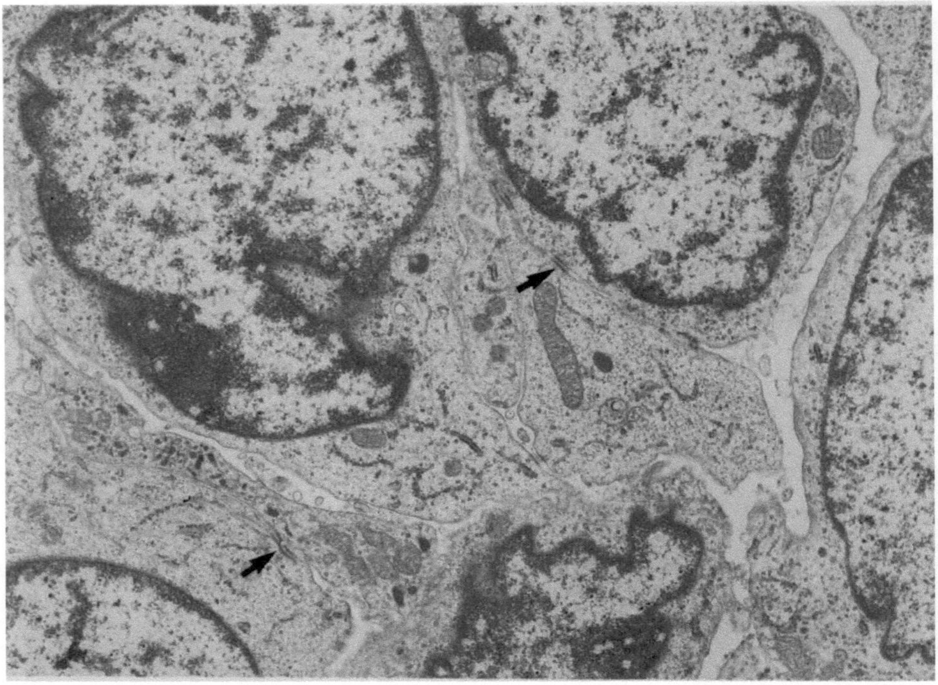

Fig. 12. Neuroectodermal tumor (case 2). Several irregular cell processes are seen and cell junctions are identified (*arrows*). (×8200)

the annulate lamellae did not have any identifiable association with the Golgi apparatus, nuclei, or cytoplasmic membrane. Annulate lamellae have been described in a PNET (SUN and WHITE 1979), in culture neuroblastomas (GOLDSTEIN 1971), and also in other types of tumors (WATANABE et al. 1977; TSCHANG et al. 1978). Therefore, these structures are not specific for PNET. To our knowledge, annulate lamellae have not been reported in Ewing's sarcoma.

There are reports in the literature of PNETs showing a positive reaction to NSE but lacking ultrastructural evidence of neural differentiation. These tumors are classified as poorly differentiated PNETs (SCHMIDT et al. 1987). One case from our files fulfilled this criterion: a primary small cell neoplasm of bone which by light and electron microscopy was indistinguishable from Ewing's sarcoma, but which displayed a positive reaction to NSE (Fig. 17). Whether this neoplasm should be classified as a PNET is open to question. We prefer to designate a tumor as a PNET when neural differentiation is demonstrated by both immunohistochemistry and electron microscopy.

5 Other Small Round Cell Tumors

Described below is a group of other tumors that should be differentiated from Ewing's sarcoma and PNET of bone.

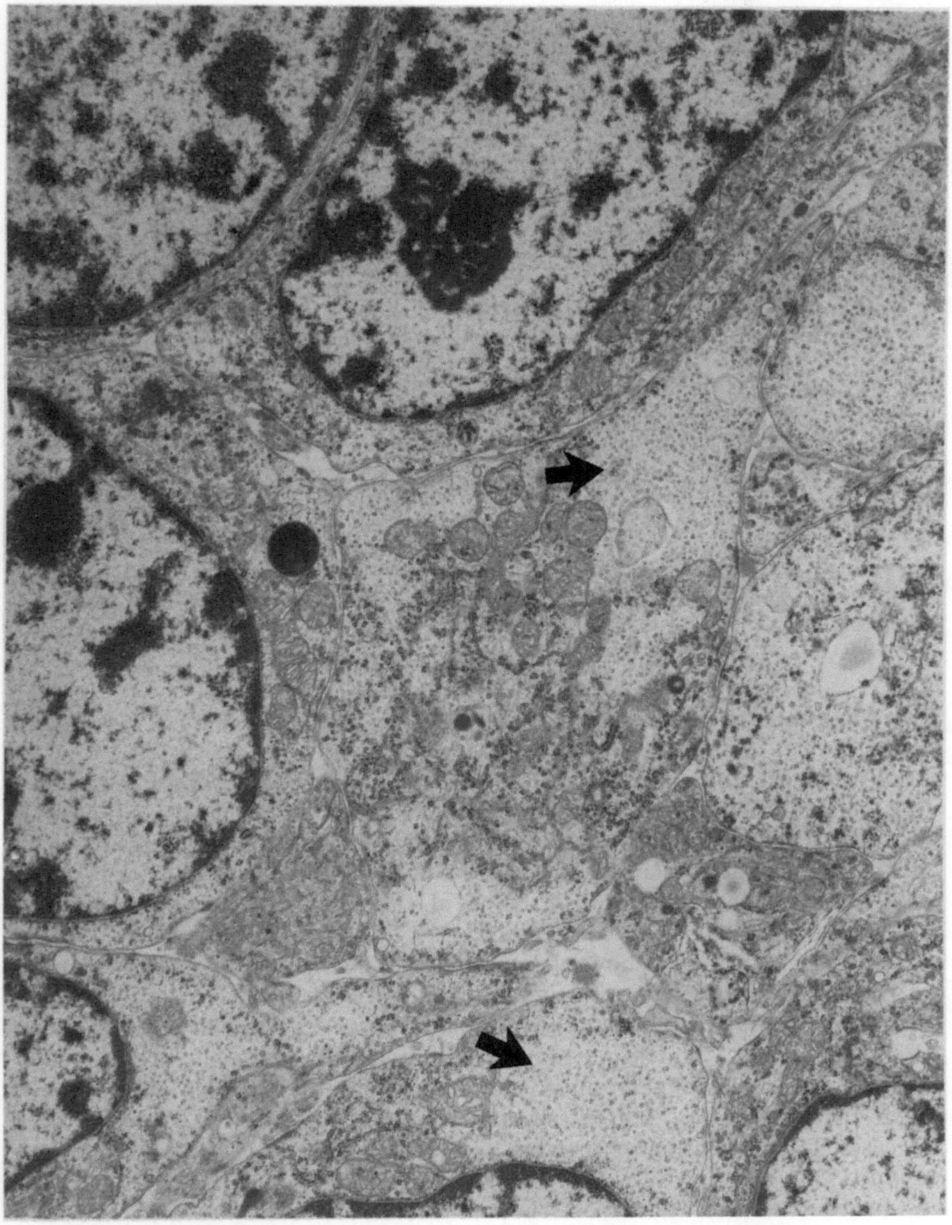

Fig. 13. Neuroectodermal tumor (case 3). Area of rosette formation. The cell nuclei are disposed peripherally and the center contains numerous cell processes. Abundant glycogen is present (*arrows*). (×12500)

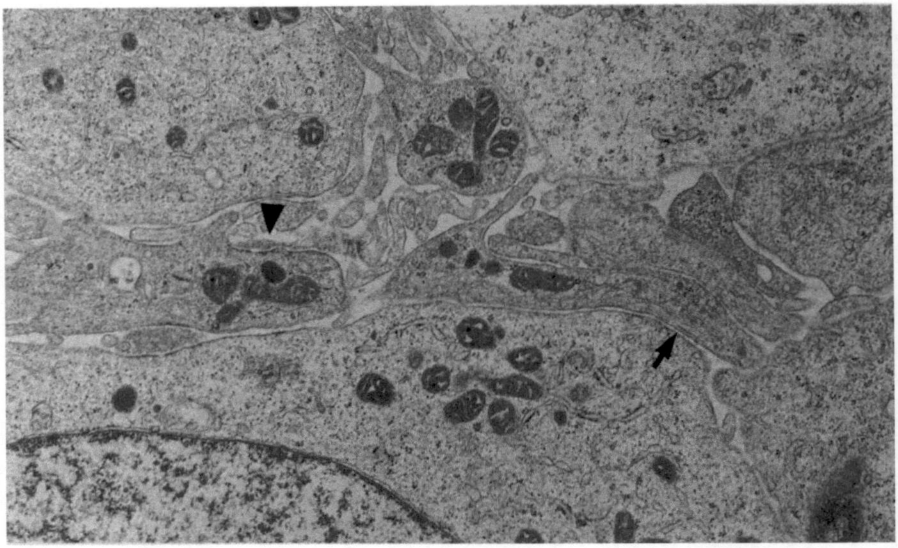

Fig. 14. Cell processes from case 1. Microtubules are identified in some of the processes (*arrow*). Basal-like lamina was noted in this case (*arrowhead*) and in other areas it was more prominent. (×12500)

5.1 Metastatic Neuroblastoma

Bone metastases in classic neuroblastoma are rare as an initial clinical manifestation. The undifferentiated tumors may lack Homer-Wright rosettes and distinction from other round cell tumors may be impossible on histological grounds alone. NSE and neurofilament triplet proteins are positive in most cases (TSOKOS et al. 1984; OSBORN et al. 1986; MUKAI et al. 1986). Vimentin has only occasionally been positive (MACKAY and ORDONEZ 1987; AZUMI and BATTIFORA 1987).

Electron microscopy shows variability in the cell morphology. The presence of true neuritic processes with numerous microtubules and typical dense core granules is quite characteristic (TRICHE and ASKIN 1983; MIERAU et al. 1985) (Fig. 18). In PNET, the degree of neural differentiation is usually not so prominent as that in classic neuroblastoma. The presence of glycogen does not preclude the diagnosis of neuroblastoma, since it is present in as many as 50% of cases, in some instances in large amounts (YUNIS et al. 1979; TRICHE and ASKIN 1983).

In classic neuroblastoma, catecholamine levels are usually elevated; in PNET on the other hand, elevated levels are seen in rare instances (VOSS et al. 1984).

5.2 Embryonal Rhabdomyosarcoma

Embryonal rhabdomyosarcoma should always be considered in the differential diagnosis of undifferentiated small cell tumors of soft tissue. This is not a major

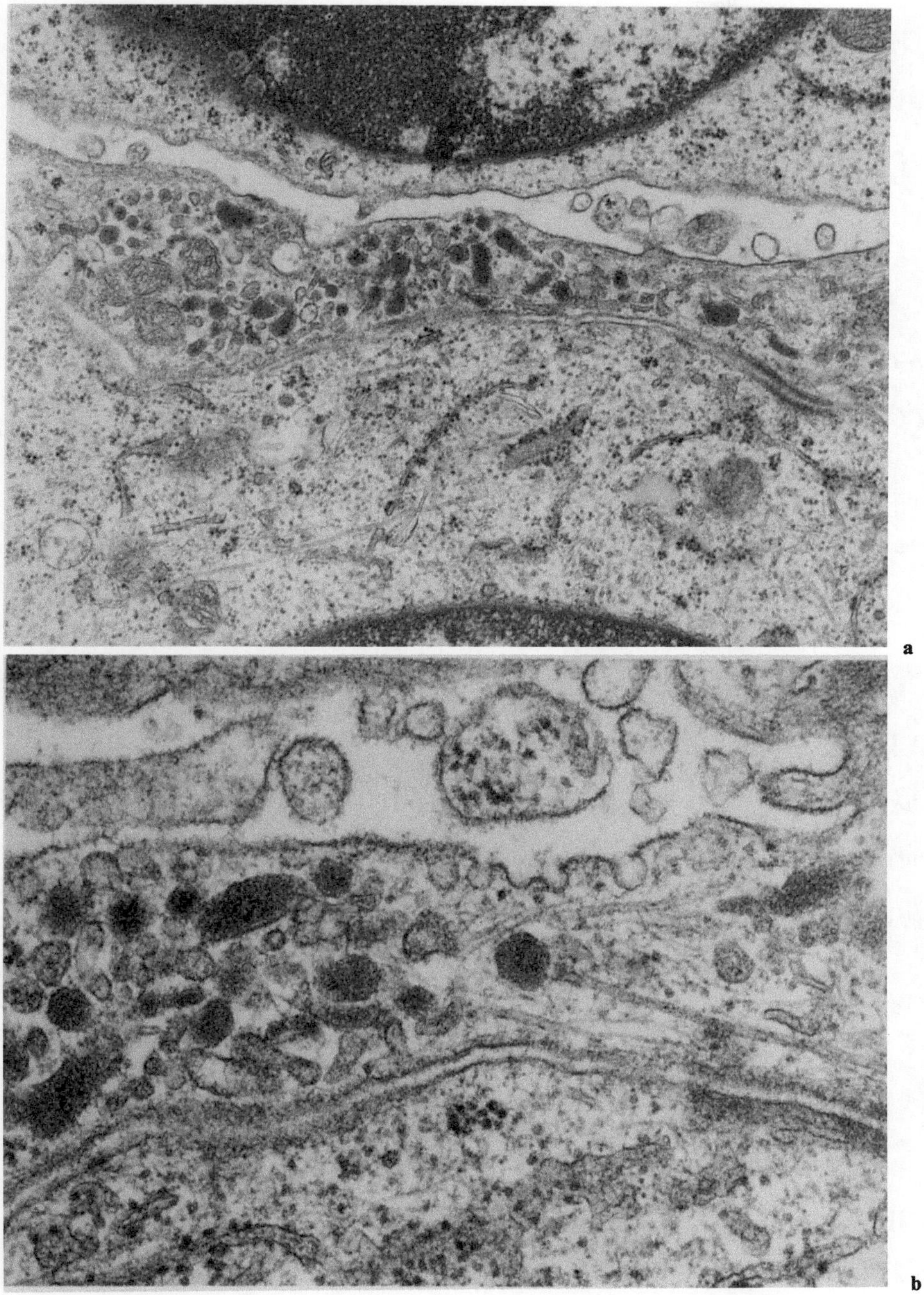

Fig. 15.a Higher magnification of cell process shown in Fig. 12 (case 2). There are numerous electron-dense granules and also microtubules. A desmosome-like junction is noted. (×50000). **b** Another cell process of case 2 containing microtubules and electron-dense granules. Pinocytotic vesicles are also noted. (×65000)

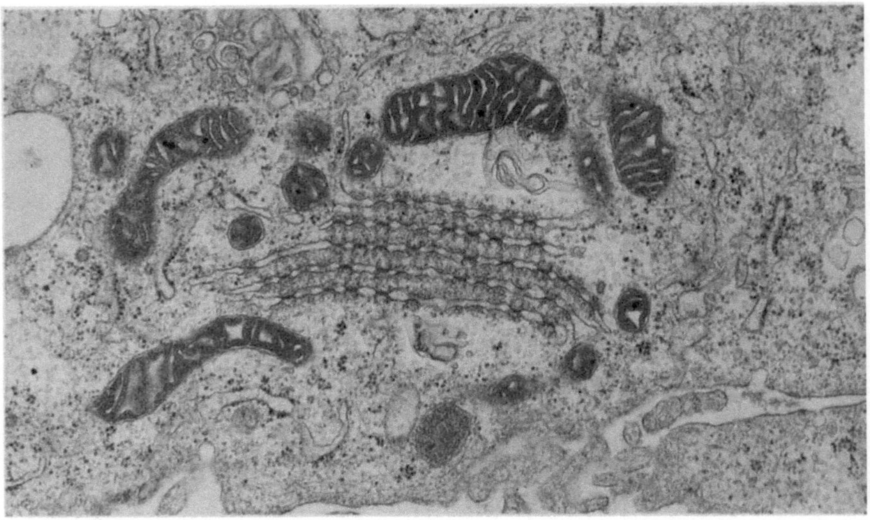

Fig. 16. Annulate lamellae from case 1. They were noted in a few cells. (× 25000)

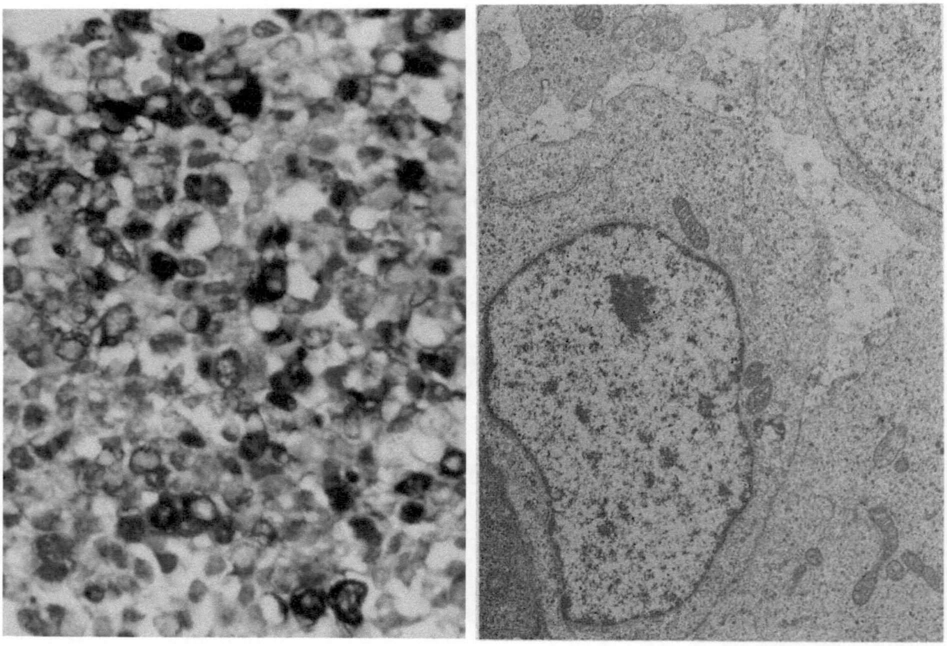

a b

Fig. 17 a, b. Probable PNET of bone. Twelve-year-old male with a small round cell tumor of fibula that morphologically resembled Ewing's sarcoma. **a** NSE reaction in the tumor cells: approximately 10% of the cells were NSE positive. (× 400). **b** Poorly differentiated cells with sparse organelles. There are a few short blunt processes, but no long projections with microtubules or dense granules are seen. (× 6500)

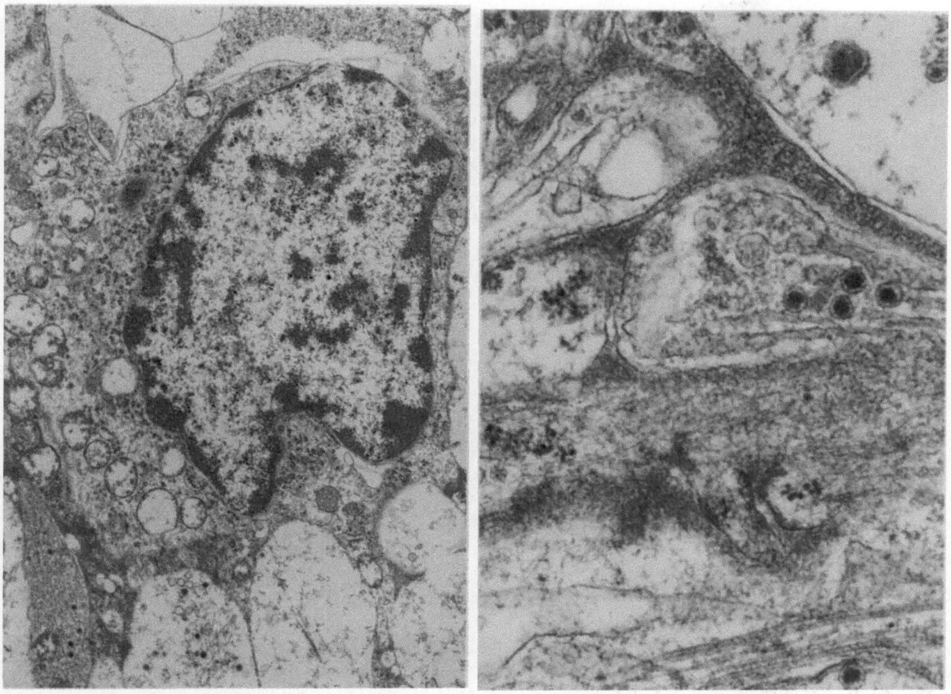

a b

Fig. 18a, b. Classic neuroblastoma. **a** Tumor cell, numerous dense core granules, and a neuritic process (*left lower corner*). (×8250). **b** Neuritic processes containing several typical dense core granules and microtubules. (×40000)

problem in bone tumors, because a rhabdomyosarcoma primary in bone is exceedingly rare (SCHAJOWICZ 1981; DAHLIN and UNNI 1986). Antibodies against different muscle constituents, including myoglobin and desmin, are useful for the diagnosis of rhabdomyosarcoma (MIERAU et al. 1985; EUSEBI et al. 1986). Some authors have found that more than 95% of these tumors are desmin positive (ALTMANNSBERGER et al. 1985). However, electron microscopy seems to be the most reliable way to diagnose a poorly differentiated rhabdomyosarcoma. The presence of thick myosin filaments with attached ribosomes disposed in a single file is considered the minimal criteria for the ultrastructural diagnosis of this tumor (MIERAU et al. 1985; ERLANDSON 1987). Other morphological features of rhabdomyosarcoma include alternating thick and thin filaments, z-substance, glycogen, and basement membrane (Fig. 19) (ERLANDSON 1987).

5.3 Non-Hodgkin's Lymphoma

The use of cell surface immunomarkers on cryostat sections is an important diagnostic method to distinguish this tumor from Ewing's sarcoma and PNET (PATTERSON 1985). Antibodies that react with human leukocytes (LCA) in paraffin sections can yield more than 80% of positive results (MIERAU et al. 1985).

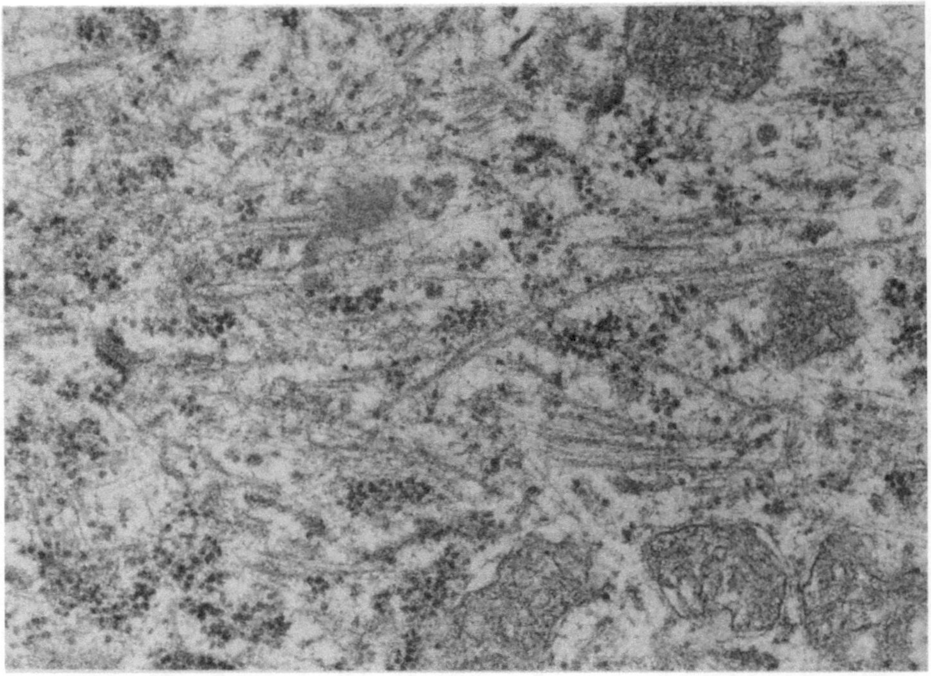

Fig. 19. Poorly differentiated rhabdomyosarcoma. High power view of the cytoplasm showing parallel arrays of alternating thick and thin filaments, with scattered aggregates of ribosomes. (× 50000)

Except for rare instances, lymphoma cells lack cell junctions and their cytoplasm contains numerous polyribosomes, mitochondria, and occasional rough endoplasmic reticulum (MIERAU et al. 1985) (Fig. 20). Although usually absent, glycogen can occasionally be identified. There is another small group of undifferentiated small cell sarcomas that lack any specific characteristic either by immunohistochemistry or electron microscopy. They are referred to as sarcomas of undetermined histogenesis (ERLANDSON 1987).

6 Conclusions

In this study of small round cell tumors of bone, the techniques of immunohistochemistry and electron microscopy were evaluated with the purpose of differentiating Ewing's sarcomas from neuroectodermal tumors.

At the present time there are no specific immunomarkers available for the diagnosis of Ewing's sarcoma. The expression of vimentin in the tumor cells indicates a predominantly mesenchymal phenotype. By electron microscopy, the cells are poorly differentiated, with primitive cell junctions and glycogen. Immunohistochemistry and electron microscopy are very useful in the diagnosis of Ewing's sarcoma because they help to rule out other diagnostic possibilities.

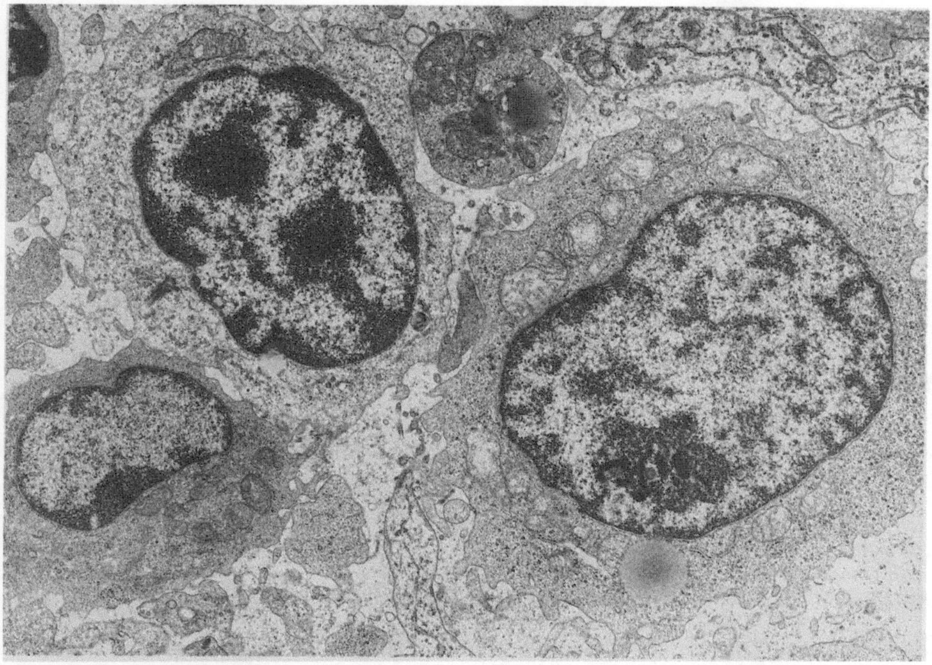

Fig. 20. Non-Hodgkin's lymphoma. The lymphoid cells show mild pleomorphism and the cytoplasm contains numerous polyribosomes, some mitochondria, and an occasional lipid droplet. Short cytoplasmic process are seen. No cell junctions were noted in the tumor. (×7500)

The presence of glycogen by itself is not significant because it also can be observed in neural tumors, rhabdomyosarcoma, and rarely in lymphoma.

In peripheral PNETs, the immunomarkers presently available are not highly specific for these lesions. A positive NSE reaction should be interpreted with caution and in combination with electron microscopy. The problem is that NSE also reacts with nonneural tumors, including rhabdomyosarcoma, and more recently lymphoma (Rabkin et al. 1987). NSE should be used together with a panel of other immunomarkers as a screening procedure in the diagnosis of small cell neoplasms. Synaptophysin was found recently to be a sensitive marker for neuroendocrine tumors (Miettinen 1987) and PNETs, but some overlap with Ewing's sarcoma was observed (Swanson et al. 1987).

Electron microscopy remains the most important technique for the diagnosis of PNET. The identification of numerous cell processes with microtubules and dense core granules is an indication of neural differentiation and helps to distinguish this tumor from Ewing's sarcoma and other small cell neoplasms of bone and soft tissue.

The presence of cytokeratin in Ewing's sarcoma, as demonstrated by us and by others (Moll et al. 1987; Greco et al. 1988), as well as neurofilaments (Moll et al. 1987), raises questions about the origin of this lesion. It is possible that Ewing's sarcoma derives from primitive multipotential cells that may show a variable expression of differentiation, as proposed by some authors (Moll et al. 1987). Some investigators have shown that in certain conditions in tissue culture, Ewing's sarcoma demonstrates neural differentiation (CAVAZZANA et al. 1987b).

The origin of PNET is not know. Further studies are needed to determine whether PNET is a separate entity or part of the spectrum of neural differentiation of Ewing's sarcoma (YUNIS 1986).

Acknowledgments. The author would like to thank Mr. Alexander Joseph and Ms. Lucy Clements for their valuable technical assistance and Ms. Hilda Castro for typing the manuscript.

References

Akhtar M, Ali MA, Sabbah R (1985) Aspiration cytology of Ewing's sarcoma. Light and electron microscopic correlations. Cancer 56:2051–2060

Aleshire SL, Glick AD, Cruz VE, Bradley CA, Parl FF (1985) Neuroblastoma in adults. Arch Pathol Lab Med 109:352–356

Altmannsberger M, Weber K, Droste R, Osborn M (1985) Desmin is a specific marker for rhabdomyosarcoma of human and rat origin. Am J Pathol 118:85–95

Angervall L, Enzinger FM (1975) Extraskeletal neoplasm resembling Ewing's sarcoma. Cancer 36:240–251

Askin FB, Rosai J, Sibley RK, Dehner LP, McAlister WH (1979) Malignant small cell tumor of the thoraco-pulmonary region in childhood. A distinctive clinicopathologic entity of uncertain histogenesis. Cancer 43:2438–2451

Ayala AG, Mackay B (1977): Ewing's sarcoma: an ultrastructural study. In: Management of primary bone and soft tissue Tumors: a collection of papers presented at the twenty-first annual Clinical Conference on Cancer, 1976, at the University of Texas System Cancer Center, M.D. Anderson Hospital and Tumor Institute, Houston, Texas. Chicago: Year Book Medical Publishers, 1977

Azumi N, Battifora H (1987) The distribution of vimentin and keratin in epithelial and nonepithelial neoplasms. A comprehensive immunohistochemical study on formalin- and alcohol-fixed tumors. Am J Clin Pathol 88:286–296

Bailey P, Cushing H (1926) A classification of the gliomata. In: Bailey P, Cushing H (eds) A classification of the tumors of the glioma group on a histogenetic basis with a correlated study of prognosis. J.B. Lippincott, Philadelphia, pp 53–95

Cavazzana AO, Navarro S, Triche T, Llombart-Bosch A (1987a) Ewing's sarcoma and peripheral neuroepithelioma compared (abstract). Lab Invest 56:12A

Cavazzana AO, Miser JS, Jefferson J, Triche TJ (1987b) Experimental evidence for a neural origin of Ewing's sarcoma of bone. Am J Pathol 127:507–518

Dahlin DC, Unni K (1986) Bone tumors. General aspects and data on 8,542 cases. Charles C. Thomas, Springfield, pp 322–336

Dehner LP (1986) Peripheral and central primitive neuroectodermal tumors. A nosologic concept seeking a consensus. Arch Pathol Lab Med 110:997–1005

Dickmann PS, Liotta LA, Triche TJ (1982) Ewing's sarcoma: characterization in established cultures and evidence of its histogenesis. Lab Invest 47:375–382

Donner LR, Ayala AG, Mackay B (1987) Ewing's sarcoma and peripheral neuroepithelioma: a comparative study (abstract). Lab Invest 56:19A

Enzinger FM, Weiss SW (1988) Soft tissue tumors. C.V. Mosby, St. Louis

Erlandson RA (1983) Case report #8. Ultrastruct Pathol 5:323:328

Erlandson RA (1987) The ultrastructural distinction between rhabdomyosarcoma and other undifferentiated "sarcomas". Ultrastruct Pathol 11:83–101

Eusebi V, Ceccarelli C, Gorza L, Schiaffino S, Bussolati G (1986) Immunocytochemistry of rhabdomyosarcoma. The use of four different markers. Am J Surg Pathol 10:293–299

Ewing J (1921) Diffuse endothelioma of bone. Proc New York Pathol Soc 21:17–24

Ewing J (1924) Further report on endothelial myeloma. Proc New York Pathol Soc 24:93–101

Gillespie JJ, Roth LM, Wills ER, Einhorn LH, Willman J (1979) Extraskeletal Ewing's sarcoma. Histologic and ultrastructural observation in 3 cases. Am J Surg Pathol 3:99–108
Goldstein MN (1971) Annulate lamellae in cultured human neuroblastoma cells. Cancer Res 31:209–213
Greco MA, Steiner GC, Fazzini E (1988) Ewing's sarcoma with epithelial differentiation: fine structural and immunocytochemical study. Ultrastruct Pathol 12:317–325
Harvey W, Squier MV, Duance VC, Pritchard J (1982) A biological and immunohistological study of collagen synthesis in Ewing's sarcoma. Br J Cancer 46:848–855
Hashimoto H, Enjoji M, Nakajima T, Kiryu H, Daimaru Y (1983) Malignant neuroepithelioma (peripheral neuroblastoma). A clinicopathologic study of 15 cases. Am J Surg Pathol 7:309–318
Hsu SM, Raine L, Fanger H (1981) Use of avidin-biotin-peroxidase complex (ABC) in immunoperoxidase techniques. A comparison between ABC and unlabelled (PAP) procedures. J Histochem Cytochem 29:557–580
Huntrakoon M (1987) Extraskeletal Ewing's sarcoma. Ultrastruct Pathol 11:411–419
Jaffe HL (1958) Tumors and tumorous conditions of the bones and joints. Lea and Febiger, Philadelphia, pp 350–368
Jaffe R, Santamaria M, Yunis EJ, Tannery NH, Agostini RM, Medina J, Goodman M (1984) The neuroectodermal tumor of bone. Am J Surg Pathol 8:885–898
Jeffree GM (1974) Enzyme of round cell tumors in bone and soft tissues: a histochemical survey. J Pathol 113:101–115
Kawaguchi K, Koike M (1986) Neuron-specific enolase and leu-7 immunoreacitve small round cell neoplasm. The relationship to Ewing's sarcoma in bone and soft tissue. Am J Clin Pathol 86:79–83
Kissane JM, Askin PB, Foulkes M, Stratton LB, Shirley SF (1983) Ewing's sarcoma of bone: clinicopathologic aspects of 303 cases from the intergroup Ewing's sarcoma study. Hum Pathol 14:773–779
Linnoila RI, Tsokos M, Triche TJ, Marangos PJ, Chandra RS (1986) Evidence for neural origin and PAS-positive variants of the malignant small cell tumor of thoracopulmonary region (Askin tumor). Am J Surg Pathol 10:124–133
Llombart-Bosch A, Blache R, Peydro-Olaya A (1982) Round cell sarcomas of bone and their differential diagnosis (with particular emphasis on Ewing's sarcoma and reticulosarcoma). A study of 233 tumors with optical and electron microscopic techniques. Pathol Annu 17:113–145
Llombart-Bosch A, Perez-Bacete M, Triche TJ (1986) Immunohistochemical analysis of Ewing's tumors and their differential diagnosis with other small round blue cell sarcomas of childhood and adolescence. Verh Dtsch Ges Pathol 70:321–324
Lloyd RV, Warner TF (1984) Immunohistochemistry of neuron-specific enolase. In: DeLellis RA (ed) Advances in immunohistochemistry. Masson Publishing USA, Inc. New York. pp 127–140
Loning T, Liebsch J, Delling G (1985) Osteosarcomas and Ewing's sarcomas. Comparative immunocytochemical investigation of filamentous proteins and cell membrane determinants. Virchows Arch [A] 407:323–336
Mackay B, Luna MA, Butler JJ (1976) Neuroblastoma. Electron microscopic observation of nine cases. Cancer 37:1334–1351
Mackay B, Ordonez NG (1987) Adult neuroblastoma of bone: a case report. Ultrastruct Pathol 11:455–464
Mahoney JP, Alexander RW (1978) Ewing's sarcoma: a light and electron microscopic study of 21 cases. Am J Surg Pathol 2:283–297
Maletz N, McMorrow LE, Greco MA, Wolman SR (1986) Ewing's sarcoma. Pathology, tissue culture and cytogenetics. Cancer 58:252–257
Mierau GW (1985) Extraskeletal Ewing's sarcoma (peripheral neuroepithelioma). Ultrastruct Pathol 9:91–98
Mierau GW, Berry PJ, Orsini EN (1985) Small round cell neoplasms: Can electron microscopy and immunohistochemical studies accurately classify them? Ultrastruct Pathol 9:99–111
Miettinen M (1987) Synaptophysin and neurofilament proteins as markers for neuroendocrine tumors. Arch Pathol Lab Med 111:813–818
Miettinen M, Lehto VP, Virtanen I (1982) Histogenesis of Ewing's sarcoma. An evaluation of intermediate filaments and endothelial cell markers. Virchows Arch [Cell Pathol] 41:277–284
Moll R, Lee I, Gould VE, Berndt R, Roessner A, Franke WW (1987) Immunocytochemical analysis of Ewing's tumors. Patterns of expressions of intermediate filaments and desmosomal proteins indicate cell type heterogeneity and pluripotential differentiation. Am J Pathol 127:288–304

Mukai M, Torikata C, Iri H et al. (1986) Expressions of neurofilament triplet proteins in human neurol tumors: an immunohistochemical study of paraganglioma, gangioneuroma, gangioneuroblastoma and neuroblastoma. Am J Pathol 122:28–35

Nakajima T, Watanabe S, Sato Y, Kameya T, Hirota T, Shimosato Y (1982) An immunoperoxidase study of S100 protein distribution in normal and neoplastic tissue. Am J Surg Pathol 6:715–727

Nakayama I, Moriuchi A, Taira Y, Takahara O, Itoga O, Tsuda N (1977) Fine structural study of annulate lamellae complexes in human tumors. Acta Pathol Jpn 27:25–39.

Nascimento AG, Unni KK, Pritchard DJ, Cooper KL, Dahlin DC (1980) A clinicopathologic study of 20 cases of large-cell (atypical) Ewing's sarcoma of bone. Am J Surg Pathol 4:29–36

Navas-Palacios JJ, Aparicio-Duque R, Valdes MD (1984) On the histogenesis of Ewing's sarcoma. An ultrastructural immunohistochemical and cytochemical study. Cancer 53:1882–1901

Nesland JM, Sobrinho-Simoes MA, Holm R, Johannessen JV (1985) Primitive neuroectodermal tumor (peripheral neuroblastoma) Ultrastruct Pathol 9:59–64

Osborn M, Dirk T, Kaser H, Weber K, Altmannsberger M (1986) Immunohistochemical localization of neurofilaments and neuron-specific enolase in 29 cases of neuroblastoma. Am J Pathol 122:433–442

Pahlman S, Esscher T, Nilsson K (1986) Expression of γ-subunit of enolase, neuron-specific enolase, in human non-neuroendocrine tumors and derived cell lines. Lab Invest 54:554–560

Patterson SD (1985) Immunologic techniques in the evaluation of lymphoma. Ultrastruct Pathol 9:195–208

Povysil C, Matejovsky Z (1977) Ultrastructure of Ewing's sarcoma. Virchows Arch [A] 374:303–316

Rabkin MS, Hammond ME, Kjeldsberg CR (1987) Clinical, morphologic and immunologic characterization of malignant lymphomas expressing neuron-specific enolase (abstract). Am J Clin Pathol 88:528–529

Roessner A, Voss B, Rauterberg J, Immenkamp M, Grundmann E (1982) Biologic characterization of human bone tumors. Ewing's sarcoma. A comparative electron and immunofluorescence microscopic study. J Cancer Res Clin Oncol 104:171–180

Schajowicz F (1981) Tumors and tumor-like lesions of bone and joints. Springer, New York, pp 244–267

Schmidt D, Mackay B, Ayala AG (1982) Ewing's sarcoma with neuroblastoma-like features. Ultrastruct Pathol 3:143–151

Schmidt D, Harms D, Burdach S (1985) Malignant peripheral neuroectodermal tumors of childhood and adolescence. Virchows Arch [A] 406:351–365

Schmidt D, Harms D, Pilon VA (1987) Small-cell pediatric tumors. Histology, immunohistochemistry and electron microscopy. Clin Lab Med 7:63–89

Seemayer TA, Thelmo WL, Bolande RP, Wiglesworth FW (1975) Peripheral neuroectodermal tumors. Perspect Pediatr Pathol 2:151–172

Steiner GC, Graham S, Lewis MM (1988) Malignant round cell tumor of bone with neural differentiation (neuroectodermal tumor). Ultrastruct Pathol 12:505–512

Stout AP (1918) A tumor of ulnar nerve. Proc New York Pathol Soc 18:2–12

Sun CN, White HJ (1979) Annulate lamellae in human tumor cells. Tissue Cell 11:139–146

Swanson PE, Wick MR, Hagen KA, Dehner LP (1987) Synapyophysin in small round cell tumors (abstract). Am J Clin Pathol 88:523

Takahashi K, Sato T, Kojima M (1976) Cytological characterization and histogenesis of Ewing's sarcoma. Acta Pathol Jpn 26:167–190

Thomas P, Battifora H, Manderino GL, Patrick J (1987) A monoclonal antibody against neuron-specific enolase. Immunohistochemical comparison with a polyclonal antiserum. Am J Clin Pathol 88:146–152

Triche TJ, Askin FB (1983) Neuroblastoma and the differential diagnosis of small-, round-, blue-cell tumors. Hum Pathol 14:569–595

Triche TJ, Tsokos M, Linnoila I, Marangos PJ, Chandra R (1985) NSE in neuroblastoma and other round cell tumors of childhood. Adv Neuroblastoma Res 295–317

Tschang T, Kasin JV, Parnell D, Kraus FT (1978) Annulate lamellae in human malignant tumors. A report of three cases. Arch Pathol Lab Med 102:426–430

Tsokos M, Linnoila RI, Chandra RS, Triche TJ (1984) Neuron-specific enolase in the diagnosis of neuroblastoma and other small, round-cell tumors in children. Hum Pathol 15:575–584

Ushigome S, Takakuwa T, Takagi M, Sato Y (1984) Neuroblastoma (or poorly differentiated ganglioneuroblastoma) arising from the left tenth rib and probably involving the left ninth rib. Case report 263. Skel Radiol 11:151–154

Vinores SA, Bonnin JM, Rubenstein LJ, Marangos DJ (1984) Immunohistochemical demonstration of neuron-specific enolase in neoplasms of the CNS and other tissues. Arch Pathol Lab Med 108:536–540

Voss BL, Pysher TJ, Humphrey GB (1984) Peripheral neuroepithelioma of childhood. Cancer 54:3059–3064

Watanabe S, Berard CW, Triche TJ (1977) Annulate lamellae in four cases of diffuse lymphocytic lymphoma. J Natl Cancer Inst 58:777–779

Weiss SW, Langloss JM, Enzinger FM (1983) Value of S100 protein in the diagnosis of soft tissue tumors with particular reference to benign and malignant Schwann cell tumors. Lab Invest 49:299–308

Wilson BS, Lloyd RV (1984) Detection of chromogranin in neuroendocrine cells with a monoclonal antibody. Am J Pathol 115:458–468

Yunis EJ (1986) Ewing's sarcoma and related small round cell neoplasms in children. Am J Surg Pathol 10 [Suppl 1]:54–62

Yunis EJ, Agostini RM, Walpusk JA, Hubbard JD (1979) Glycogen in neuroblastoma. A light and electron microscopic study of 40 cases. Am J Surg Pathol 3:313–323

Immunohistological Demonstration of Osteonectin in Normal Bone Tissue and in Bone Tumors

A. Schulz and G. Jundt

1	Introduction	31
2	Materials and Methods	32
2.1	Tissues Studied	32
2.2	Antibodies	32
2.3	Protein Blot	33
2.4	Immunohistochemistry	33
2.5	Immunoelectron Microscopy	33
3	Results	34
3.1	Protein Blots	34
3.2	Immunohistochemistry of Osteonectin in Bone Matrix-Forming Tissue	36
3.3	Tissues Free of Bone Matrix	36
3.3.1	Cartilage	36
3.3.2	Other Tissues	36
3.4	Immunoelectron Microscopy of Osteonectin in Osteoblasts and Osteoid	38
3.5	Immunohistochemical Studies in Bone Tumors and Tumor-like Lesions	38
3.5.1	Tumor-like Lesions	38
3.5.2	Benign Bone Tumors	42
3.5.3	Osteosarcomas	42
3.5.4	Non-Bone-Forming Skeletal Tumors	45
3.6	Soft Tissue Tumors	45
4	Discussion	45
4.1	Osteonectin as a Constituent of Bone Matrix Proteins	45
4.2	Functional Aspects of Osteonectin	50
4.3	Osteonectin as a Marker Protein of Osteoblasts	51
4.4	Osteonectin Antibodies in Bone-Forming Tumors	51
5	Summary	52
	References	53

1 Introduction

The principal protein component of bone matrix is type-I collagen. Although it is the only type of collagen present it is not bone specific because it is also found in nonmineralizing connective tissue of the skin, lung, liver, eyes, and tendons (Church 1981; Gay and Rhodes 1980; von der Mark 1981). Therefore the specific quality of bone matrix as a mineralizing connective tissue is probably due to its 10% noncollagenous protein content. Based on this assumption a noncollagenous protein was extracted from fetal bovine bone that showed binding properties for collagen as well as for hydroxyapatite (the main mineral constituent of bone) and was therefore named osteonectin (Termine et al. 1981).

Initially, osteonectin was regarded as a bone-specific protein according to the investigations of TERMINE and associates (1981). It was therefore an obvious conclusion that osteonectin is produced by osteoblasts. Conversely this would mean that the immunohistochemical demonstration of intracellular osteonectin speaks for an osteoblastic differentiation of the respective cells.

To check the importance of osteonectin as a cellular differentiation marker for osteoblasts, immunocytochemical studies with antibodies against human (hON) and bovine (bON) osteonectin were performed on bone matrix-forming human callus tissue. Production, secretion, and extracellular distribution of osteonectin at the ultrastructural level were demonstrated by immunoelectron microscopy of the normal osteoblast and freshly deposited bone matrix in human callus tissue.

The immunohistochemical studies of tumors were performed on benign and malignant bone tumors for the presence of osteonectin. Mesenchymal tumors without bone formation served as controls. To ensure that cellular immunoreactivity was due to the presence of osteonectin we studied osteosarcoma tissue by protein blot after SDS polyacrylamide gel electrophoresis (SDS-PAGE).

Osteosarcoma, the malignant variant of the osteoblastic lineage, was of particular interest in this context. Depending on their histological pattern and their matrix production, osteosarcomas were subdivided into the following types: osteoblastic, fibroblastic, chondroblastic, anaplastic, small cell, and telangiectatic (HUVOS 1979; MARTIN et al. 1982; DAHLIN and UNNI 1986). If osteoid production by the tumor cells can be demonstrated histologically, there will be no problem in a firm classification of a tumor as an osteosarcoma. Diagnosis becomes difficult, however, if the tumor shows no matrix production, or if matrix production is scanty and hard to recognize. In such cases the immunohistochemical demonstration of osteonectin would be an important and helpful tool for establishing the definite diagnosis of osteosarcoma. To elucidate whether osteonectin immunohistochemistry would meet this requirement we investigated a number of osteosarcomas of varying degrees of differentiation.

2 Materials and Methods

2.1 Tissues Studied

Bone matrix-forming tissue obtained at surgery from eight patients was investigated (4 × callus, 3 × reactive bone formation, 1 × myositis ossificans).

From the group of bone-forming tumors and tumor-like lesions, two cases of fibrous dysplasia, three osteoid osteomas, and 13 osteosarcomas were studied. Further primary skeletal tumors were one chondromyxoid fibroma, one chondroblastoma, three chondrosarcomas, and four Ewing's sarcomas. The group of soft tissue tumors included two fibrosarcomas, one rhabdomyosarcoma, one leiomyosarcoma, and one meningeal sarcoma.

2.2 Antibodies

Antibodies were raised in rabbits, as previously described (TERMINE 1981). Their specificity was determined in the Ouchterlony test with purified osteonectin. Antibodies against both hON and bON were supplied by J.D. TERMINE and his colleagues P. GEHRON-ROBEY and L.W. FISHER from the NIH, Bethesda, Maryland, USA. We are greatly indebted for this generous gift.

2.3 Protein Blot

Osteosarcoma tissue was homogenized in proteinase-inhibiting buffer (TERMINE 1981), ultracentrifuged (70000 g), and the cytosol fraction lyophilized. The lyophilisate was separated by SDS-PAGE according to LAEMMLI (1970) (collection gel: 3.5% acrylamide; separation gel: 12.5% acrylamide). One gel portion was stained with Coomassie Blue R-250. From the other gel portion the proteins were electrophoretically transferred to nitrocellulose film (TOWBIN et al. 1979). After saturation with 3% bovine serum albumin and 10% horse serum (Gibco) the nitrocellulose paper was incubated with antiosteonectin 1:1000. The immune reaction was developed by the streptavidin-biotin-peroxidase complex method (Amersham, Braunschweig, FRG) and 4-chloro-1-naphthol as chromogen.

2.4 Immunohistochemistry

All studies were performed on formalin-fixed material (4% buffered formalin) after embedding in paraffin. If necessary, the specimens were decalcified in EDTA solution (10%) or acids (Ossafixona by Röhm Pharma, Weinheim, FRG). Either the PAP technique (STERNBERGER 1979; VAN NOORDEN and POLAK 1983) or the ABC method (HSU et al. 1984) was used. The DAB development was slightly modified (STRAUS 1982). Identical results were obtained with both methods. The sections were incubated overnight at 4° C with the primary antibody after optimal antibody dilution (1:1200) had been tested in preceding experiments. To reveal antigenic sites possibly masked by the preparation technique or by complex protein composition of the bone tissue, the sections were additionally treated with the enzymes trypsin (incubation for 30 min at 37° C in a solution of 100 mg trypsin and 160 mg $CaCl_2$ in 100 ml aqua dest, pH 7.8, according to BROZMAN 1978), hyaluronidase (incubation for 30 min at 37° C, 30 IU/section, according to TUNG et al. 1985), and collagenase (incubation for 30 min at 37° C in a solution of 0.25 collagenase in PBS, modified according to PAUL 1979).

2.5 Immunoelectron Microscopy

The tissue was reduced to particles measuring 0.5–1.0 mm in diameter immediately after surgical excision, fixed in PBS containing 1% glutaraldehyde and

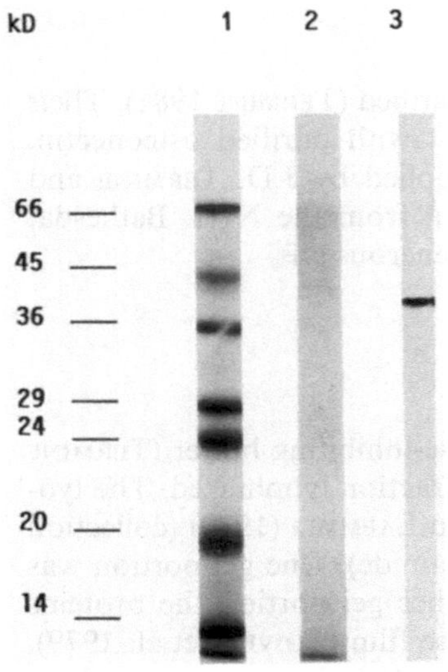

Fig. 1. Protein blot following SDS-PAGE of the cytosolic osteosarcoma fraction. *Lane 1:* marker proteins (Comassie). *Lane 2:* cytosolic osteosarcoma fraction (Coomassie). *Lane 3:* protein blot incubated with antiosteonectin showing a positive reaction at approximately 38 kD

2.0% picric acid for 3 h at room temperature, washed in PBS, and stored. Embedding was done in Lowicryl-K4M (Plano, Marburg, FRG) which was polymerized under UV light at −15° C in a refrigerator box (ROTH 1983). Ultrathin sections were cut with diamond knives and taken up on Formvar-coated copper–palladium nets.

Incubation with the primary antibodies (dilution 1:10 to 1:50 in 1% ovalbumin solution in PBS) was performed for 2 h at room temperature. After washing with PBS the ultrathin sections were incubated with a protein A–gold solution (15-nm gold particles) or a secondary antibody against rabbit immunoglobulin coupled with 15-nm gold particles (Janssen, Beerse, Belgium) for 1 h (ROTH 1983; SCHULZ et al. 1986; ROMANOWSKI et al. 1987). Subsequent contrasting of the sections was performed with 5% uranyl acetate in distilled water for 5 min and with 0.4% lead citrate for 20 s. In parallel with the processing for immunoelectron microscopy the tumor tissue was embedded in a low viscosity synthetic resin mixture for conventional transmission electron microscopy (SCHULZ 1977).

3 Results

3.1 Protein Blots

The protein blots of the cytosolic fraction of osteosarcomas revealed a strong immunoreactivity at approximately 38 kD (Fig. 1). A weaker band was also observed at 66 kD, probably resulting from deposition on albumin. This corre-

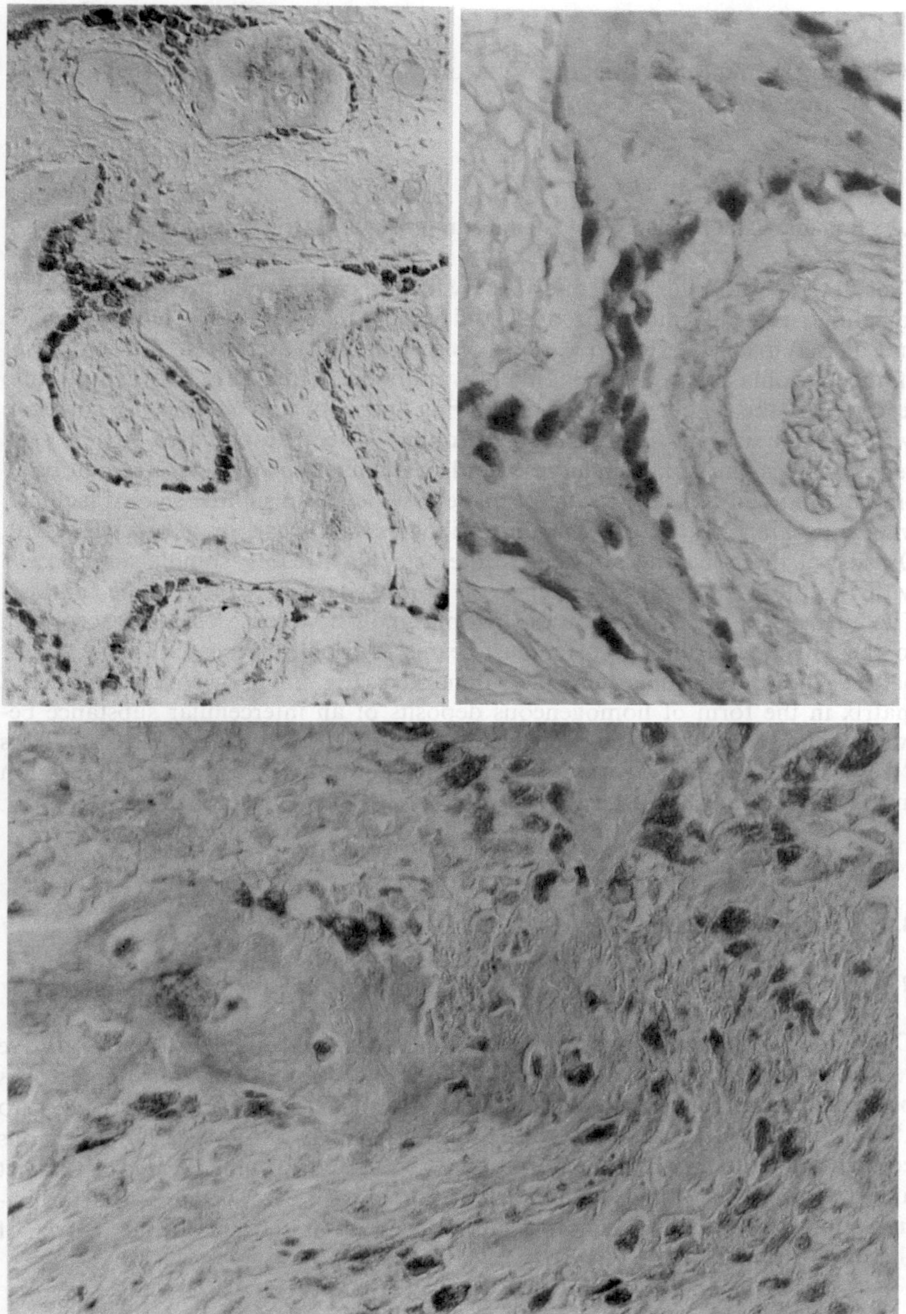

a b

c

Fig. 2 a–c. Immunohistochemistry of osteonectin in bone matrix-forming tissue (callus). **a** Intensive marking of osteoblast seams at trabecular bone surfaces (×112). **b** Marking of osteoblasts and young osteocytes in newly formed bone trabeculae (×300). **c** Immature bone matrix-forming tissue with intensive marking of osteoblasts and osteocytes. Presumable osteoprogenitor cells adjacent to bony surfaces are stained with varying intensity (×399). Antiosteonectin, PAP, no counterstaining, Nomarski

sponds to the molecular weight of osteonectin as previously reported (Fisher and Termine 1985).

3.2 Immunohistochemistry of Osteonectin in Bone Matrix-Forming Tissue

The material of callus and myositis ossificans consists mainly of trabecular, sometimes centrally mineralized osteoid with osteoblast seams on the surface and densely packed osteocytes. An intense granular reaction of the cytoplasm of the osteoblasts was seen with both antibodies (Fig. 2a). The cytoplasmic reaction of the osteocytes was of varying intensity and seemed to correlate with the cell size and cell location. "Young" osteocytes situated close to the osteoid trabecular surface in large, roundish lacunae showed a stronger antibody binding than did centrally located, smaller osteocytes in spindle-shaped lacunae, where marking by the osteonectin antibodies was weak or absent (Fig. 2b). Outside of the bone and adjacent to the osteoblast seams, spindle-shaped cells with the morphological appearance of fibroblasts were found to be marked. The intensity of the marking in the cytoplasm of these cells decreased according to their distance from the osteoblast seams. Fibroblasts located in the center between bone trabeculae remained unmarked (Fig. 2c). Formation of osteoid matrix in the form of homogeneous deposits of an intercellular substance between rounding cells was especially observed in early stage callus tissue. This "fresh" matrix formation was also accompanied by an intense antibody reaction in the respective cells (Fig. 2c).

3.3 Tissues Free of Bone Matrix

3.3.1 Cartilage

Chondrocytes and cartilaginous intercellular substance failed to show a positive reaction with osteonectin antibodies with the exception of the transitional zones between chondroid and osteoid tissue, the so-called chondroid bone (Beresford 1981). In these zones, where the chondroid matrix exhibits a homogeneous condensation in H&E stained sections, the chondrocytes revealed a distinct and sometimes very intense granular reaction of their cytoplasm. After trypsination an osteonectin marking was also apparent in the chondroid matrix of these transitional zones (Fig. 3).

3.3.2 Other Tissues

Interstitial connective tissue from various body regions, adipose tissue, and smooth and skeletal muscle were additionally investigated as bone matrix-free controls. Here the reactions with osteonectin antibodies were completely negative, in the cells as well as in the intercellular spaces (Table 1).

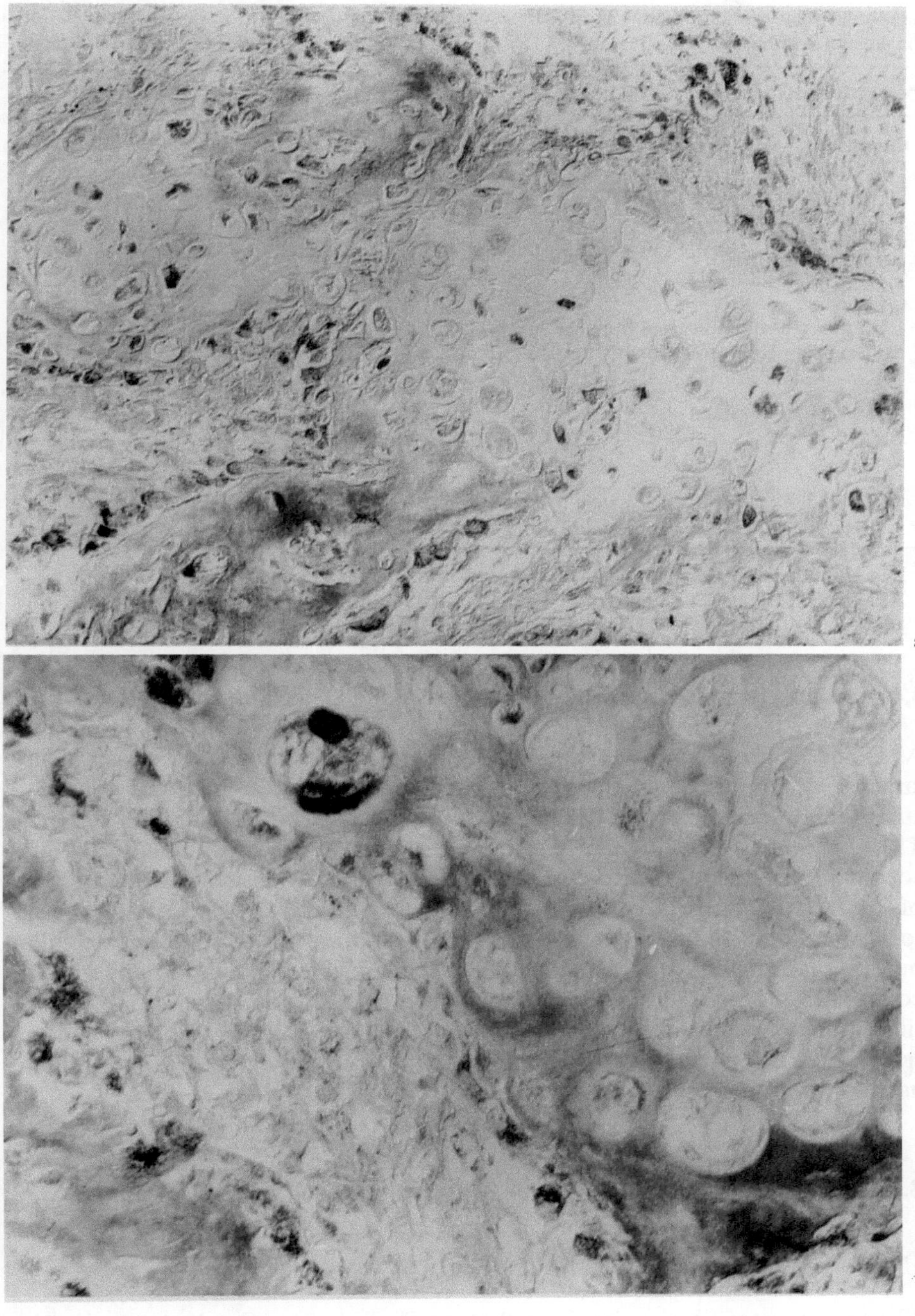

a

b

Fig. 3. a Callus tissue showing a transition between cartilage and bone, so-called chondroid bone, which is diffusely marked by the osteonectin antibody (×112). **b** Chondrocytes are likewise occasionally marked when lying in these areas of mineralizing chondroid bone (×300). Antiosteonectin, PAP, no counterstaining, Nomarski

Table 1. Survey of immunohistochemical results with osteonectin antibodies in skeletal and nonskeletal soft tissues

Positive for osteonectin	Negative of osteonectin
Bone tissue	Endosteal lining cells (nonfunctioning osteoprogenitor cells)
Osteoblasts	Old (quiescent) osteocytes
Developing osteoprogenitor cells	Chondroblasts, chondrocytes
Young active osteocytes	Cartilaginous matrix
Osteoid[a]	Nonskeletal matrix
Mineralized bone[b]	Stromal connective tissue
Cartilage	Fibroblasts
Chondrocytes of chondroid bone	Collagenous intercellular substance
Mineralizing chondroid bone matrix	Smooth muscle tissue
	Striated muscle tissue
	Fat cells
	Nerves

[a] Reaction intensified after trypsination of paraffin-embedded tissue
[b] Reaction positive after demineralization and trypsination

3.4 Immunoelectron Microscopy of Osteonectin in Osteoblasts and Osteoid

As a sign of protein synthesis and secretion, active osteoblasts possess a dense lamellar system of rough endoplasmic reticulum (rER) and usually several vesicular Golgi fields (Fig. 4). Occasional osteonectin marking is found in the rER. The intracellular marking becomes more distinct after the accumulation of glycoprotein in secretory vacuoles, which are frequently present in the vicinity of the Golgy fields (Fig. 5). Expulsion of osteonectin takes place after the secretory vacuoles have fused with the basement membrane of the cell. Extracellular marking is not found immediately subcellular in the aggregation zone of the collagen fibrils but only in the deeper osteoid maturation zone, where mineralization of the bone matrix also sets in (Fig. 6a). The osteonectin antibodies concentrate in the densification zones of the matrix, which, after contrasting, present as amorphous converings of the collagen fibrils (Fig. 6b).

3.5 Immunohistochemical Studies in Bone Tumors and Tumor-like Lesions

3.5.1 Tumor-like Lesions

The two cases of fibrous dysplasia that we studied showed a distinctly positive reaction with the osteonectin antibodies. This reaction occurred chiefly in cells immediately adjacent to newly formed woven bone or cells located within the trabeculae of woven bone. The reaction differed in degree, sometimes covering

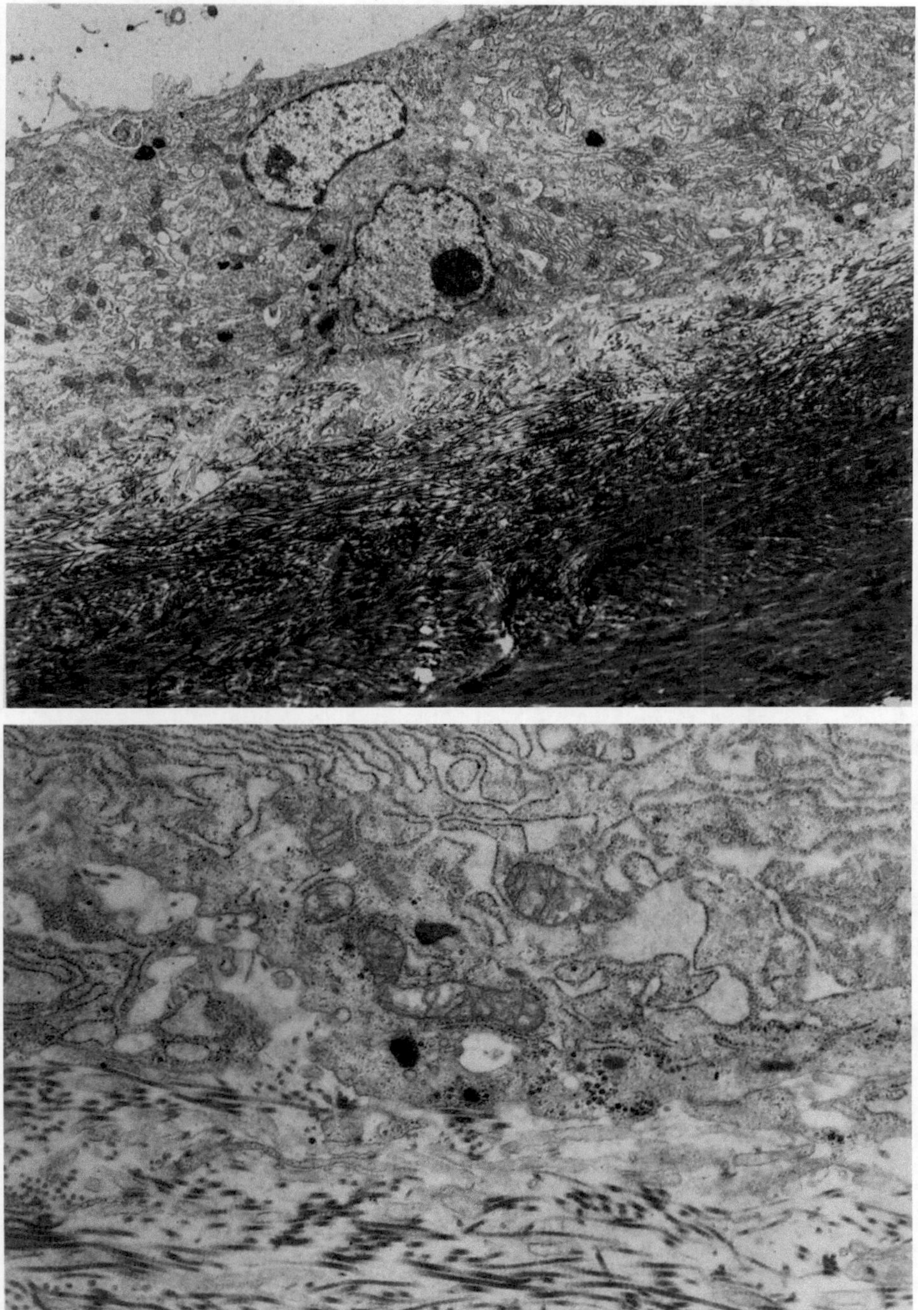

a

b

Fig. 4. a Electron photomicrograph of actively bone-forming osteoblasts on bone matrix still lacking mineralization (× 5800). **b** Interface between an actively matrix-producing osteoblast and the underlying osteoid only visible by its collagenous components (× 1500)

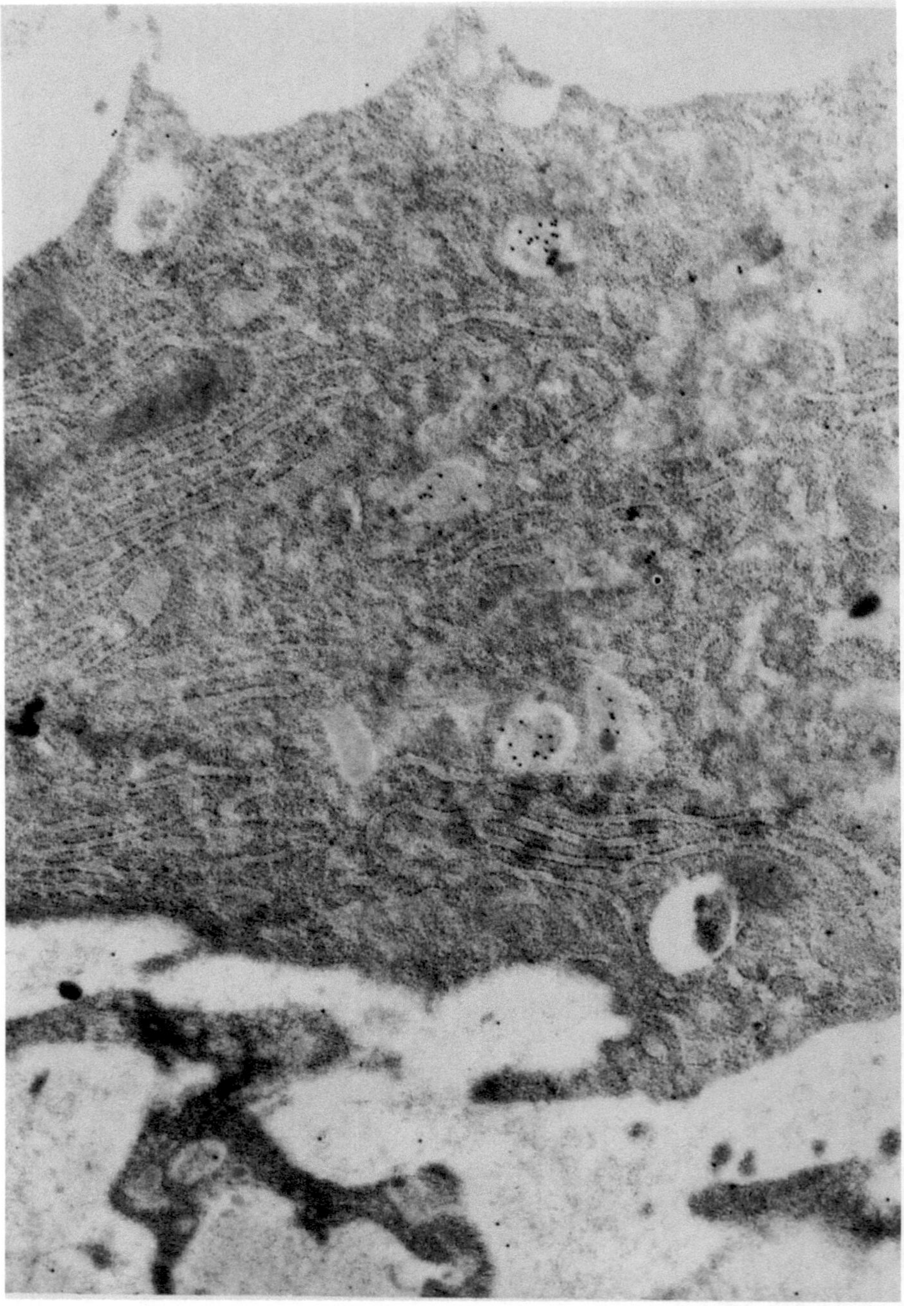

Fig. 5. Immunoelectron microscopy of osteonectin: Intracellular accumulation of osteonectin in vesicles, as shown by gold particles (× 18 000)

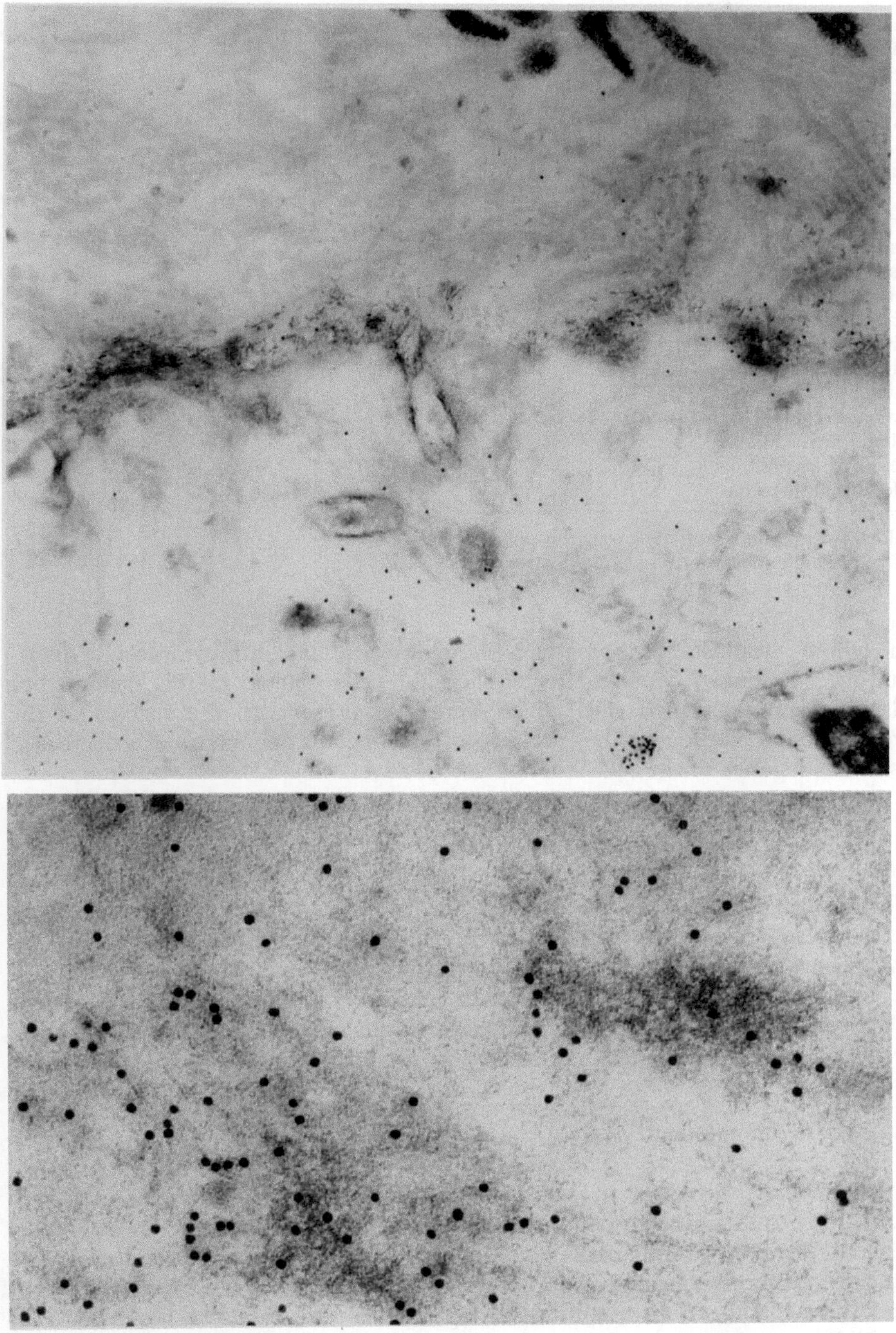

Fig. 6 a, b. Immunoelectron microscopy of osteonectin. **a** No marking of immature collagen fibrils just below the osteoblast, increasing immunoreactivity in the mature osteoid (×15000). **b** Concentration of immunoreactivity in amorphous deposits of bone matrix being considered as coating of collagen fibrils by noncollagenous bone proteins (×80000)

Table 2. Immunohistochemical results with osteonectin antibodies in skeletal and nonskeletal tumors

Tumor diagnosis	Immunohistochemical proof of osteonectin	
	Positive cases	Total cases
Osteosarcoma	13	13
Osteoid osteoma	3	3
Fibrous dysplasia	2 (focal)	2
Chondroblastoma	0[a]	1
Chondromyxoid fibroma	0	1
Chondrosarcoma	0[a]	3
Ewing's sarcoma	0	4
Fribrosarcoma	0	2
Rhabdomyosarcoma	0	1
Leiomyosarcoma	0	1
Meningeal sarcoma	0	1

[a] Positive immunoreactivity occurring only in areas of beginning mineralization

the whole cytoplasm and sometimes showing a granular intracytoplasmic distribution. Not only the cuboid, osteoblast-like cells reacted in this fashion but also the spindle-shaped cells which were also present on the surface of the woven bone trabeculae. The intensity of osteonectin demonstration decreased with the distance of the cells from woven bone.

3.5.2 Benign Bone Tumors

The three osteoid osteomas were also positive. Nearly all cuboid osteoblastic cells around the newly formed trabeculae of the spongiosa revealed intense cytoplasmic staining (Fig. 7). At low magnification it gave the impression of a band-like seam around the trabeculae. Definitely positive reactions were also observed in oval to spindle-shaped cells located centrally in the nidus area, whereas the multinucleated giant cells were completely negative.

3.5.3 Osteosarcomas

Thirteen osteosarcomas in various stages of differentiation were studied. According to their main component the tumors were subtyped as follows: osteoblastic, fibroblastic, and anaplastic (Fig. 8). All osteosarcomas reacted positively with the antibody against hON and bON. The intensity of the reaction differed and showed a clear-cut quantitative dependence (number of marked cells) on the differentiation of the tumor tissue. The classical osteoblastic osteosarcomas, being composed of tumor cells and matrix components in nearly equal quantities, revealed a strongly positive marking of malignant osteoblasts in the immedi-

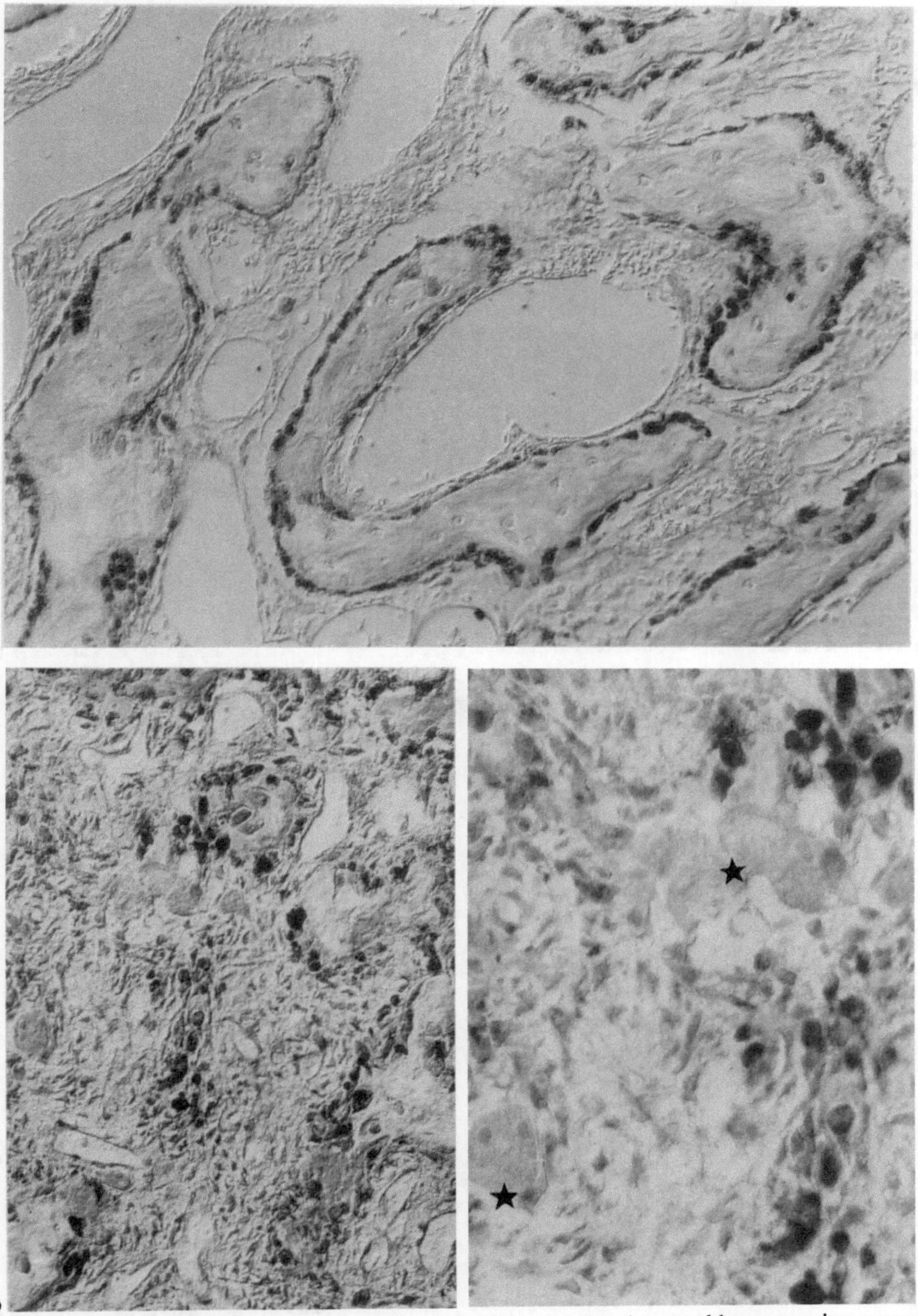

a

b

c

Fig. 7a–c. Osteonectin in osteoid osteoma. **a** Positive reaction in osteoblasts covering woven bone trabeculae of the peripheral zone (×112). **b** Nidus area with positively reacting osteoblasts in early stages of differentiation (×112). **c** Nidus area with positively reacting osteoblasts but negative osteoclastic giant cells (*) (×300). Antiosteonectin, PAP, no counterstaining, Nomarski

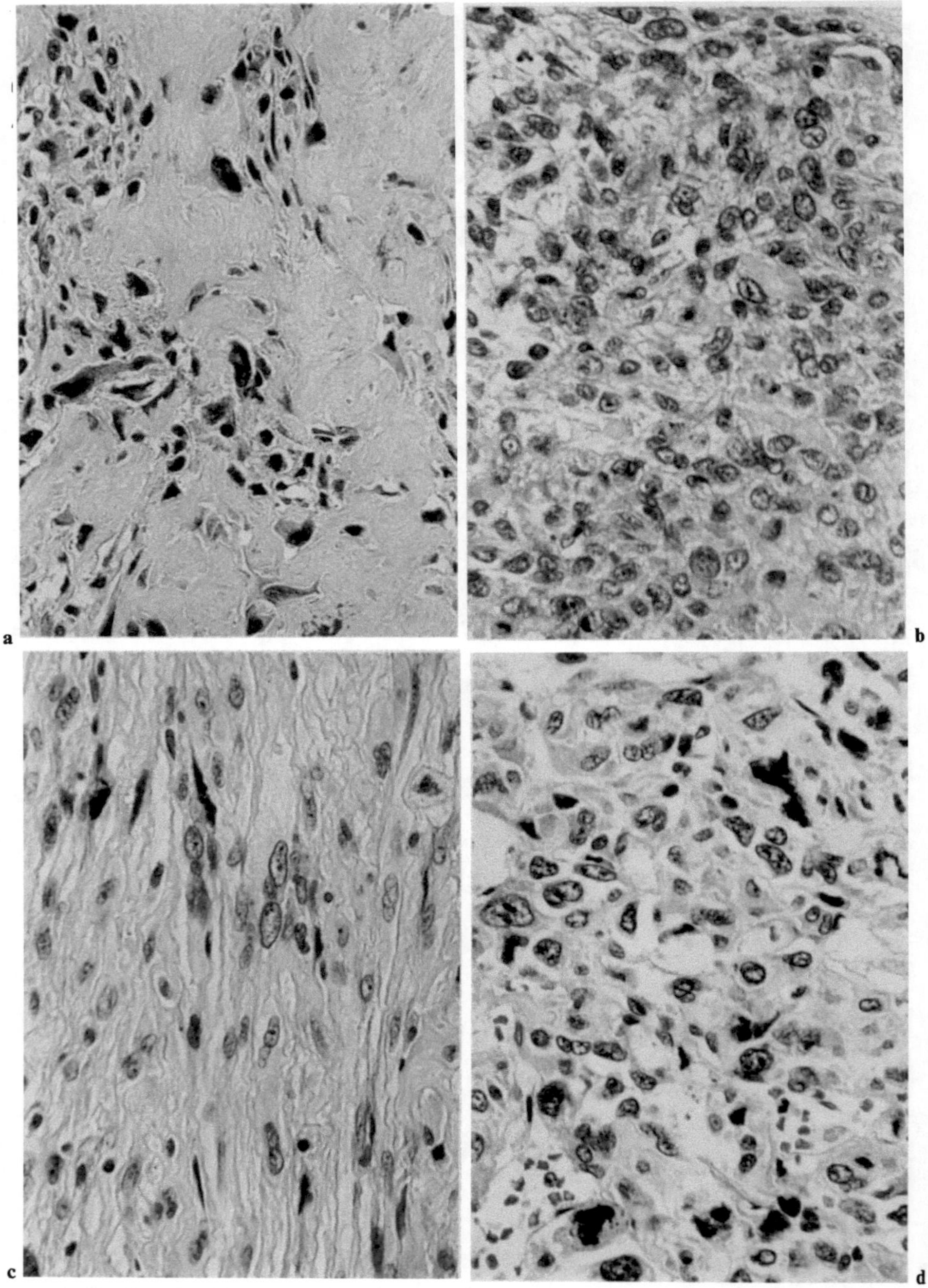

Fig. 8a–d. Histological pattern of different types of osteosarcoma. **a** Classical osteosarcoma with nearly equal parts of atypical osteoblasts and matrix components. **b** Osteoblastic osteosarcoma with scanty matrix production. **c** Fibroblastic osteosarcoma. **d** Anaplastic osteosarcoma with atypical pleomorphic osteoblasts. (H & E, × 300)

ate surroundings of osteoid islands within the tumor tissue (Fig. 9a, b). A topographically unordered and rather disseminated marking was seen in the tumor cells of osteoblastic osteosarcomas with still clearly discernible but less pronounced osteoid formation of the diffuse interstitial osteoid deposition type (Fig. 9c).

The non-matrix-forming tumors also showed a positive reaction. In the anaplastic tumor type, some hyperploid tumor osteoblasts with giant nuclei were found to display a strong marking of the frequently broad cytoplasm. In addition there was also a gradual difference in the cytoplasmic marking of the atypical osteoblastic tumor cells (Fig. 10): The non-matrix-forming fibroblastic type likewise showed a disseminated and intense cytoplasmic marking of some tumor cells. On the other hand, there were also numerous other tumor cells in which the intensity of the cytoplasmic immune reaction was distinctly weaker and of gradual difference (Fig. 11).

3.5.4. Non-Bone-Forming Skeletal Tumors

All other investigated skeletal tumors were negative. None of the Ewing's sarcomas showed a positive tumor cell reaction. The chondromatous tumors were likewise negative but presented a special feature: Whereas the chondromatous tumor portions were also completely negative, single positively reacting cells located near the mineralization zones were seen in the chondroblastoma segments that consisted in part of fibroblastic spindle-shaped cells. The immediately adjacent multinucleated osteoclastic giant cells were negative.

The chondrosarcomas also revealed no marking of tumor cells. They were negative, as was the chondroid matrix. However, chondrocytes with a positive cytoplasmic reaction were observed in those matrix zones that already displayed an osteoid-like staining behavior under the light microscope. This reaction was also found in the chondromatous portions of the osteosarcomas.

3.6 Soft Tissue Tumors

Independent from their morphological differentiation all soft tissues tumors were negative. These findings were also confirmed after prior treatment with enzymes.

4 Discussion

4.1 Osteonectin as a Constituent of Bone Matrix Proteins

Osteoblasts differ from other connective tissue cells by their ability to form bone matrix. Ninety percent of the latter consists of type I collagen, the remaining 10% of noncollagenous proteins. The bone matrix stores calcium salts in

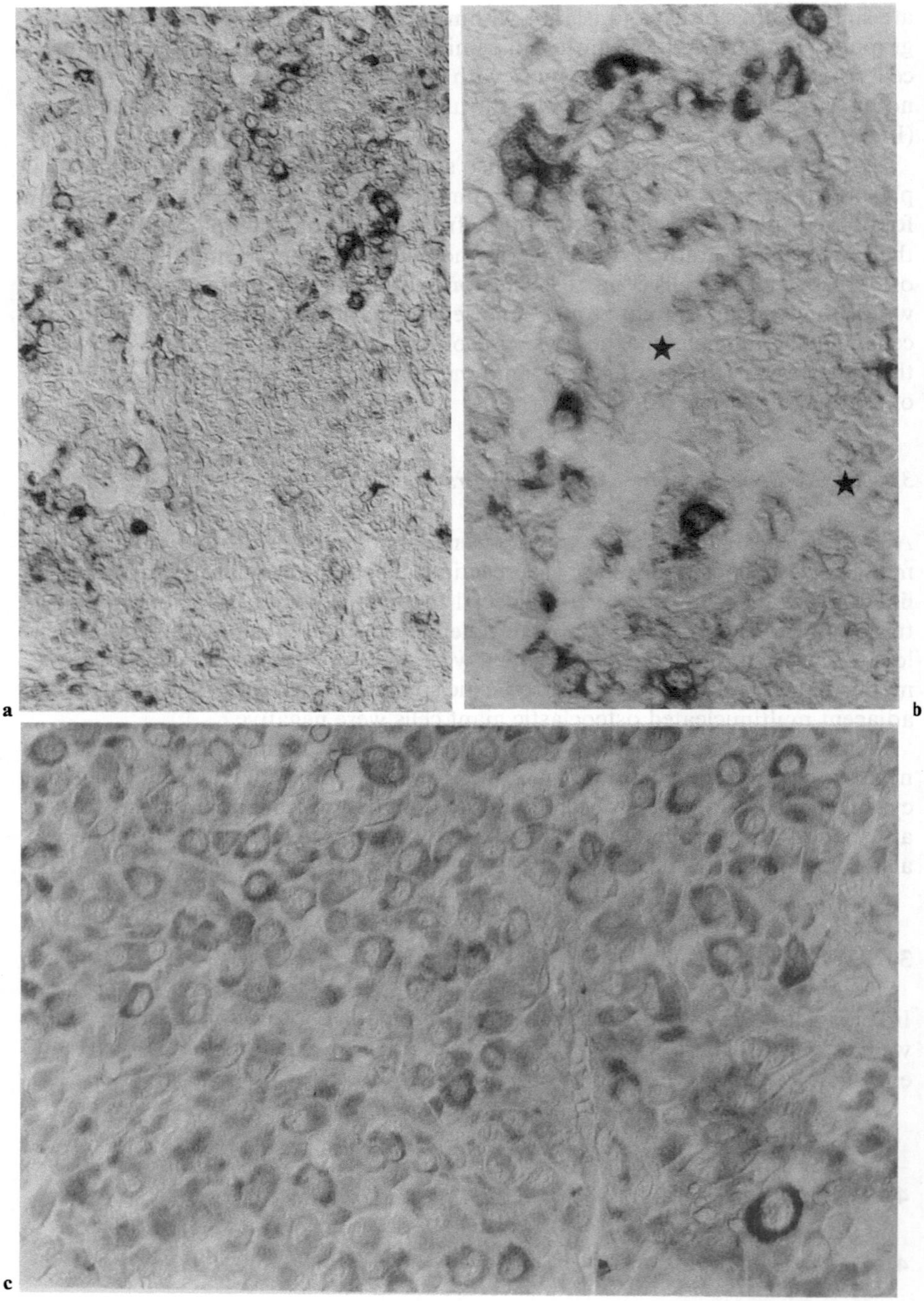

Fig. 9 a–c. Osteonectin in osteoblastic osteosarcoma. **a** Classical osteosarcoma with intensively marked atypical osteoblasts adjacent to osteoid islands (×112). **b** Higher magnification of classical osteosarcoma showing positive osteoblasts but no immunoreactivity in tumor osteoid (*) (×300). **c** Weaker marking of most of the tumor cells in osteoblastic osteosarcoma with scanty matrix production (×300). Antiosteonectin, ABC, no counterstaining, Nomarski

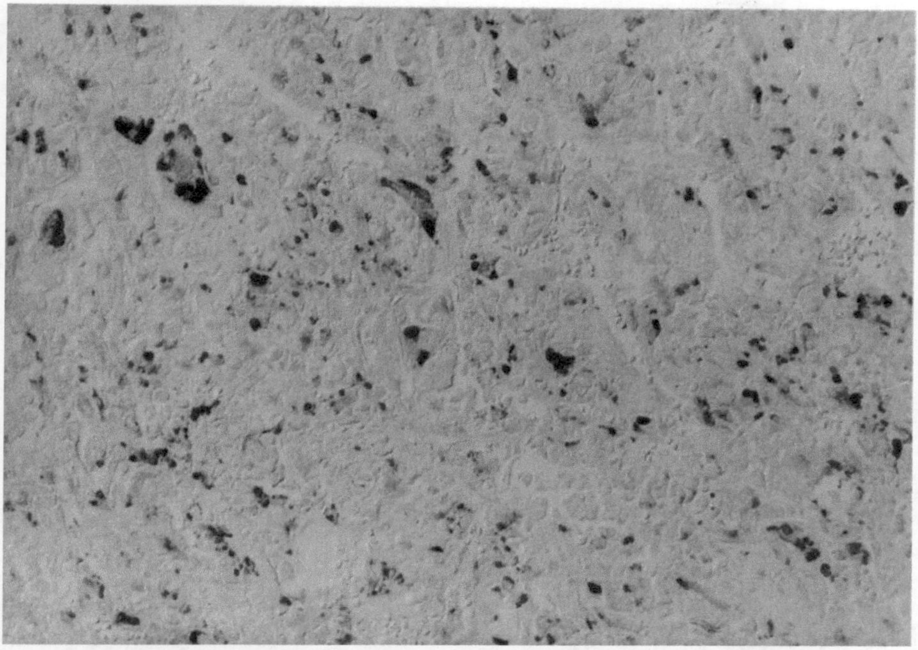

a

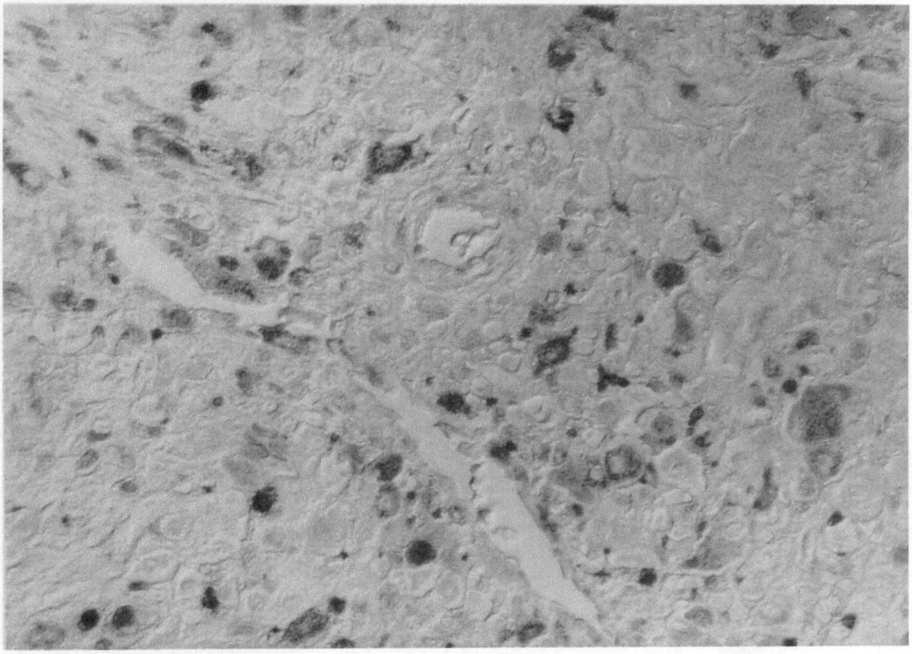

b

Fig. 10a, b. Osteonectin in anaplastic osteosarcoma. **a** Strong immunoreactivity in disseminated tumor cells (×112). **b** Gradual difference of the cytoplasmic marking of atypical pleomorphic osteoblasts (×300). Antiosteonectin, ABC, no counterstaining, Nomarski

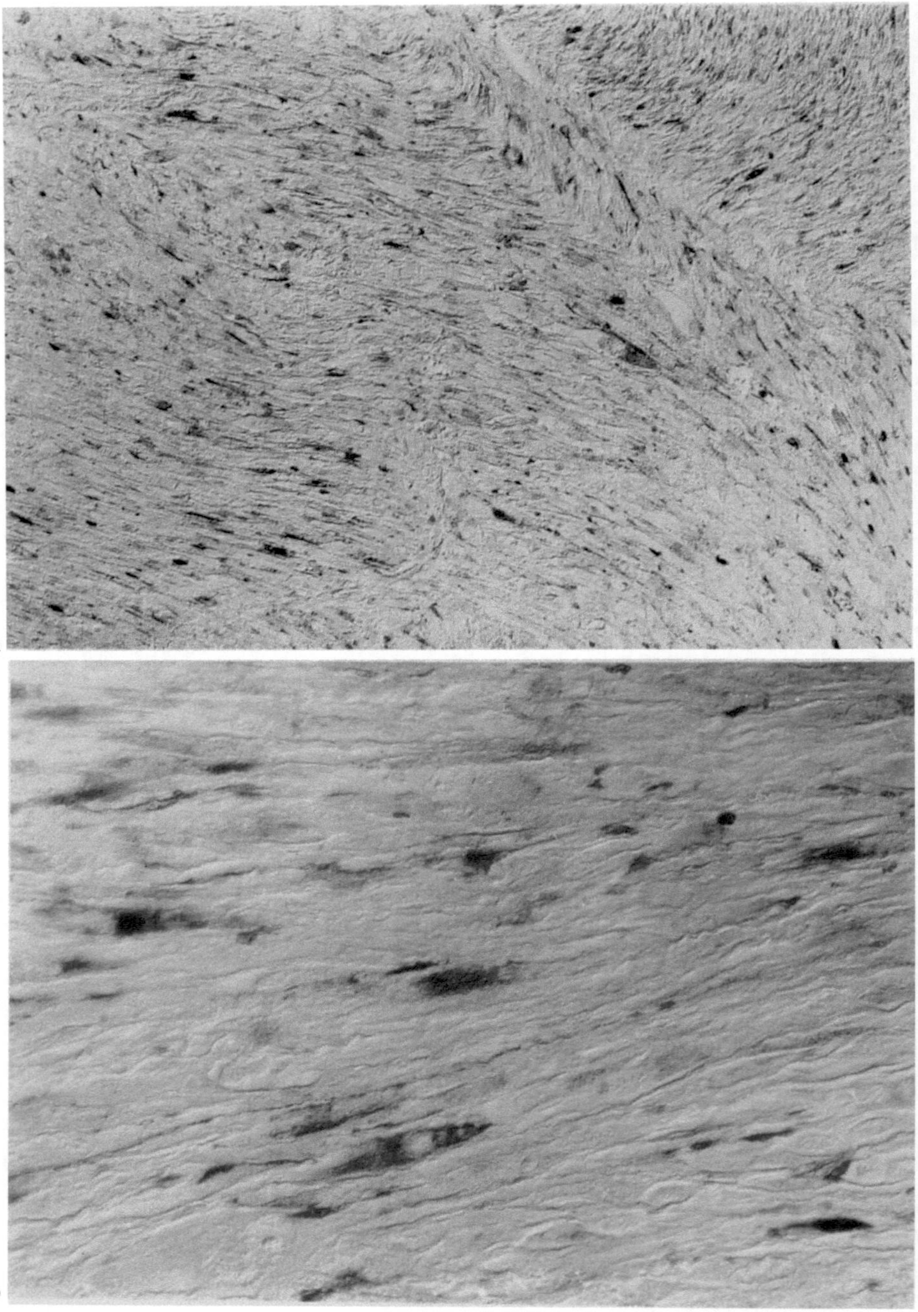

Fig. 11 a, b. Osteonectin in fibroblastic osteosarcoma. **a** Moderate immunoreactivity of numerous fibroblastic tumor cells (× 112). **b** Distinct cytoplasmic staining of spindle-shaped tumor cells (× 300). Antiosteonectin, ABC, no counterstaining, Nomarski

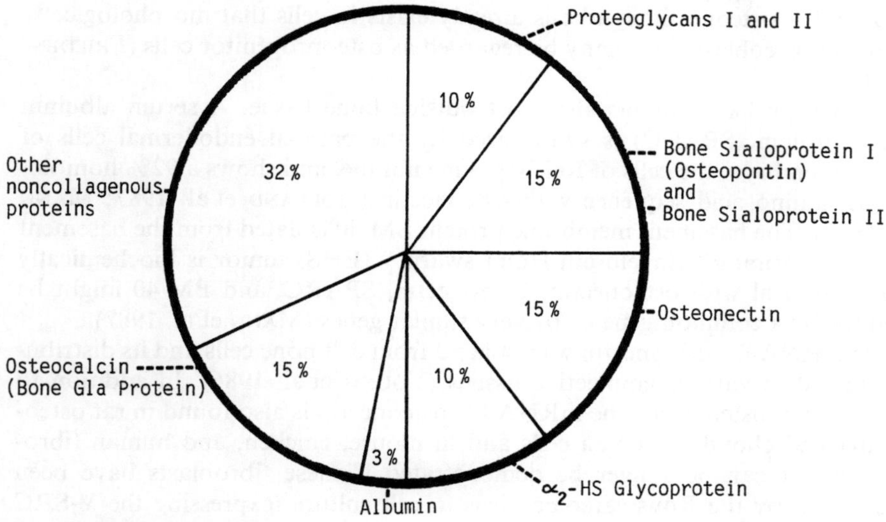

Fig. 12. Distribution of NCPs in developing bone (according to TERMINE 1987)

the form of hydroxyapatite, thus forming the mineralized bone. Only with the isolation of the noncollagenous matrix proteins did it become possible to ascertain the bone-specific components of this specialized connective tissue matrix. These proteins must therefore be regarded as a specific cellular product of the osteoblasts, whereas the collagenous bone constituents in the form of type I collagen are also found in many, other connective tissue (FISHER and TERMINE 1985; VON DER MARK 1981).

The noncollagenous bone proteins (NCPs) have been classified. Their quantitative distribution (Fig. 12) relates to newly formed human and bovine bone tissue since these matrix proteins are increasingly converted to low molecular derivatives in completely mineralized bone after weeks and months (FISHER and TERMINE 1985). With regard to quantity, the major members of the NCP family are osteonectin (TERMINE et al. 1981), osteocalcin (PRICE et al. 1976), and the bone sialoproteins I and II (FISHER et al. 1983b). The small bone proteoglycans I and II account for less than 1% of the NCPs demonstrable in mature bone (FISHER et al. 1983a). The amount of those bone matrix proteins that exert an inductive effect on osteoblasts, such as bone morphogenic protein (NAKAGAWA and URIST 1977), is also small. Non-bone-specific serum proteins, such as α_2-HS glycoprotein, albumin, transferrin, and IgG, account for a larger share.

One of the main components of the NCPs is osteonectin. It has a molecular weight of 38000 daltons (SDS-PAGE), is a phosphorylated glycoprotein, and was isolated from bovine bone tissue in 1981 (TERMINE et al. 1981). Antibodies against osteonectin have been used successfully for the characterization of bovine and human bone cell cultures (WHITSON et al. 1984; GEHRON ROBEY and TERMINE 1985), in a study of dental tissue (TUNG et al. 1985), and in reactive bone lesions (JUNDT et al. 1987). In this context it has been shown that the capability for osteonectin synthesis already exists in cells that morphologically are not yet osteoblasts but many be regarded as osteoprogenitor cells (FRIEDENSTEIN 1973).

Osteonectin-like proteins also exist outside bone tissue. A serum albumin binding protein (SPARC) is synthesized by the parietal endodermal cells of the mouse embryo, the cells of Reichert's membrane, and shows a 92% homology of its amino acid sequence with osteonectin (HOLLAND et al. 1987; MANN et al. 1987). The basement membrane protein BM 40 isolated from the basement membrane forming "Engelbreth-Holm swarm" (EHS) tumor is biochemically largely identical with osteonectin. Osteonectin, SPARC, and BM 40 might be coded for by a common gene or by very similar genes (MANN et al. 1987).

The mRNA for osteonectin was isolated from calf bone cells and its distribution studied in various connective tissues (YOUNG et al. 1986). In addition to its presence in osteoblasts, the mRNA for osteonectin is also found in rat osteosarcoma and chondrosarcoma cells and in mouse, chicken, and human fibroblasts, but it can no longer be demonstrated if these fibroblasts have been transformed by the Rous sarcoma virus in cell culture (expressing the V-SRC oncogen, YOUNG et al. 1986). "Osteonectin-like products" have also been found in serum, where they are platelet associated (FISHER et al. 1987). The importance of the presence of osteonectin mRNA or osteonectin-like products in nonosteogenic tissues is not clear. Our own negative immunohistochemical findings seem to indicate that osteonectin is formed in tissues other than bone only under special conditions (cell culture) or in extremely low quantity (fibroblasts), and that, it is possibly destroyed at once by proteolysis (YOUNG et al. 1986) and eludes immunohistochemical detection. This is confirmed by the results of a radioimmunological determination of tissue levels of osteonectin, revealing a 500- to 1000-fold higher concentration of osteonectin in bone (10000–15000 ng osteonectin per 100 μg protein) in comparison with numerous soft tissues (3–22 ng osteonectin per 100 μg protein) (GEHRON-ROBEY et al. 1987).

4.2 Functional Aspects of Osteonectin

The functional importance of osteonectin in bone is unknown. It was found to have a strong affinity for calcium hydroxyapatite molecules as well as for collagen fibrils, thus linking the two structures. For this reason it was given the name osteonectin. Its probable function is to maintain bone structure by contributing to the stabilization of the hydroxyapatite molecule and to its organization at the fibrillar collagen matrix (FISHER and TERMINE 1985). Our electron microscopic results support this view: Osteonectin is present in the mature bone matrix, which is called osteoid. Together with other noncollagenous bone matrix constituents it seems to envelop the collagen fibrils. This envelope has already been observed, on a purely electron microscopic basis, as a maturation process of the osteoid prior to the onset of mineralization (FORNASIER 1981). No osteonectin marking is detectable in the direct subcellular osteoblast attachment zone of the matrix where the aggregation of collagen fibrils from the procollagen molecules takes place. The fact that osteonectin marking occurs first in the next deeper layer of the matrix permits the conclusion that the in vitro affinity of osteonectin for collagen (FISHER and TERMINE 1985) alone is not sufficient to cause binding to the collagen portion of the bone matrix but that interaction with other noncollagenous bone matrix components is required (SCHULZ et al. 1987). This is also confirmed by the immunoelectron microscopic observation of BONNUCCI et al. (1986) that osteonectin marking is stronger in mineralized than in nonmineralized bone matrix.

4.3 Osteonectin as a Marker Protein of Osteoblasts

Osteonectin is present in bone cells (osteoblasts, osteocytes) if active matrix synthesis takes place. The finding that reactivity with osteonectin antibodies was also observed in cells of fibroblastic appearance seems to call for a different interpretation. These spindle-shaped cells are always seen in close proximity to an osteoblastic seam. This topographical relation to active matrix-producing osteoblasts and the decreasing intensity of osteonectin reactivity with increasing distance from the bone surface leads to a assumption that these spindle-shaped cells are newly recruited precursor cells of osteoblasts. They probably represent an intermediate stage between the so-called determined osteoprogenitor cells (FRIEDENSTEIN 1973) and completely developed active osteoblasts.

4.4 Osteonectin Antibodies in Bone-Forming Tumors

Even under pathological conditions osteoblasts usually retain their ability to form osteoid. This permits their definite morphological identification. But if this ability is incompletely developed, as may be the case in malignant bone tumors, it can be very difficult to classify a tumor as being an osteosarcoma, because these tumors can in some of their segments mimic the picture of other mesenchymal tumors such as fibrosarcoma, malignant fibrous histiocytoma, synovial sarcoma, or chondrosarcoma. This problem arises in particular if the diagnosis must be established on the basis of a biopsy, as has recently been proposed in some therapeutic plans (ROSEN et al. 1982; WINKLER et al. 1984). It would therefore be helpful to have other indicators available that might demonstrate the osteoblastic origin of a tumor, in addition to purely morphological criteria.

Immunohistochemical studies with antibodies against type I collagen have shown that these collagen types are not only demonstrable in osteosarcomas but also in other tumors. In addition, osteosarcoma cells seem not only to lose their ability to produce osteoid but also the ability to synthesize type I collagen. Therefore they react in fibrosarcomatous areas, for instance, only with antibodies against type III collagen (REMBERGER and GAY 1977; ROESSNER et al. 1983). Attempts to produce antibodies against osteosarcoma cells did result in antibodies, but these reacted not only with osteosarcomas but also with other soft tissue tumors (BRULAND et al. 1986). Antibodies against noncollagenous bone proteins such as osteonectin apparently do not pose these problems because they have only been demonstrated so far in osteoblastic cells (TERMINE et al. 1981; WHITSON et al. 1984; JUNDT et al. 1987). These results prompted us to investigate whether osteonectin antibodies would also be suitable marker for benign and malignant osteoblastic tumor cells.

Our results show that all the ostersarcomas we studied did react with the osteonectin antibody. That this immunoreactivity was indeed due to the presence of osteonectin could be demonstrated in the protein blot. A positive immunohistochemical reaction was not only found in the osteoid-producing tumor parts but also in the fibrosarcomatous and pleomorphic areas. All soft tissue tumors of similar morphological structure but different histogenesis were negative. There were two exceptions, however, that concerned the cartilage tumors. The chondroblastoma as well as some of the chondrosarcomas displayed areas with foci of a positive osteonectin reaction. These areas also showed light microscopic particularities. In the chondroblastoma, spindly oval cells in the neighborhood of mineralized areas were positive. The same feature has been observed in reactive bone lesion (callus) in morphologically similar cells which are located in the neighborhood of newly formed trabeculae and are probably determined osteoprogenitor cells (DOPCs) (FRIEDENSTEIN 1973). Since chondroblastomas often show mineralized areas and sometimes also formation of new bone (GRAVANIS and GIANSANTI 1971; DAHLIN and UNNI 1986) it may be assumed that the spindle-shaped oval cells that reacted positively with antiosteonectin are DOPC-like cells. In the chondrosarcomas, chondrocyte-like tumor cells surrounded by an osteoid-like matrix were seen on light microscopy. It was only in those areas in which the transition of chondrosarcoma tissue of mineralizing "chondroid" bone occurs (BERESFORD 1981) that a sometimes strong osteonectin marking was observed. This indicates a "switch-over" of cellular metabolism to the production of bone matrix proteins, similar to the process of enchondral ossification. This switch-over can also be proven by the fact that a combination of cartilage-specific type II collagen and bone typical type I collagen occurs in chondroid bone (BERESFORD 1981).

Despite these two exceptions it can be stated that the demonstration of osteonectin in tumors has proved to be a valuable further parameter in the diagnosis of bone-forming tumors, in particular of osteosarcomas. In combination with the light microscopic findings, a positive osteonectin reaction makes it possible for the pathologist to classify a malignant tumor as an osteosarcoma even if only scanty material is available.

5 Summary

Osteonectin is a noncollagenous protein of bone which is believed to be bone specific, since its concentration in bone tissue is 500- to 1000-fold higher than in other connective tissues. Immunohistochemistry with polyclonal osteonectin antibodies shows a highly specific marking of actively matrix-producing osteoblasts. Osteonectin is involved in the process of osteoid maturation and mineralization. Immunohistochemistry of osteonectin antibodies proved to be a valuable tool in the diagnosis of bone tumors. Since osteonectin production seems to be an early event in the differentiation of cells of the osteoblastic lineage, immunoreactivity of osteonectin antibodies is observed in types of osteosarcoma lacking osteoid production (anaplastic, fibroblastic) while corresponding types of soft tissue tumors remain unstained.

References

Beresford WA (1981) Chondroid bone, secondary cartilage and mataplasia. Urban and Schwarzenberg, Baltimore

Bonnucci E, Bianco P, Hayashi Y, Termine JD (1986) Ultrastructural immunohistochemical localization of non-collagenous proteins in bone, cartilage and developing enamel. In: Ali SY (ed) Cell mediated calcification and matrix vesicles. Elsevier, Amsterdam, pp 33–38

Brozman M (1978) Immunohistochemical analysis of formaldehyde- and trypsin- or pepsin-treated material. Acta Histochem 63:251–260

Bruland O, Fodstad O, Fundernd S, Pihl A (1986) New monoclonal antibodies specific for human sacromas. Int J Cancer 38:27–31

Church RL (1981) Chromosome mapping of connective tissue proteins. Int Rev Connect Tiss Res 9:99–150

Dahlin DC, Unni KK (1986) Bone tumors, 4th edn. Charles C. Thomas, Springfield

Fisher LW, Termine JD (1985) Noncollagenous proteins influencing the local mechanisms of calcification. Clin Orthop 200:362–385

Fisher LW, Termine JD, Dejter SW Jr et al. (1983a) Proteoglycans of developing bone. J Biol Chem 258:6588–6594

Fisher LW, Whitson SW, Avioli LV, Termine JD (1983b) Matrix sialoprotein of developing bone. J Biol Chem 258:12723–12727

Fisher LW, Hawkins GR, Tuross N, Termine JD (1987) Purification and partial characterization of small proteoglycans I and II, bone sialoproteins I and II, and osteonectin from the mineral compartment of developing human bone. J Biol Chem 262:9702–9708

Fornasier VL (1981) Transmission electron microscopy. Studies of osteoid maturation. In: Jee WS, Parifitt AM (eds) Bone histomorphometry. Armour Montagu, Levallois, France, pp 103–108

Friedenstein AJ (1973) Determined and inducible osteogenic precursor cells. In: Hard tissue growth, repair, and mineralization (CIBA Foundation Symposium), Blackwell, London, pp 169–185

Gay S, Rhodes RK (1980) Immunohistochemical demonstration of the genetically-distinct collagen types in human skeletal tissues. Metab Bone Dis Rel Res 2:97–101

Gehron Robey P, Termine JD (1985) Human bone cells in vitro. Calcif Tissue Int 37:453–460

Gehron Robey P, Fisher LW, Stubbs JT, Termine JD (1987) Biosynthesis of osteonectin and a small proteoglycan (PG-II) by connective tissue cells in vitro. Development and diseases of cartilage and bone matrix, pp 115–125

Gravanis MB, Giansanti JS (1971) Benign chondroblastoma. Report of four cases with a discussion of the presence of ossification. Am J Clin Pathol 55:624–631

Holland PWH, Harper SJ, McVey JH, Hogan BLM (1987) In vito expression of mRNA for the Ca^{++}-binding protein SPARC (osteonectin) revealed by in situ hybridization. J Cell Biol 105:473–482

Hsu SM, Raine L, Fanger H (1984) Use of avidin-biotin peroxidase complex (ABC) in immunoperoxidase techniques: a comparison between ABC and unlabeled antibody (PAP) procedures. J Histochem Cytochem 29:577–580

Huvos AG (1979) Bone tumors. WB Saunders, Philadelphia

Jundt G, Berghäuser K-H, Termine JD, Schulz A (1987) Osteonectin – a differentiation marker of bone cells. Cell Tissue Res 248:409–415

Laemmli UK (1970) Cleavage of structural proteins during the assembly of the head of bacteriophage T4. Nature 227:680–685

Mann K, Deutzmann R, Paulsson M, Timpl R (1987) Solubilization of protein BM-40 from a basement membrane tumor with chelating agents and evidence for its identity with osteonectin and SPARC. FEBS Lett 218:167

Martin SE, Dwyer A, Kissane JM, Costa J (1982) Small-cell osteosarcoma. Cancer 50:990–996

Nakagawa M, Urist MR (1977) Chondrogenesis in tissue cultures of muscle under the influence of a diffusible component of bone matrix. Proc Soc Exp Biol Med 154:568–572

Paul J (1979) Zell- und Gewebekulturen (translated and adapted by Maurer S and Maurer R). de Gruyter, Berlin, pp 219–220

Price PA, Otsuka AS, Poser JW, Kristaponis J, Raman N (1976) Characterization of a -carboxyglutamic acid-containing protein from bone. Proc Natl Acad Sci USA 73:1447–1451

Remberger K, Gay S (1977) Immunohistochemical demonstration of different collagen types in the normal epiphyseal plate and in benign and malignant tumors of bone and cartilage. Z Krebsforsch 90:95–106

Roessner A, Voss B, Rauterberg J, Immenkamp M, Gundermann E (1983) Biologic characterization of human bone tumors. J Cancer Res Clin Oncol 106:234–239

Romanowski R, Jundt G, Altmannsberger M, Schulz A (1987) Immunelektronenmikroskopie von Zell- und Matrixantigenen in Knorpel- und Knochentumoren. Verh Dtsch Ges Pathol 71:394

Rosen G, Caparros B, Huvos AG et al. (1982) Preoperative chemotherapy for osteogenic sarcoma: selection of postoperative adjuvant chemotherapy based on the response of the primary tumor to preoperative chemotherapy. Cancer 49:1221–1230

Roth J (1983) The colloidal gold marker system for light and electron microscopic cytochemistry. In: Bullock GR, Petrusz P (eds) Techniques in immunocytochemistry, vol 2. Academic, London, pp 217–284

Schulz A (1977) A reliable method of preparing undecalcified human bone biopsies for electron microscopic investigation. Micr Acta 80:7–18

Schulz A, Jeckel HM, Berghäuser K-H, Jundt G (1986) Bildung und Abgabe von CEA durch Coloncarcinom-Zellen – Ultrastrukturell-immunocytochemische Untersuchungen mit der Protein-A-Gold Methode. Verh Dtsch Ges Pathol 70:269–273

Schulz A, Romanowski R, Jundt G, Berghäuser K-H (1987) Immunoelectron microscopy of cell and matrix antigens in bone cells and bone tumors. Calcif Tissue Int 41 [Suppl 2]:18

Sternberger LA (1979) Immunocytochemistry, 2nd edn. Wiley, New York

Straus W (1982) Imidazole increases the sensitivity of the cytochemical reaction for peroxidase with diamino-benzidine at a neutral pH. J Histochem Cytochem 30:491–493

Termine JD (1987) Noncollagenous proteins of enamel and bone. Calcif Tissue Int 41 [Suppl 2]:810

Termine JD, Kleinman HK, Whitson SW, Conn KM, McGarvey ML, Martin GR (1981) Osteonectin, a bone-specific protein linking mineral to collagen. Cell 26:99–105

Towbin H, Staehelin T, Gordon J (1979) Electrophoretic transfer of proteins from polyacrylamid gels to nitrocellulose sheets: procedure and some applications. Proc Natl Acad Sci USA 76:4350–4354

Tung PS, Domenicucci C, Wasi S, Sodek J (1985) Specific immunohistochemical localization of osteonectin and collagen types I and III in fetal and adult porcine dental tissues. J Histochem Cytochem 33:531–540

van Noorden S, Polak JM (1983) Immunocytochemistry today – techniques and practice. In: Polak JM, van Noorden D (eds) Immunocytochemistry. Wright PSG, Bristol, pp 11–42

von der Mark K (1981) Localization of collagen types in tissues. Int Rev Connect Tissue Res 9:265–324

Whitson SW, Harrison W, Dunlap Mk, Bowers DE Jr, Fisher LW, Robey PG, Termine JD (1984) Fetal bovine bone cells synthesize bone-specific matrix proteins. J Cell Biol 99:607–614

Winkler K, Beron G, Kotz R et al. (1984) Neoadjuvant chemotherapy for osteogenic sarcoma: results of a cooperative German Austrian study. J Clin Oncol 2:614–624

Young MF, Bolander ME, Day AA, Ramis CI, Gehron Robey P, Yamada Y, Termine JD (1986) Osteonectin mRNA: distribution in normal and transformed cells. Nucleic Acids Res 14:4483–4497

Note added in proof: Meanwhile osteonectin/SPARC/BM-40 immunoreactivity has been demonstrated in decidua and some carcinomas. WEWER UM, ALBRECHTSEN R, FISHER LW, YOUNG ME, TERMINE JD (1988) Am J Pathol 132:345–355

Tumor Bone Formation in Different Osteosarcomas: Topological, Biochemical, and Histochemical Analyses

J. ALTHOFF, P. QUINT, H.J. HÖHLING, A. ROESSNER, and E. GRUNDMANN

1	Introduction	55
2	Enchondral Bone Formation	56
2.1	Morphology and Histology of the Epiphyseal Growth Plate	56
2.2	Biochemical Analyses of the Epiphyseal Growth Plate	58
2.2.1	Topological Distribution of the Extractable Compounds	61
3	Bone Formation in Osteosarcomas	66
3.1	Clinical Aspects	66
3.2	Histological and Biochemical Analyses of Osteosarcomas	67
3.2.1	Morphological and Histological Description of Large Tumor Samples	67
3.2.2	Biochemical Data	70
3.3	Zonal Combined Biochemical and Histological Analyses	77
3.3.1	Zonal Morphological and Histological Characterization	77
3.3.2	Zonal Biochemical Characterization	79
4	Comparison of Hard Tissue Formation in Osteosarcomas with Physiological Bone Formation	84
	References	88

1 Introduction

Generally osteosarcomas show a pattern of considerable heterogeneity. Areas with osteoblastic cells are very often surrounded by fibroblastic areas, and anaplastic, telangiectatic, and small cell areas are present. On the basis of their different morphology and histology DAHLIN and UNNI (1977) have introduced several subentities within osteosarcomas. Studies by GRUNDMANN et al. (1981) and ROESSNER (1984) have substantiated the value of a cytogenetic approach. During the growth of tumor bone, several morphological types of differentiation, probably caused by different metabolic processes, can be observed in the same tumor, but little is known about the related biochemical changes. For a better understanding of this pathological bone formation occurring during tumor growth, it is important to study physiological bone formation. This may be done in different model systems, such as mineralizing avian tendons (ALTHOFF et al. 1977, 1978; QUINT et al. 1977; HÖHLING et al. 1976), dentinogenesis (LINDE et al. 1981), organ cultures (URIST et al. 1983; RATH et al. 1981; ALTHOFF et al. 1988), and enchondral ossification occurring in the epiphyseal growth plate (WUTHIER 1969; SCHMIDT et al. 1978; ALTHOFF et al. 1982).

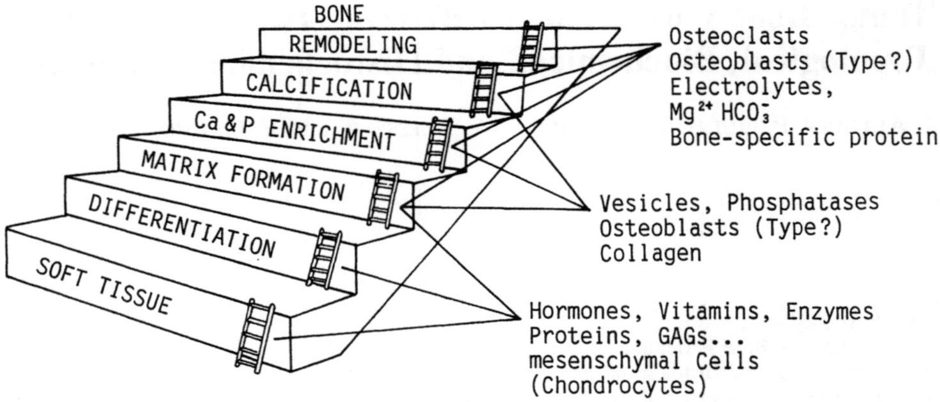

Fig. 1. Scheme symbolizing the different steps of bone formation. Different types of cells, producing characteristic metabolites, are involved in this sophisticated process

The multiple steps of bone formation (Fig. 1) are a very complex process which is not yet fully understood. The complexity is reflected by the morphology of the epiphyseal growth plate. This complexity, revealed by the arrangement of different types of cells within a comparatively small area (Fig. 2), suggests that this type of bone formation would be an appropriate model for comparison with pathological bone formation in osteosarcomas.

2 Enchondral Bone Formation

2.1 Morphology and Histology of the Epiphyseal Growth Plate

The epiphyseal growth plate can be divided into different zones based on morphological criteria such as cell shape. While a good agreement is reached concerning the definition of the different zones for the unipolar growth plate, problems arise when defining the zones of the bipolar growth plate (SCHLÜTER 1978). The problem is whether the different morphological zones are also characterized by different biochemical processes which finally result in the formation of bone. Some of the most important cell types found in the epiphyseal growth plate will be described.

Cartilage contains chondrocytes. These cells produce a proteoglycan-rich matrix as well as collagen type II, among other important proteins (growth factors etc.). The cartilage itself can be divided into different zones: the resting zone, the proliferating zone, zones of palisades, and the hypertrophic zone. In these zones the chondrocytes obviously operate in a cartilage-producing way; however, when they begin to hypertrophy they do change metabolism. When the chondrocytes have reached a maximal hypertrophy a new type of

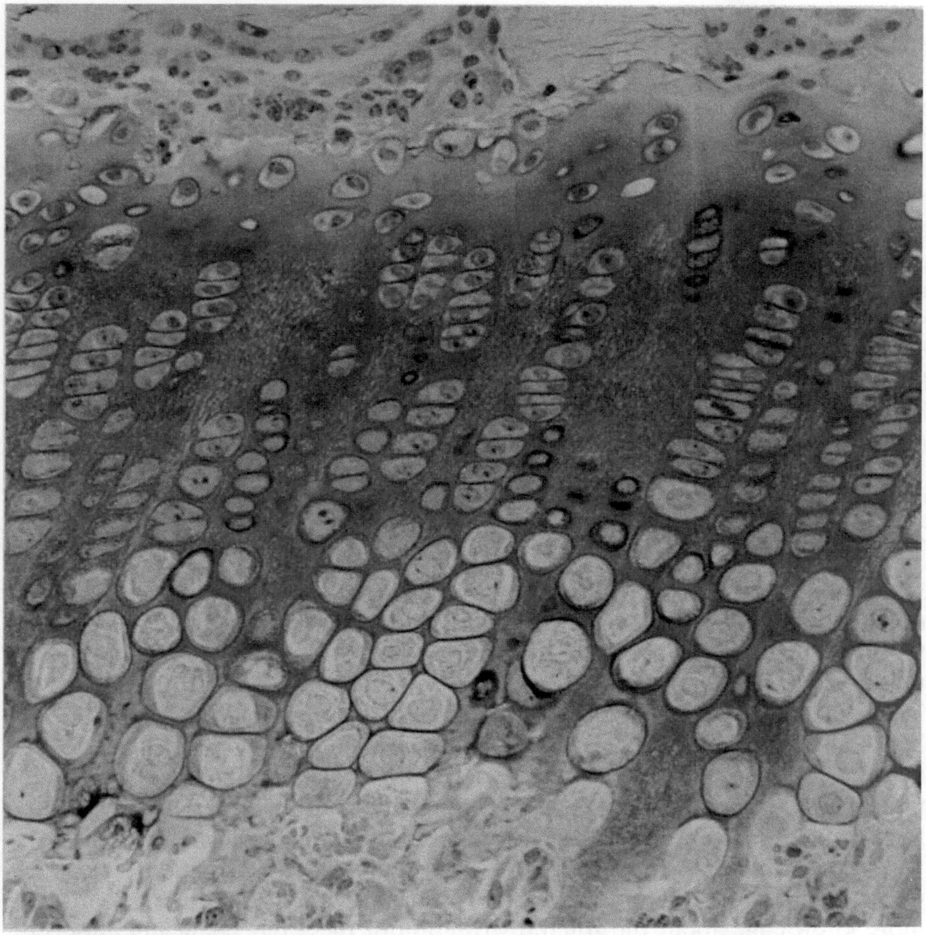

Fig. 2. Epiphyseal cartilage of the guinea pig tibia with differentiating chondrocytes: The hypertrophic cartilage undergoes calcification and osteoblasts are visible

cell can be observed: the chondroclast. Chondroclasts digest the transverse chondronic walls surrounding the chondrocytes. A large number of chondrocytes seem to die; however, a considerable number of cells are present at sites of primary calcification. In this area at the end of the cartilage many blood vessels invade the cartilage accompanied by mineral deposition, the blood supply of cartilage being comparatively poor. Primary calcification develops along the longitudinal septae and is obviously carried out metabolically by the osteoblasts developing along them. This primary calcification is also known as cartilage calcification.

When cartilage calcification has reached a high density, another cell type can be found: osteoclasts. These cells metabolize the calcified cartilage and at the same time osteoblasts, probably different from the osteoblasts at sites of cartilage mineralization (JONES et al. 1988), form the trabecular bone. Some of the osteoblasts are immured in the newly formed trabecular bone and are then characterized as osteocytes. This zone is called the remodeling zone, due to the fact that the primary bone or primary spongiosa is transformed into the final trabecular bone. When trabecular bone formation is completed the bone marrow is formed; this process will not be described here. In the calcifying areas the structure of the matrix changes. The osteoblasts produce collagen type I, and the bone matrix contains proteoglycans which differ in amount and structure from those in cartilage. When bone remodeling is finished, the number of osteoclasts decreases. In the final trabecular bone, however, there are still some osteoclasts always accompanied by a certain number of osteoblasts. The osteoblasts are connected with osteocytes by gap junctions. In healthy trabecular bone a steady state exists between bone degradation and bone formation. This balance can be disturbed by hormonal influences, calcium, magnesium, and phosphorus deficiency, causing bone diseases.

2.2 Biochemical Analyses of the Epiphyseal Growth Plate

Some questions concerning the biochemical process occurring during enchondral ossification have been answered by the studies of WUTHIER (1969). BOYDE and SHAPIRO (1980) have carried out qualitative and KREFTING et al. (1980) quantitative electron microprobe analyses of the epiphyseal growth plate. These authors investigated the distribution of some important elements such as Ca, P, Mg, Na, and K. Besides this more inorganic approach, it is of general interest to attain more knowledge about the biochemical organic components. Alkaline phosphatase is an important enzyme for bone formation, as is acid phosphatase for bone remodeling (REDDI 1981). Mg^{2+} is a cofactor of the alkaline phosphatase and probably has a regulatory effect on the process of mineral formation (ALTHOFF et al. 1978; QUINT et al. 1980). Thus it was of great interest to obtain more knowledge about the zonal distribution of these biochemically important components, probably gaining some insights into enchondral bone formation.

By cutting a continuous series of cryostat sections through the bipolar epiphyseal growth plate of the porcine proximal ulna, from the epiphyseal mineralized region to the metaphyseal zone of bone remodeling, it should be possible to combine morphological results with biochemical data. In a repeated sequence sections were chosen for light microscopy in order to compare the biochemical analyses directly with the morphological results. The procedure of tissue preparation and analysis will be described briefly.

Longitudinal slices of the growth plate were frozen in liquid nitrogen and trimmed to blocks (2 × 2 × 4 mm) under the same conditions. Serial 5 or 10 μm thick frozen sections were cut in a cryomicrotome proceeding from the epiphyseal bone into the metaphysis (Fig. 3). For the biochemical analyses pooled frozen sections were transferred into an extraction solution containing isotonic NH_4Cl concentration buffered to pH 8.0. After extraction and centrifugation the supernatants and the sediments were analyzed. In the supernatants, nuclease, acid phosphatase activity, alkaline phosphatase activity, protein, inorganic and

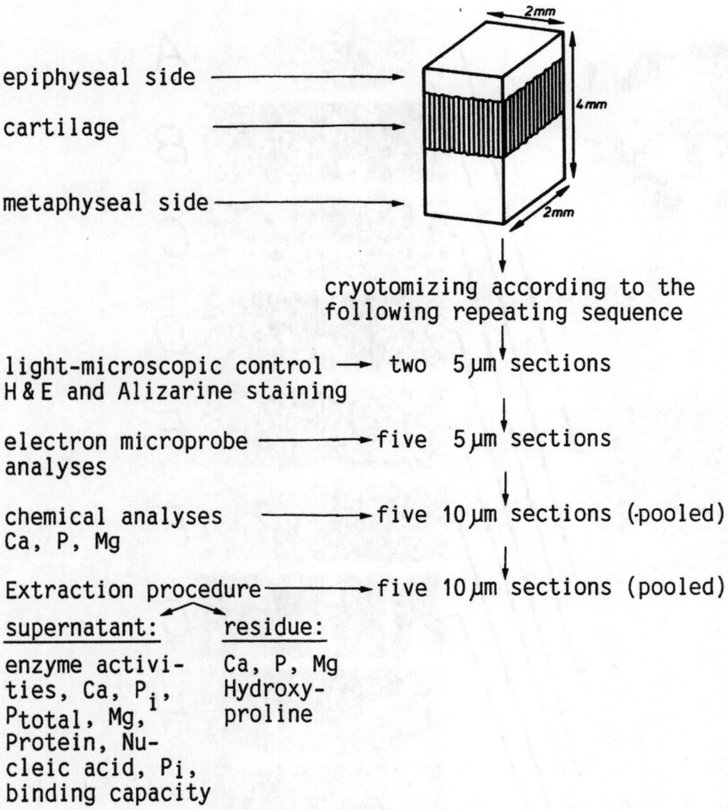

Fig. 3. Flow diagram of the slicing procedure, demonstrating the distribution of the cross-sections for the different analyses

organic phosphorus, calcium, magnesium, sodium, and potassium were determined. In the sediments calcium, phosphorus, magnesium, and collagen via hydroxyproline were determined.

In Fig. 4 (left) a longitudinal section of a porcine proximal ulna is shown. Higher magnification micrographs of transverse sections for different levels through this growth plate are marked by lines to indicate the levels of the growth plate at which the topological analyses were carried out (Fig. 4, right). They demonstrate the different morphological characteristics of each zone. Here only those results are reported which were obtained from the analyses of the diaphyseal part of the growth plate. The epiphyseal side is smaller but gave similar results.

Zone A: The zone of resting cells (germinative zone) contains relatively few small cells; it extends for some 50–80 μm in a longitudinal direction.

Zone B: The proliferative zone contains cells which are still small but more numerous; they are arranged in pairs of four or eight proceeding towards the

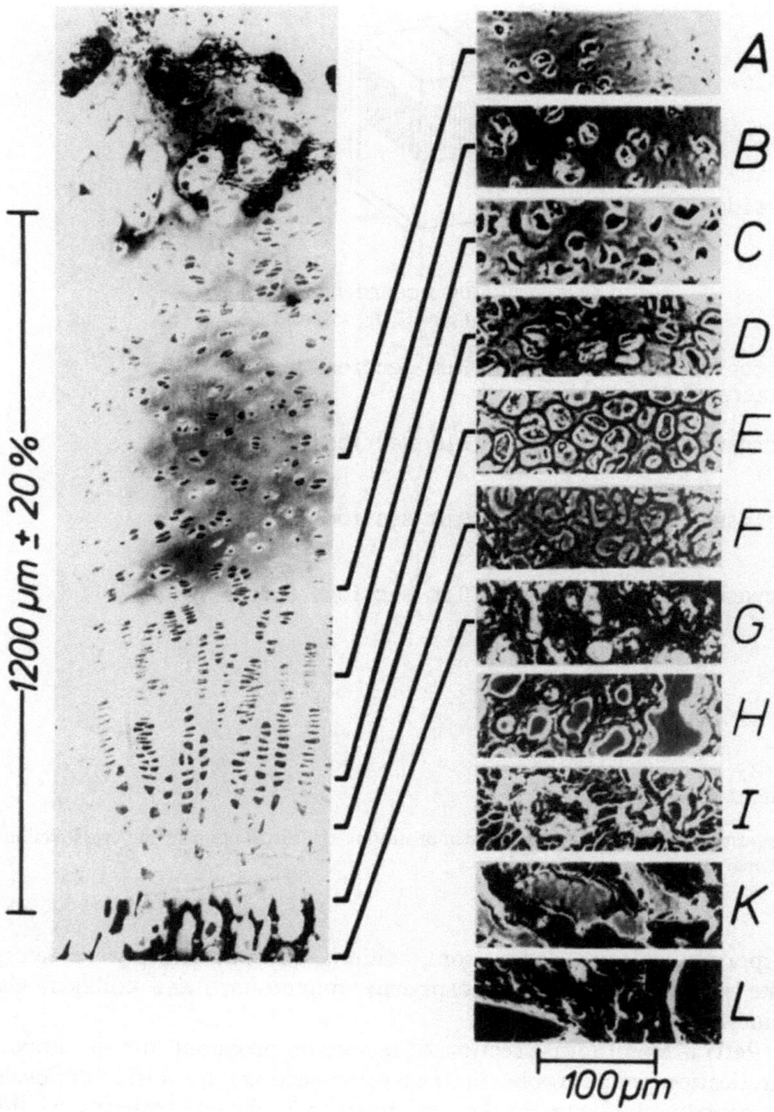

Fig. 4. *Left:* Longitudinal section of a 10-week-old porcine proximal ulna epiphyseal growth plate (mainly the unmineralized part of the bipolar growth plate). *Right:* The coordinated cross-sections (metaphyseal part) of the different zones being analyzed

diaphysis. The size of the cells increases continuously towards the edge of the proliferative zone. In this region the cells are more densely packed and a group arrangement could no longer be observed. Zone B extends for 200–500 µm.

Zone C: The upper columnar cell zone contains cells which have formed longitudinal rows more or less of the same size. Zone C extends for some 90–100 µm.

Zone D: We included in zone D cells which still have a typical elliptical form. Zone D extends for some 100–130 μm.

Zone E: In this zone the hypertrophy of the cartilage cells increases rapidly, finally reaching a relatively rounded form. This zone extends for 160–190 μm.

Zone F: This zone contains cells of maximal hypertrophy which already show signs of degeneration; it extends for some 180–210 μm and may contain some traces of calcified cartilage, caused by the slightly arched structure of the growth plate.

Zone G: Primary calcification was observed in this zone. The mineralized longitudinal septum between neighboring longitudinal rows of cells can be seen. This zone extends for some 170–190 μm.

Zone H: In this zone the calcification of the longitudinal septum is nearly completed. The structure of the septum is altered by the incorporated mineral. Bone formation is commencing. The zone extends for 100–130 μm.

Zone I: In this zone high cellular activity promoting bone formation is observed; the calcification has reached a high density. No structural elements of the longitudinal septum are detected. The zone extends for 180–210 μm.

Zone K: In this zone bone remodeling occurs, as indicated by the formation of trabeculae, extending for 360–400 μm. At the end of this zone typical trabecular bone can be recognized.

Zone L: This zone contains pure trabecular bone; bone formation seems to be completed.

The total extent of the diaphyseal side of the plate analyzed was about 2.3 mm, the extent of the unmineralized diaphyseal part being about 800 μm while the extent of the unmineralized part on the epiphyseal side was about 400 μm. The data given here are the average values calculated from five different animals and vary within ±20%.

2.2.1 Topological Distribution of the Extractable Compounds

Typical results of the topochemical analyses are summarized in Figs. 5 and 6. Zones A–L correspond to those which have just been characterized morphologically.

The enzyme activites and the extracted electrolyte concentrations are given in relative values, taking the highest value found as 100%. The 100% values are summarized in Table 1. The main results which can be derived from Figs. 5 and 6 (and Table 1) are the following: No remarkable enzyme activity could be extracted from the cartilage zone A (resting zone). At the end of this zone the inorganic phosphate-binding capacity showed a maximum; it fell sharply to zero in zone D. The nucleic acid content distinctly increased in the proliferative zone (zone B), with a peak at the beginning of zone C (upper columnar zone), and then fell continuously, except for some variations in zones E and

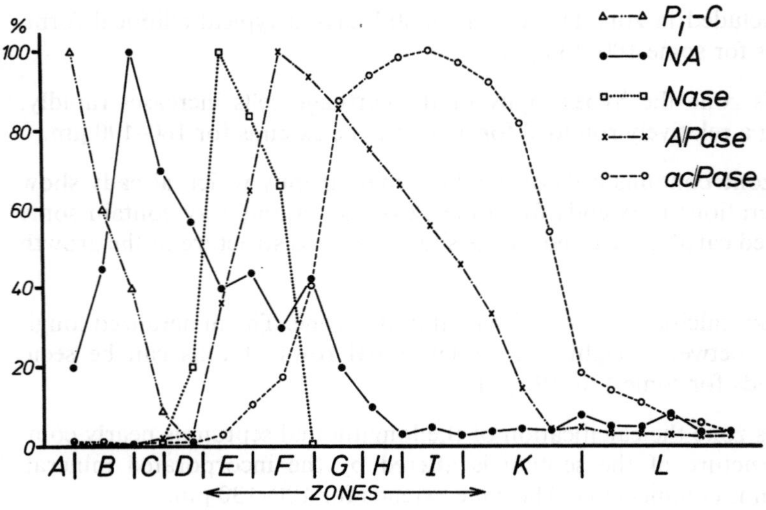

Fig. 5. Graphic presentation of extracted organic compounds and enzymes from the different zones of a 10-week-old porcine proximal ulna epiphyseal growth plate (only the metaphyseal part of the bipolar growth plate). The values given are relative values, taking the highest found values as 100%. *P_i-C*, P_i binding capacity; *NA*, nucleic acid; *Nase*, nuclease activity; *APase*, alkaline phosphatase activity; *acPase*, acid phosphatase activity

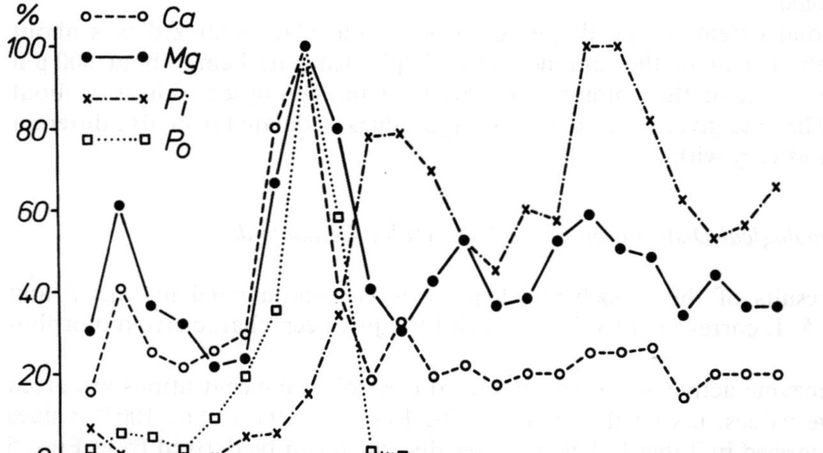

Fig. 6. Graphic presentation of extracted ions from the different zones of a 10-week-old porcine proximal ulna epiphyseal growth plate (corresponding to Fig. 5; only the metaphyseal part of the bipolar growth plate). The values given are relative values, taking the highest found values as 100%. P_i, inorganic phosphorus; P_o, organic phosphorus

Table 1. Maximal values of the extracted compounds in the different zones of the growth plate

P_i binding capacity[a]	6.1	Zone A
Nucleic acid[b]	87	Zone C
Nuclease activity[c]	0.074	Zone E
APase activity[c]	0.70	Zone F
Organic phosphorus[d]	5.7	Zone F
Ca^{2+} [d]	2.3	Zone F
Mg^{2+} [d]	0.13	Zone F
acPase activity[c]	0.25	Zone I
Inorganic phosphate[d]	2.4	Zone K

[a] nmol per ml per µg
[b] µg per 100 mg extracted dry mass
[c] Units per mg extracted nucleic acid
[d] % extracted dry weight
APase, alkaline phosphatase; acPase, acid phosphatase

F (beginning and maximal hypertrophy), down to a constant level in the region of bone remodeling (zone I). Measurable amounts of a nuclease activity could be detected in zone D, where the first signs of cell hypertrophy could be observed, and peaked in zone E where the increase in cell size was very rapid.

A sharp increase in alkaline phosphatase activity followed and overlapped with the nuclease activity. A maximum alkaline phosphatase activity was found in zone F, the zone of maximal hypertrophy and cell degeneration, just in front of the mineralization area. It is possible that some slices contain calcified material due to the slightly arched growth plates. The first increase in acid phosphatase activity was also measurable in zone F (maximum hypertrophy); this increase continued in zones G and H, and peaked with a broad maximum in zone I.

The Ca and Mg content (probably mainly ions), which could be extracted form the sections with the buffer as well as the extracted organic phosphorus showed a strong correlation with the alkaline phosphatase activity since they all peaked together in zone F (maximum hypertrophy).

The maximum value for inorganic phosphorus was found in zone K (bone remodeling), but there was also a peak in zones G and H_0 and it increased simultaneously with the acid phosphatase activity. Mg was also analyzed by electron microprobe analysis. Since the freezing conditions in this project to avoid an intra-extracellular exchange of the mobile elements were not optimal, the intracellular concentrations must be interpreted with caution and are not included in Table 2. Better freezing conditions could be achieved for the proximal growth plate of the tibia of rats, and results of an intra- and extracellular distribution for Ca and P (and S) were reported by Krefting et al. (1980). It should be mentioned that a good agreement exists for the extracellular Ca, P, and S contents between the tibia growth plate and the porcine growth plate of this project.

The results for calcium, magnesium, and phosphorus are summarized in Table 2. Taking the total amount of Ca of the germinative and proliferative zones (zones A and B), the concentration (per dry weight) is about 0.6%, corre-

Table 2. Total amount of elements relevant for the calcification process

Zone	Ca[a]	Mg[a]	P[a]	S_{intra} [b]	S_{extra} [b]	P_{intra} [b]	P_{extra} [b]
A	0.3	0.1	0.2	0.7	3.5	5.0	0.1
B	0.9	0.1	0.7	0.8	4.0	5.0	0.1
C	2.2	0.2	1.2	0.7	3.2	4.0	0.2
D	1.9	0.2	1.2	0.7	2.7	4.0	0.2
E	4.2	0.2	2.4	0.6	2.1	4.0	0.4
F	6.7	0.3	3.3	0.6	0.3	n.m.	9.0
G	10.2	0.4	4.6	n.m.	0.6	n.m.	6.0
H	17.6	0.5	7.5	n.m.	0.2	n.m.	12.0
I	19.8	0.5	8.8	n.m.	0.2	n.m.	12.0
K	13.1	0.5	6.6	n.m.	0.1	n.m.	12.0

[a] Chemical analyses %Wt
[b] Electron microprobe analyses %Wt
n.m., not measured

sponding to about 58 mM/kg wet weight, assuming a water content of 67% for the tissue. The total Ca content steadily increased up to about 7% in zone F (zone of maximum hypertrophy).

It is important to discuss the chosen extraction procedure. The cryostat sections are 10 μm thick. Assuming an average cell diameter of about 20 μm, each cell would be cut by this procedure. Thus, the slicing is comparable with mechanical homogenization, and consequently the buffer treatment yielded an extract containing intra- and extracellular material. In order to keep the enzymes and the electrolytes in their physiological state as far as possible, no detergents were used; rather an extraction under mild conditions with isotonic salt solutions, was preferred. The slightly alkaline medium of pH 8.0 was chosen to avoid a dissolution of apatite, which is easily soluble at pH 7.0. Furthermore this pH value causes a reduction (about 20%) in the activity of the neutral proteases present in these areas of the growth plate. Data obtained by electron probe microanalysis showed that the extracellular Ca content remained relatively constant in the germinative and proliferative areas of the growth plate, ranging around 0.7% (58 mM/kg wet weight, for 68% water).

The extracellular P content in these zones lies in the range of 0.1%–0.2% (19–20 mM/kg wet weight for 67% tissue water). The product of the contents of extracellular Ca and P is established within 580–1160 mM^2. The ion product for Ca^{2+} and P_i, which is necessary for an in vitro mineralization in a collagen-rich matrix, centers around 2 mM (FLEISCH and NEUMAN 1961). Therefore the concentration of Ca and phosphate is already much higher in those zones which are far away from the mineralization front. However, this may imply that a great reservoir, especially for Ca, already exists in the unmineralized regions; nevertheless, we will have to explain how the system keeps Ca and phosphate in such a state that mineral nucleation is prevented until a stimulus for the nucleation is given in the hypertrophic zone.

A maximum of extractable Ca and Mg is detectable in zone F (maximum hypertrophy) (Fig. 6). The proliferation rate in the top region of the cell columns (zone D) is still very high. The extracted nucleic acid content showed a maximum value here (Schmidt et al. 1978). A distinct increase in nuclease activity in zone E (hypertrophy) may be associated with a change in cell metabolism. Although the cells become strongly hypertrophic they are still very productive and several enzymes can be detected. Schmidt et al. (1978) found the highest lysozyme activity of the epiphyseal growth plate in this zone; and high activities of β-glucuronidase, cathepsin, alkaline phosphatase, and acid phosphatase were found in this region by Granda and Posner (1971). Due to the relatively high resolution of the topological analyses, it was possible to differentiate between the zonal distribution of the enzymes. It was shown that the nuclease activity is found first and is followed shortly after, and coincidentally, by an increase in alkaline phosphatase activity; the acid phosphatase increase occurs at a later stage. If the resolution of the topological analytical technique had been been less, these enzyme activities would have been detected at the same site.

With regard to the sequence of the enzyme activities there is good reason to assume that nuclease activity is connected with the splitting of phosphodiester linkages in DNA and RNA when they are released into the extracellular space together with the onset of degeneration of some chondrocytes. Thus, the nuclease activity would produce phosphomonoesters which are known to be inhibitors of the calcification process (Blumenthal et al. 1977).

In the adjacent region of maximum hypertrophy and cell erosion (zone F) alkaline phosphatase activity showed a distinct maximum accompanied by a peak in buffer extractable organically bound phosphorus, Mg, and Ca (Fig. 6). The extracted Ca^{2+} in this region obviously does not originate from dissoluted apatite, or a peak for extractable P_i would be present at the same site. Mg^{2+} and Ca^{2+} can form soluble 1:1 complexes with the phosphoesters. The Mg–phosphomonoester complexes in particular are good substrates for the alkaline phosphatases of mineralizing collagen-rich systems and can be split in this region (Althoff et al. 1978). The controlling function of Mg during the calcification process has been discussed elsewhere (Quint et al. 1980).

With regard to the special slope of alkaline phosphatase activity in the calcified regions of the growth plate, it is possible that a second alkaline phosphatase activity exists, indicated by the shoulder of the curve in the zones H, I, and K (Fig. 5).

At the end of zone F (maximum hypertrophy) organically bound phosphorus has disappeared; the intercolumnar cartilage matrix becomes more and more calcified. It may be that alkaline phosphatase causes the liberation of orthophosphate in the right locations, resulting in mineralization.

The increase in acid phosphatase activity and the simultaneous increase in extractable inorganic phosphate indicate the first signs of bone remodeling (Reddi 1981) due to osteoclastic activity. It is interesting to note that the total Ca and P content is high in zones H, I, and L (cartilage mineralization – bone formation). In the zone of bone remodeling (zone K), however, Ca is reduced to 13% and P to 7%.

With regard to the formation of trabecular bone, a process in which osteoclastic activities are involved, the mineralized intercolumnar cartilage matrix has to be catabolized. This mechanism is, of course, different from the process of primary cartilage mineralization. Comparing these results with the distribution and activity of the matrix vesicles, it seems important to note that the zone in which most of the matrix vesicles appear (Anderson 1967; Bonucci 1967; Ali 1976) and become mineralized coincides with zone F (zone of maximum cell hypertrophy), in which alkaline phosphatase activity, buffer extractable organically bound phosphate, and extractable Ca and Mg have a maximum. Thus, these data show that topological analyses with relatively high resolution may reflect the chronology of enchondral ossification.

3 Bone Formation in Osteosarcomas

3.1 Clinical Aspects

On the basis of the information obtained by the analyses of enchondral ossification, it is possible that by comparison with tumor bone formation similarities to or differences from physiological bone formation will be revelaed. By applying the combined analytical procedure as described for the study of enchondral bone formation, bone tumor samples were sliced and analyzed according to the repeating sequence as shwon in Fig. 7. Four histologically different types of osteosarcoma were selected from the material collected in the Bone Tumor Registry of Westphalia FRG (Knochengeschwulstregister Westfalen).

Case 1. A female patient born in 1934 presented for the first time in February 1982 with pain in the right hip region. Roentgenological examination revealed extensive osteolysis in the right hip joint, protruding towards the soft tissues. Surgical biopsy resulted in the histological diagnosis of a typical osteoblastic osteosarcoma.

Case 2. A 46-year-old female patient was first diagnosed in 1965, with a tumor in the left tibial head which was removed surgically. In 1973, a spontaneous fracture of the tibial head occurred with tumor recurrence. In 1977, tumor foci were found near the second lumbar vertebra, and in February 1981 near the eighth thoracic vertebra. In March 1981, a focus was found in the skull. In March 1982, amputation of the left leg was performed for a local recurrence. The histological diagnosis was a small cell sclerosing osteosarcoma. Detailed clinical and morphological data of this rare case are published elsewhere (Roessner et al. 1985).

Case 3. A male patient born in 1956. A lesion was found in the distal area of the left femur in February 1982 and roentgenological examination suggested a typical parosteal osteosarcoma. Histology confirmed this diagnosis: well differentiated parosteal osteosarcoma grade I (Huvos 1979).

Case 4. A young male patient, born in 1969, complained for the first time in February 1982 about pain in the area of the left distal humerus. Roentgenolog-

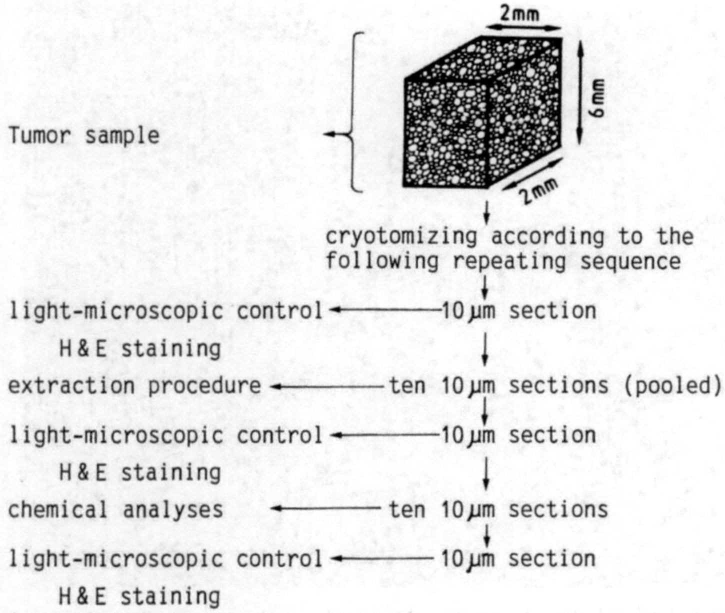

Fig. 7. Flow diagram showing the sequence of transverse slicing for the topological analysis of tumor samples

ical examination suggested an osteosarcoma; surgical biopsy confirmed the diagnosis of a highly malignant anaplastic osteosarcoma.

3.2 Histological and Biochemical Analyses of Osteosarcomas

3.2.1 *Morphological and Histological Description of Large Tumor Samples*

For routine light microscopy, tissue samples were fixed in 10% formol and embedded in paraffin. The sections were stained with H&E, VAN GIESON, LADEWIG, and AZAN.

Typical osteoblastic osteosarcoma (*case 1*). In poorly differentiated areas spindle-shaped or round cells are densely packed, and only small bundles of collagenous material were found in interstitial spaces. Only a few extracellular deposits seem to consist of osteoid-like material. A large part of the tumor, however, is composed of primitive osteoid trabeculae, and many cells are immured like osteocytes in the osteoid deposits (Fig. 8). In several scattered foci the tumor has a sclerosing appearence.

Small cell sclerosing osteosarcoma (*case 2*). The features of the small cell sclerosing osteosarcoma differ considerably on the light microscopic level. In the anaplastic areas of this tumor small, round, densely packed tumor cells show a

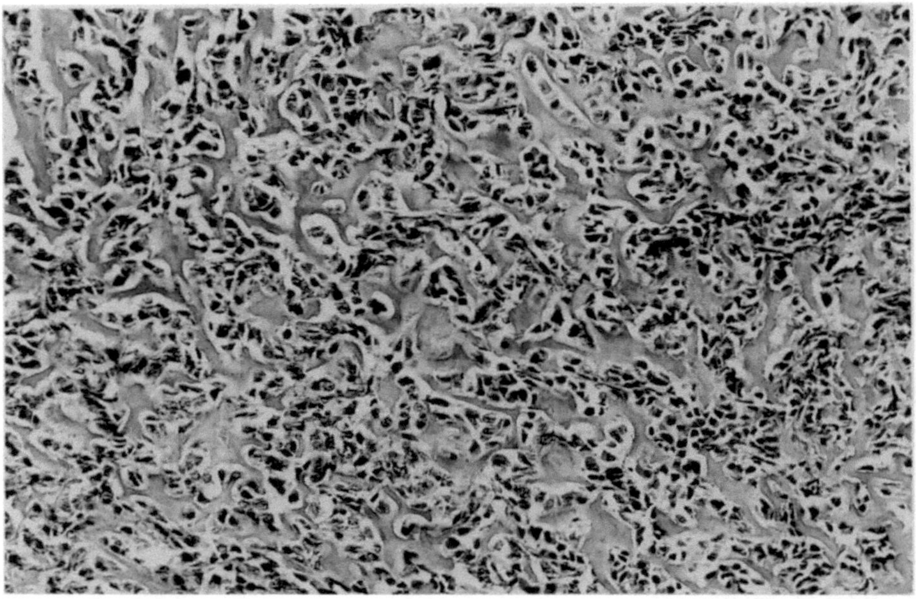

Fig. 8. Histology of a typical osteoblastic osteosarcoma. Many polymorphic tumor cells are immured as osteocytes in primitive, poorly differentiated osteoid trabeculae. (× 136)

small cytoplasmic rim, and a striking resemblance to the cells of Ewing's sarcoma. Stained with Best carmin they are strongly positive, which indicates a high content of cytoplasmic glycogeneous granules. Only scattered foci of osteoid deposits are distributed in the anaplastic areas between these cells. In more highly differentiated samples the amount of sclerosing osteoid trabeculae appears considerably increased, and more tumor cells appear as immured osteocytes in these trabeculae. However, there are still large areas between the osteoid trabeculae where only anaplastic round cells are observed (Fig. 9). In some areas of the sclerosing osteosarcomas, sclerosis is so advanced as to leave only a few scattered minor foci of round tumor cells. Some bone trabeculae even show a lamellated pattern.

Parosteal osteosarcoma (*case 3*). This osteosarcoma reveals a very typical pattern. When compared with the tumor cells of highly malignant osteosarcoma, the cells in parosteal osteosarcoma are considerably less polymorphic. The tumor is partly composed of collagenous, fiber-rich tissue with spindle-shaped, fibroblast-like tumor cells. Mitoses are infrequent in these areas. In other regions the tumor contains bone trabeculae that are remarkably well differentiated, and lamellated bone structures are observed in most instances (Fig. 10).

Anaplastic osteosarcoma (*case 4*). This osteosarcoma is composed of polymorphic cells with large hyperchromatic nuclei. Mitoses are very frequent. Only a few collagen fibers are observed in the interstitial spaces (Fig. 11). Osteoid for-

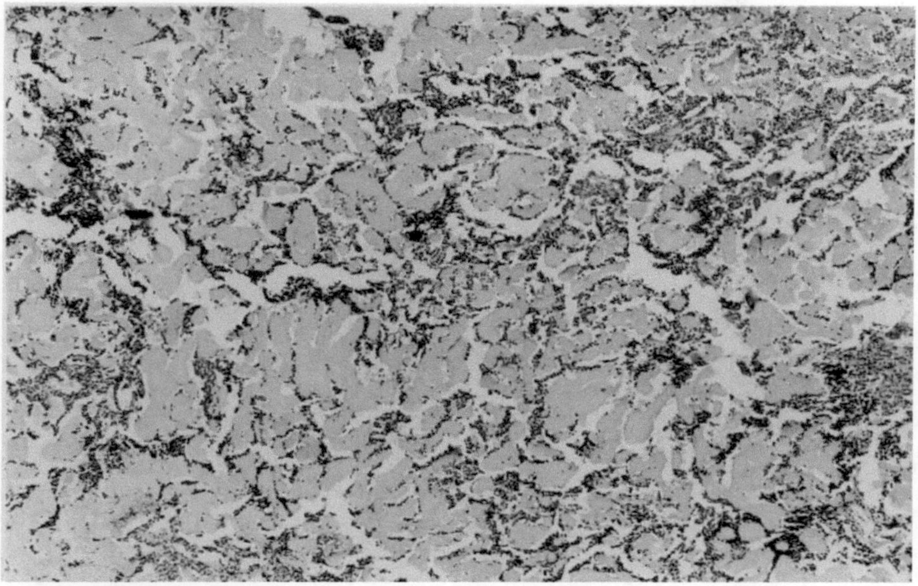

Fig. 9. Small cell sclerosing osteosarcoma with clusters of round cells similar to Ewing's sarcoma cells among large osteoid trabeculae. (× 56)

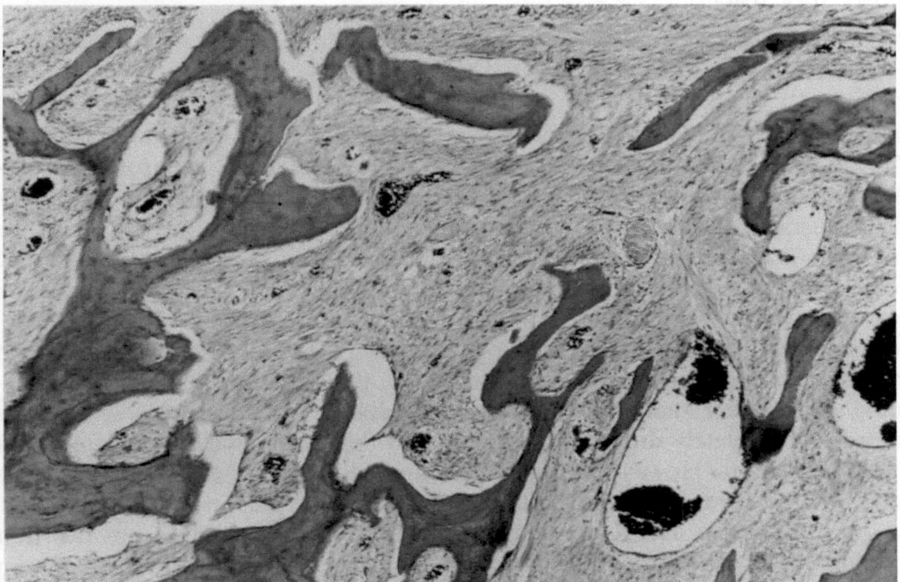

Fig. 10. Parosteal osteosarcoma with remarkably well differentiated lamellated bone trabeculae. Fiber-rich fibroblastic stroma. (× 56)

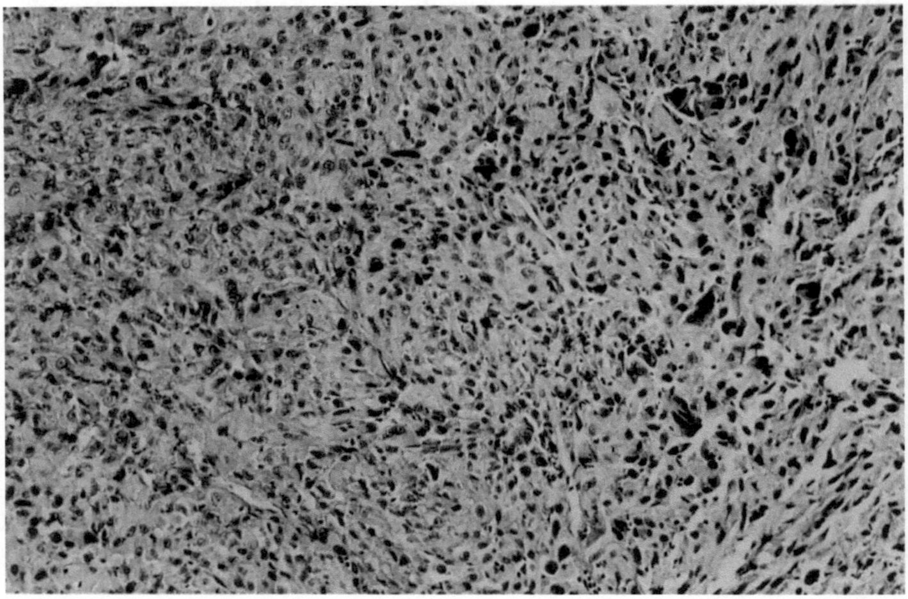

Fig. 11. Densely packed polymorphic tumor cells in anaplastic osteosarcoma. No osteoid formation is detectable in this tumor region. (×136)

mation is visible in only a few foci in connection with an increased alkaline phosphatase reaction.

3.2.2 Biochemical Data

Table 3 shows the data obtained by the analyses of some important elements. The highest extractable amount of Ca and P_i were found in the parosteal osteosarcoma. This was expected since with this tumor bone formation resembles the formation of healthy trabecular bone in the epiphyseal growth plate. In those zones in the growth plate high remodeling activity can be observed and the amount of extracted Ca and P_i is relatively high. The small cell, sclerosing osteosarcoma also shows high amounts of extractable Ca and P_i. The osteoblastic osteosarcoma had a Ca/P_i ratio of about 1.00. This is comparable with the primary calcification process in the growth plate. In the anaplastic osteosarcoma P_i is higher than Ca, resulting in a ratio of about 0.5. These findings suggest a completely different metabolism in this tumor when compared with the other tumors. However, Ca and P_i contents are higher than in blood. This fact is due to special metabolic effects different from those in connective tissue. As regards the Na and K contents of these osteosarcomas, it is obvious that the anaplastic osteosarcoma showed the lowest Na but the highest K content compared with the three other sarcomas. The highest Na content after buffer extraction ("bound Na") was found in the small cell sclerosing bone tumor followed by the parosteal and the osteoblastic osteosarcoma. Although it is

Table 3. Bufferextracted Ca and P_i contents (mmoles/kg fresh weight) and the resulting molar Ca/P_i ratios as well as K contents and molar K/Na ratios for the different types of osteosarcomas and degree of proliferation: (+) lowest; (++++) highest

	Case 1	Case 2	Case 3	Case 4
Ca/P_i	1.02±0.03 (21)	1.75±0.18 (18)	1.20±0.21 (23)	0.47±0.06 (27)
$Ca_{extr.}$	53±5.2 (21)	84±12 (18)	101±31 (23)	15±4.5 (27)
P_i	51±4.8 (21)	48±6.2 (18)	84±21 (23)	31±11 (27)
K	0.71±0.21 (41)	0.22±0.01 (46)	0.10±0.03 (45)	1.38±0.39 (55)
K/Na	0.69±0.18 (41)	0.49±0.09 (46)	0.23±0.03 (45)	1.31±0.14 (55)
Degree of proliferation	+++	++	+	++++

$Ca_{extr.}$: Calcium contents in the buffer extracts; P_i: inorganic phosphate in the buffer extracts; K: Kalium contents in the buffer extracts on % of the untreated dry mass; K/Na: Potassium/Sodium-molar ratios in the buffer extracts; all values (±s); number of measurements in brackets

difficult to interpret the results on the basis of these data only, the ratio K/Na can be related to the degree of malignancy (Quint et al. 1988). It is possible that in the extraction procedure the entire sample, including blood, was analyzed. The molar ratio of blood for K/Na is 0.5 and the ratios found for the four different tumors were between 0.2 and 1.3. Thus vascularization could not exert an important influence on the molar K/Na ratios. Further, using this extraction procedure it is not possible to distinguish between intra- and extracellular K and Na contents. However, when K/Na ratios were related to the amount of cells via the DNA contents a relationship between these ratios and the degree of malignancy could be found, 4.2 for highly malignant anaplastic osteosarcoma followed by osteoblastic osteosarcoma 0.7, small cell sclerosing bone tumor 0.2, and parosteal osteosarcoma 0.1. This characteristic decline suggests that mainly extracellular K and Na were measured, because in healthy resting cells the intracellular K content is relatively high when compared with the Na content. According to Zs-Nagy et al. (1987) the intracellular K content in tumor cells is about 4 times higher than in healthy cells. By changing the intra-extracellular distribution of these ions, the membrane potentials change. Such a membrane depolarization may result via a general trigger function in an increased rate of mitoses (Cone 1971). Rozengurt (1980) demonstrated that an enhanced Na influx resulted in an increased proliferation. Lukacs et al. (1983) found analogue relationships for the tumor growth.

Thus it seems to be very important to determine the amount of electrolytes in bone tumors, because a disturbed K/Na balance reflects the degree of malignancy of osteosarcoma.

Enzymes and Matrix Components. Table 4 summarizes the data obtained by biochemical analyses. The highest acid phosphatase activity was found for the

Table 4. Enzymatic activities and contents of compounds analyzed in four different types of osteosarcoma

Parameters	Case 1	Case 2	Case 3	Case 4
acPase[a]	0.49±0.10	0.25± 0.05	0.31± 0.06	0.31±0.11
APase[a]	11.00± 2.5	3.9 ± 0.79	26.9 ± 7.5	Betw. 0.0 and 3.41
APase[f]	0.24± 0.07	0.15± 0.05	0.42± 0.15	Betw. 0.0 and 0.29
β-Glucuronidase[a]	0.32± 0.11	1.9 ± 0.6	n.d.	n.d.
Proteolytic activity[a] (mean val.)	1.10	0.52	0.00	0.01
P_{total}[b]	4.72± 0.79	7.35± 2.57	8.45± 1.85	1.08±0.29
$P_{i\ extr.}$[c]	69.00±23.00	43.00± 7.2	62.00±22.00	14.00±3.5
$P_{o\ extr.}$[c]	1.6 ± 0.6	1.0	11.5 ± 4.6	36.00± 8.4
$P_{remained}$[b]	3.78± 1.18	7.09± 1.12	8.00± 1.88	0.27±0.13
Hyp_{total}[b]	3.25± 0.79	2.5 ± 0.51	4.00± 1.8	1.74±0.83
Hyp_{extr}[b]	0.01	0.01	0.01	0.46 (mean value)
$Hyp_{remained}$[b]	3.25± 0.79	2.5 ± 0.51	4.00± 1.8	1.57±0.77
$Hexosamine_{total}$[b]	0.81± 0.34	0.57± 0.12	0.18± 0.09	1.03±0.34
$Hexosamine_{extr}$[b]	0.58± 0.11	0.29± 0.11	0.02± 0.005	0.45±0.26
$Hexosamine_{remained}$[b]	0.29± 0.06	0.21± 0.09	0.16± 0.09	0.60±0.24
$Protein_{extr.}$[b]	15.5 ± 5.8	16.4 ± 5.6	26.8 ± 6.2	27.4 ±2.7
Collagen[b]	24.1 ± 5.8	18.5 ± 3.8	29.6 ±13.3	12.9 ±6.1
DNA[d]	0.50± 0.08	0.31± 0.04	0.25± 0.04	3.17±0.21
Water content[e]	76.1 ± 4.1	44.1 ± 6.2	28.8 ± 6.3	79.8 ±6.3
Calcium[e]	10.6 ± 1.0	2.75± 0.54	9.81± 0.91	0.07±0.01

[a] mU per μg DNA
[b] % dry weight
[c] mmoles per kg fresh weight
[d] μg per mg fresh weight
[e] % fresh weight
[f] Specific activity (mU per μg protein)
remained, contents in the buffer-treated sections; extr., contents in the buffer extracts; n.d., not determined

osteoblastic osteosarcoma. The other bone tumors showed acid phosphatase activities in the same range. Alkaline phosphatase activity was highest in the parosteal osteosarcoma followed by the osteoblastic, the small cell sclerosing, and the anaplastic osteosarcoma. For the anaplastic osteosarcoma there were only some areas with alkaline phosphatase activity; therefore only a range could be given in between which this activity was found. β-Glucuronidase activity is relatively high in the small cell sclerosing osteosarcoma and low in the highly malignant osteoblastic osteosarcoma. Proteolytic activity is highest in the typical osteoblastic osteosarcoma, lower in the small cell sclerosing osteosarcoma, and undetectable in the parosteal osteosarcoma. With regard to P_i (extractable inorganic phosphorus), extractable hexosamine, and DNA content (Table 4), highest values were always found in osteoblastic osteosarcomas accompanied by a high water content (76%). In contrast, the highest values of extractable protein were found in the parosteal osteosarcoma.

With regard to total phosphorus, parosteal osteosarcoma ranks first, followed by small cell sclerosing osteosarcoma; lower values are found in the typical osteoblastic osteosarcoma. For extracted organic phosphorus (P_0) the parosteal osteosarcoma shows values about ten times higher than those in typical osteoblastic osteosarcoma. Very low values are found in the small cell sclerosing osteosarcoma. The total hydroxyproline content is highest in parosteal osteosarcoma, lower in osteoblastic, and low in small cell sclerosing osteosarcoma. The total hexosamine contents are high in osteoblastic, lower in small cell sclerosing, and low in parosteal osteosarcoma.

Anaplastic osteosarcomas differ considerably from the other osteosarcoma types. Histology and morphology reveal in most areas an uncalcified matrix rich in tumor cells that fail to show the typical network of collagenous material present during the formation of bone. Corresponding with these findings, the total hydroxyproline content is low (Table 4). In contrast to the other osteosarcomas the hexosamine content is much higher. The water content of the anaplastic osteosarcoma of about 80% is comparable with that of the typical osteoblastic osteosarcoma.

Enzyme activities are generally low in this anaplastic bone tumor. No alkaline phosphatase activity was found in most of the analyzed areas of this tumor; however, in some parts of the anaplastic osteosarcoma, a distinct increase in alkaline phosphatase activity could be observed. The total phosphorus content as well as the extractable P_i content are lower than in the other three tumors, but extractable P_0 and DNA contents are highest in this anaplastic osteosarcoma. The values for extracted protein are about the same as those found in parosteal osteosarcoma.

The biochemical analyses of relatively large tumor samples reveal some characteristic differences between the bone tumors analyzed in this study. Alkaline phosphatase activity as an indicator for osteoblastic activities showed highest values for the parosteal osteosarcoma, followed by the osteoblastic osteosarcoma. When comparing these results with the morphological findings it is obvious that the osteoblasts are numerous in the parosteal as well as in the osteoblastic osteosarcoma. These osteoblasts alone form new tumor bone. This bone, however, is unphysiological, as shown by the different types being formed. For osteoblastic osteosarcoma it can be compared with the newly formed primary spongiosa during enchondral ossification; in contrast with this, the bone formed by the parosteal osteosarcoma is comparable with trabecular bone developing in the stage of bone remodeling and is probably produced by another type of osteoblast (Jones et al. 1988). However, osteoblastic osteosarcomas are not only comparable with the enchondral ossification, since there are also high proteolytic activities suggesting the presence of osteoclasts, phagocytes, and osteocytes. These biochemical findings lead to the assumption that the osteoblastic osteosarcoma includes different stages and zones of cellular differentiation, and a simple overall analysis of biochemical parameters does not reflect the high degree of heterogeneity in this type of bone tumor. This is also confirmed by the analysis of the matrix components and the composition of the bone mineral. Compared with normal bone the hexosamine contents (reflecting the amount of glycoproteins and proteoglycans) are increased and a large amount is easily extractable under isotonic conditions. These findings indicate high metabolic activity. The collagen content is in a range somewhat lower than in healthy bone, indicating that the matrix is changed pathologically. This is also reflected by the high content of water. The DNA content, the highest found for the bone-forming tumors, reveals the high proliferation rate and cell density of this tumor. The total phosphorus content is rather low compared with the other bone-forming osteosarcomas, and about 20% of the total phosphorus is extracted under isotonic conditions and most of it is organically bound phosphorus. These data reflect the intense phosphate metabolism occurring, e.g., during enhanced mitosis and calcification (ALTHOFF et al. 1982; KAKUTA et al. 1985).

By contrast with the conventional biochemical variables the content of sodium and potassium is not so heterogeneously distributed. It is possible that they reflect the state of proliferation in this tumor. By comparing the bone-forming osteosarcoma it was shown that the K/Na ratio was highest for the osteoblastic osteosarcomas (QUINT et al. 1988).

From the morphological and histological point of view, parosteal osteosarcomas seem to form a bone very similar to healthy bone. Osteoblasts and osteocytes are numerous. The number of osteoclasts is not significantly different from healthy bone. However, alkaline phosphatase activity is relatively high, reflecting a high cellular activity of the tumor osteoblasts although their number is not characteristically higher than in normal bone. These findings are supported by the results of analyses for calcium and phosphorus extracted under isotonic conditions. Even the matrix is comparable to healthy bone. The collagen and hexosamine contents do not differ much from normal bone. The DNA and water contents are relatively low. In summary, this parosteal osteosarcoma, when compared with the other bone-forming tumors investigated here, shows a high calcification activity and low osteolytic activities, pointing to a low bone remodeling activity.

The small cell sclerosing osteosarcoma shows few osteoblasts and the number of osteocytes is also low. Osteoclasts are only present in such areas where the density of small cells has reached a high value. By comparison of these findings with the biochemical data, it is clear that this type of tumor shows a great heterogeneity and abnormal nonhomogeneous bone. Although acid phosphatase, β-glucuronidase, and proteolytic activities are measurable, these lytic activities cannot derive from osteoclasts, since the number of this cell type is so low. Interestingly, the phosphorus content is relatively high. The alkaline phosphatase activity is low, pointing to low calcifying activity. These findings are confirmed by the observation of small numbers of osteoblasts. The matrix of this type of bone-forming tumor is quite different from the two discussed here. The collagen content is comparatively low and the hexosamine content is high. All these findings reveal bone formation that is not comparable with other types of controlled biomineralization processes and it is thought to be an uncontrolled process not regulated by osteoblasts, osteoclasts, and osteocytes. It is in agreement with this interpretation that the DNA content compared with parosteal osteosarcoma reveals an increased number of cells and the water content points to areas of incomplete calcification. The ratio of K/Na is extremely low, suggesting a low proliferation rate.

The anaplastic osteosarcoma is quite different from the other bone tumors being investigated here. Histologically it is composed of polymorphic cells. Mitoses are very frequent. Fibrous material is scanty. These observations may lead to the assumption that the collagen content is low. Osteoid formation cannot be recognized. From the biochemical point of view it is important to note that the alkaline phosphatase activity is very low, indicating that this type of tumor certainly does not develop towards a bone-forming tumor. The matrix shows a low collagen content. However, the hexosamine contents are very high, pointing to proteoglycan- and/or glycoprotein-rich matrix. In agreement with the morphological findings the DNA content is very high, reflecting the density of cell package. The DNA was the highest compared with the other bone tumors investigated. The water content was also highest when compared with the other tumors. These findings suggest that this anaplastic osteosarcoma is highly undifferentiated. This is also confirmed by the low phosphorus content. Interestingly, the K/Na ratio is very high. Comparing the K/Na ratios of the four different osteosarcomas of this study with their degree of proliferation it is obvious that the K/Na ratio corresponds to the degree of proliferation.

These observations reveal that the balance of Na and K metabolism is disturbed in tumors (Quint et al. 1988) and that changes in Na and K balances may reflect the metabolic state of a tissue.

Except for the K/Na ratios obtained by analyses of comparatively large tumor samples resulting in averaged values, all the other data, obtained by the different histochemical analytical procedures, revealed an extraordinary heterogeneity of the different osteosarcomas. To demonstrate this inhomogeneity, Fig. 12 and 13 show two histograms of the distribution of phosphorus and alkaline phosphatase activity obtained for the different bone-forming osteosarcomas of this study. The data were obtained from analyses of two different series of the histologically controlled slicing procedures. Measured values are entered on the abscissa, while the ordinate reflects the frequency of occurrence of the measured values. Plotting the values of two different series (Figs. 12a, 13a), it is obvious that they show different peaks for the frequency of occurrence both for P contents (Fig. 12a) and for alkaline phosphatase activity (Fig. 13a). Figures 12b and 13b summarize the values of series I and II. The shape of the curve for a single topological series as well as a comparison of the two curves illustrates the strong inhomogeneity of the chemical composition even in tissue samples of a relatively small size. Since the anaplastic osteosarcoma consists only of soft tissue, containing in most areas no alkaline phosphatase activity and low phosphorus contents, this osteosarcoma is not presented. Concerning the distribution of phosphorus, the most homogeneous bone tumor seems to be the osteoblastic osteosarcoma (case 1), while the parosteal osteosarcoma shows two different areas of distribution for phosphorus. One area is in the range of 5% and the other in the range of about 10%. This means that in one tumor differences of about 100% can be observed. An analogous histogram for the phosphorus distribution was found for small cell sclerosing osteosarcoma. Although most of the measured values were found to be in the range of about 9%, another area showed a concentration of about 5%. The

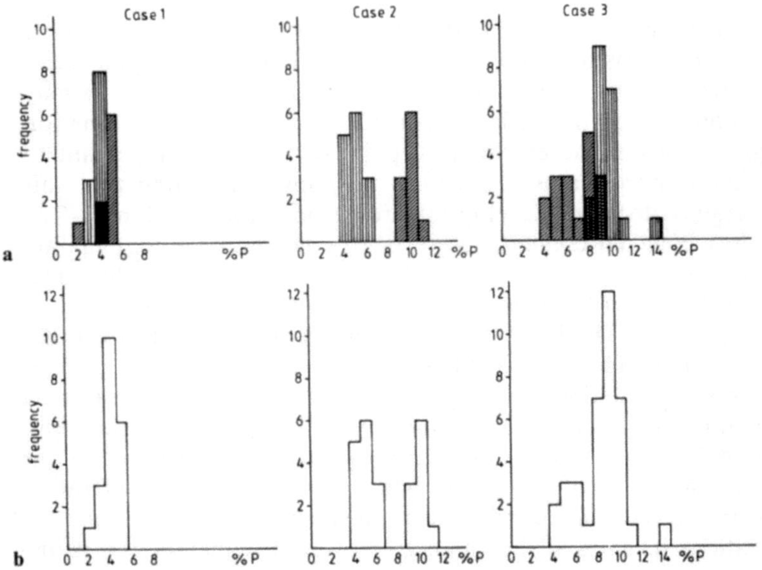

Fig. 12. a Histograms of the distribution of total phosphorus (P, % dry weight) obtained from two different series of sectioning of the different osteosarcomas. *Vertical lines*, series I; *diagonal lines*, series II; e.g., for series I case 1, eight values were found in the range of 3.5% and 4.5% P, while for series II two values were found in this range. **b** Histograms of the distribution of total phosphorus (P, % dry weight) of the different osteosarcomas, summarizing the above series I and II

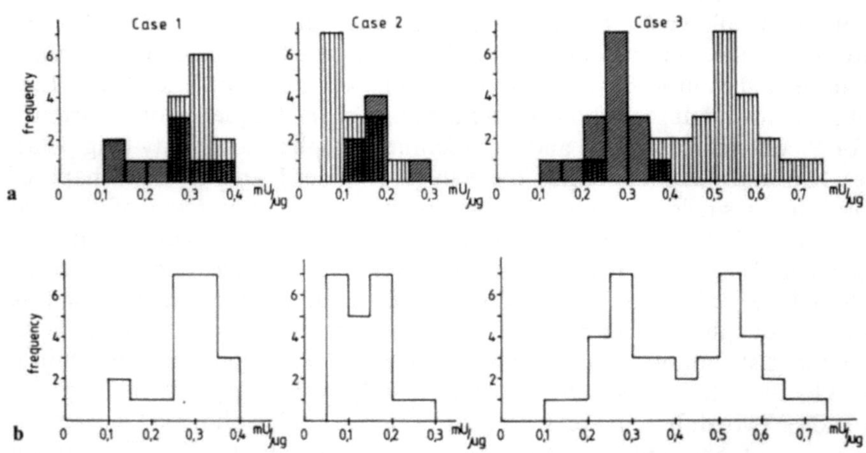

Fig. 13. a Histograms of the distribution of alkaline phosphatase activity (mU/µg protein) obtained from two different series of sectioning of the different osteosarcomas. *Vertical lines*, series I; *diagonal lines*, series II; e.g., for series I case 1 six values for alkaline phosphatase activity were found in the range of 0.3 and 0.35, while for series II only one value was found in this range. **b** Histograms of the distribution of alkaline phosphatase activity (mU/µg protein) of the different osteosarcomas, summarizing the above series I and II

osteoblastic osteosarcoma was the most homogeneous with regard to the phosphorus contents, with eight values at 4% for series I and six values for series II. However, regarding the distribution for alkaline phosphatase activity this tumor also reveals an inhomogeneity. The small cell sclerosing osteosarcoma is characterized by an even greater homogeneity concerning the distribution of alkaline phosphatase activity. For the parosteal osteosarcoma even two different mean values were found, one at about 0.3 and the other at about 0.5 mU/μg.

These findings demonstrate clearly that the bone-forming tumors are very heterogeneous, even in such small samples ($2 \times 2 \times 0.1$ mm). Therefore it is very difficult to describe bone-forming tumors on the basis of a few histological samples only. As can be deduced from these results, it was important to study the different areas of bone tumor differentiation in detail in order to relate the biochemical data directly to the morphological and histological analyses of those small tumor areas.

3.3 Zonal Combined Biochemical and Histological Analyses

3.3.1 Zonal Morphological and Histological Characterization

The osteoblastic osteosarcoma reveals morphologically and histologically different stages of differentiation. In Figs. 14a–f, some characteristically differentiated tissues are shown. Figure 14a illustrates a section of an anaplastic undifferentiated area of the osteoblastic osteosarcoma. The cells in this area of the tumor are invading the bone. Some collagenous material seems to be present. In another area (Fig. 14b) the spindle-shaped cells change into cartilage-like cells. They are surrounded by chondronic walls and show signs of hypertrophy. When they have reached a high degree of hypertrophy, calcification can be observed. Morphologically this observation suggests that the bone formation is equivalent to the enchondral ossification occurring in the epiphyseal growth plate (see Fig. 4). However, this tumor cartilage is not thoroughly arranged, resulting in a dense and undirected calcification (Fig. 14c). During this calcification process many cells are immured into the newly formed tumor bone (Fig. 14d). In a further step of tumor bone development the calcified matrix can be metabolized by osteoclastic cells (Fig. 14e) and remodeled to trabecular tumor bone (Fig. 14f).

The small cell sclerosing osteosarcoma is an infrequent type of bone tumor. However, this tumor, too, reveals areas of histologically different development. Figure 15a shows a poorly differentiated area of tumor tissue with large amounts of small obviously sclerosing cells with high lytic activity. Figure 15b, in contrast, demonstrates that areas of bone tumor tissue also exist that show no signs of greater differentiation. It can be observed that the number of osteoblasts is rather low in this type of tumor, although in the stage of calcification osteocytes are immured in the tumor bone. Only some osteoclasts are present at sites where the small cells are densely packed. It is an open question whether these small cells are able to differentiate to osteoblasts and osteocytes or whether remaining bone cells, being adapted during the tumor growth, are forming

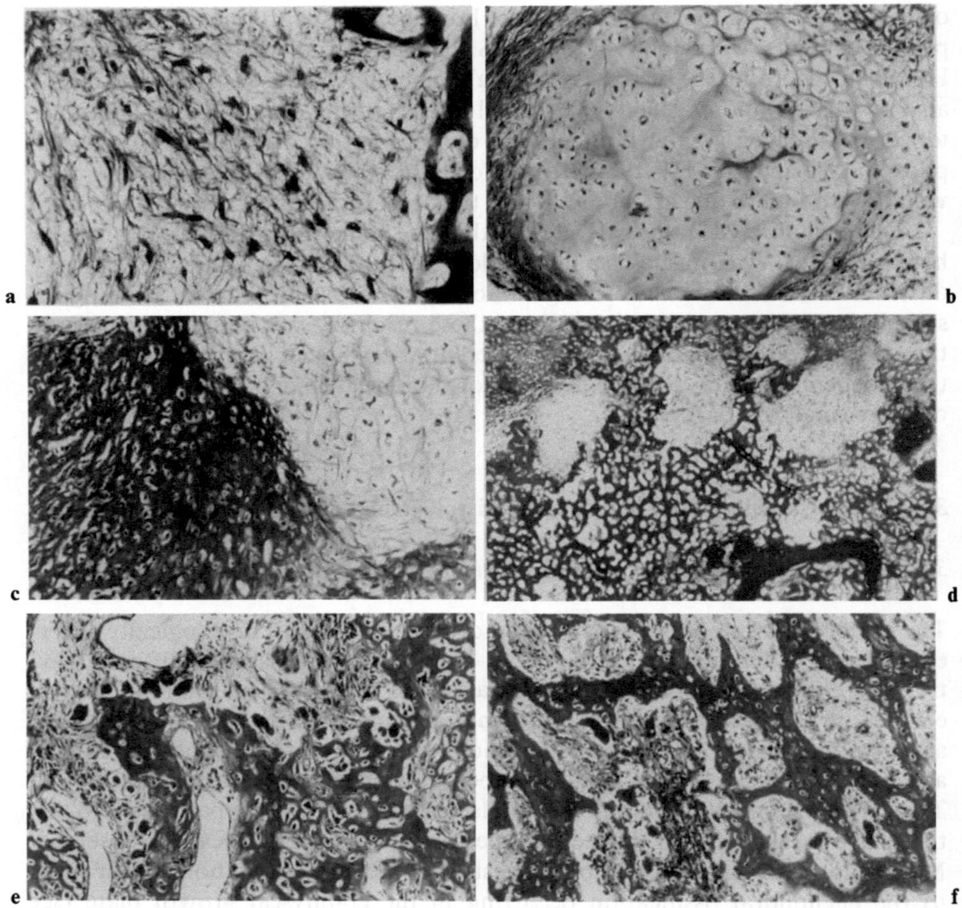

Fig. 14a–f. Uncalcified areas of tumor tissue (**a**) are sometimes surrounded by hypertrophic cartilage (**b**); the cartilage undergoes enchondral ossification (**c**) and this calcified cartilage is remodeled to tumor bone (**d–f**)

the tumor bone. The parosteal osteosarcoma is very different compared with the osteoblastic and the small cell sclerosing osteosarcoma. From the morphological point of view this tumor resembles normal healthy bone. Only some areas of this tumor reveal slight differences. The number and arrangement of osteoblasts is comparable with those found in normal bone, the distribution and arrangement of osteocytes show the same pattern. Osteoclasts are not as numerous as in healthy bone. However, there are some differences concerning the shape of bone trabeculae. In Figs. 16a and 16b two different stages of bone development illustrate that the trabeculae are of different shapes. Figure 16a shows the more undifferentiated stage, while Fig. 16b shows a mature tumor bone. The anaplastic osteosarcoma morphologically shows no signs of typical

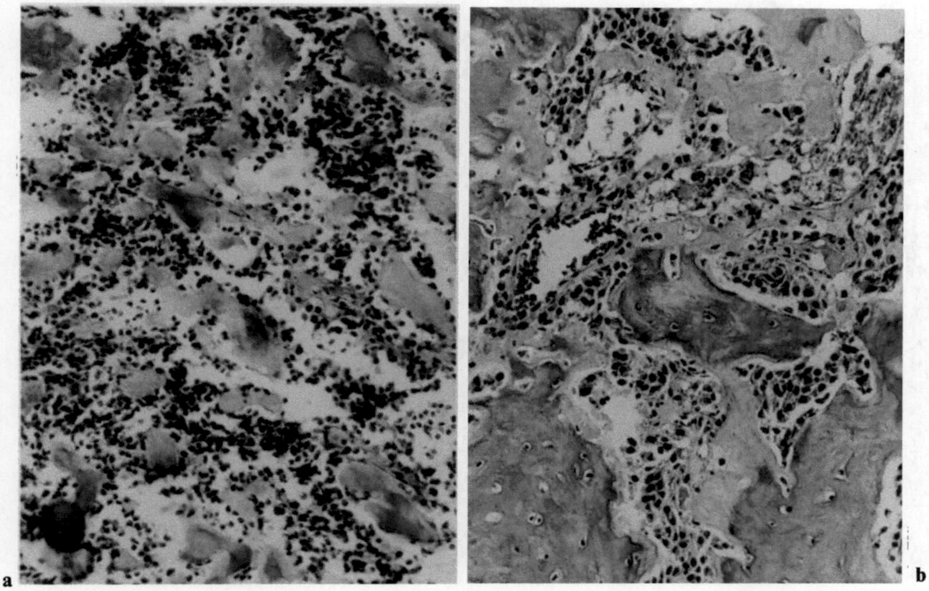

Fig. 15. a Poorly differentiated area of small cell sclerosing osteosarcoma with broad clusters of anaplastic round cells and small immature osteoid deposits (H&E, ×136). **b** Sclerosing area with broad trabeculae containing many immured osteocytes (H&E, ×136)

bone-forming osteosarcoma. In Fig. 17a the most frequent morphological pattern of this type of osteosarcoma is shown. This tumor is composed of polymorphic cells with large hyperchromatic nuclei. Mitoses are very frequent and the matrix seems to contain only a few collagenous fibers. However, in some areas of this tumor, the beginning of cell differentiation can be recognized. This differentiation is characterized by a dense package of cells. The diameter of the cells seems to increase slightly in these areas (Fig. 17b).

3.3.2 Zonal Biochemical Characterization

The morphological and histological analyses carried out in direct combination with biochemistry should demonstrate that the differences observed are reflected by the biochemical analytical data. Therefore two different stages of tumor development were chosen for a more refined analysis. One stage of tumor development represents the more undifferentiated areas and another stage the more differentiated areas of the osteosarcomas being investigated. In Table 5 the topochemical data for the highly malignant osteoblastic osteosarcoma are summarized. For the poorly differentiated areas of this tumor the proteolytic activity is relatively high, as is the alkaline phosphatase activity. High amounts of extracted inorganic phosphorus (P_i) and organically bound phosphorus (P_0) indicate elevated levels of calcification. The acid phosphatase activity is also increased, indicating that bone remodeling activity is also high. With regard

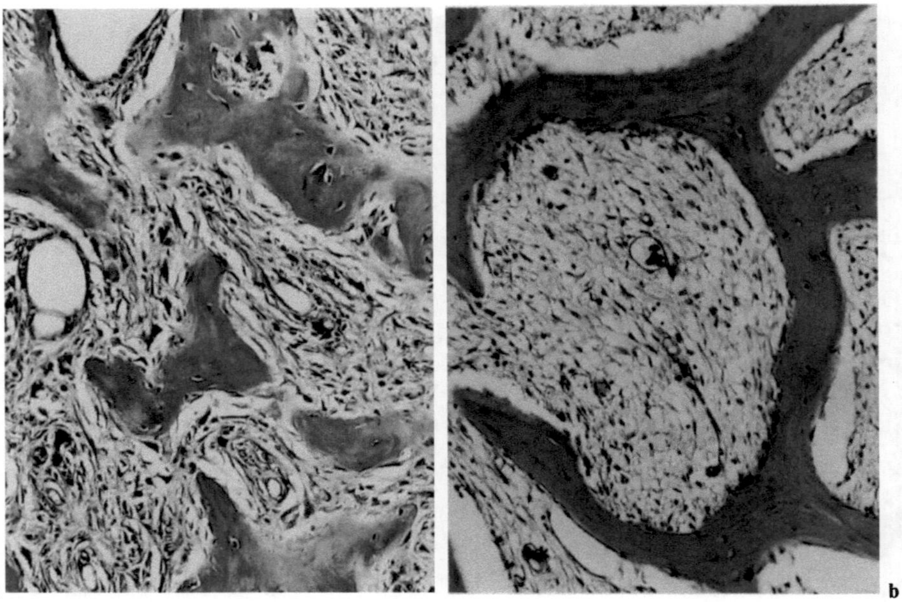

a b

Fig. 16. **a** Area of growing tumor in parosteal osteosarcoma with interwoven bone trabeculae and proliferating fibroblastic mononuclear stromal cells (H&E, ×136). **b** Area of mature tumor bone in parosteal osteosarcoma. Lamellated bone trabeculae are hardly distinguishable from normal bone formation. Fiber-rich connective tissue between bone trabeculae (H&E, ×136)

to the matrix components it is obvious that the collagen content is higher than in the zone of cartilage calcification in the epiphyseal growth plate. The total hexosamine content, reflecting the amounts of proteoglycans and glycoproteins, is comparatively high. The water content of about 80% is relatively high. The calcium content is about 4% (per dry weight) in these undifferentiated areas of the osteoblastic osteosarcoma. In the more mature regions of this bone tumor the metabolic process of calcification seems to be slower. The acid phosphatase, alkaline phosphatase, proteolytic, and β-glucuronidase activities are reduced. The extracted protein is also low and the water content is about 10% lower than in the more undifferentiated areas. However, collagen as well as the calcium and phosphorus contents are increased. These findings reflect that those areas of more differentiated tumor tissue consist of a more mature tumor bone. The biochemical data for the small cell sclerosing osteosarcoma obtained from the morphologically controlled sites reveal for the areas of lower differentiation (Table 6, Fig. 15a), a relatively high alkaline phosphatase activity suggesting a calcification process. The proteolytic activity measured here may represent the invasive phase of the tumor. The buffer extracted protein as well as the isotonically extracted hexosamine contents may reflect increased metabolic activities. The respective contents are higher than in tissue with normal bone (PUGLIARELLO et al. 1973). In the areas of sclerosing tumor bone (Table 6, Fig. 15b) alkaline phosphatase and proteolytic activities are remarkably reduced compared with those found in areas of lower differentiation. However, acid phospha-

a 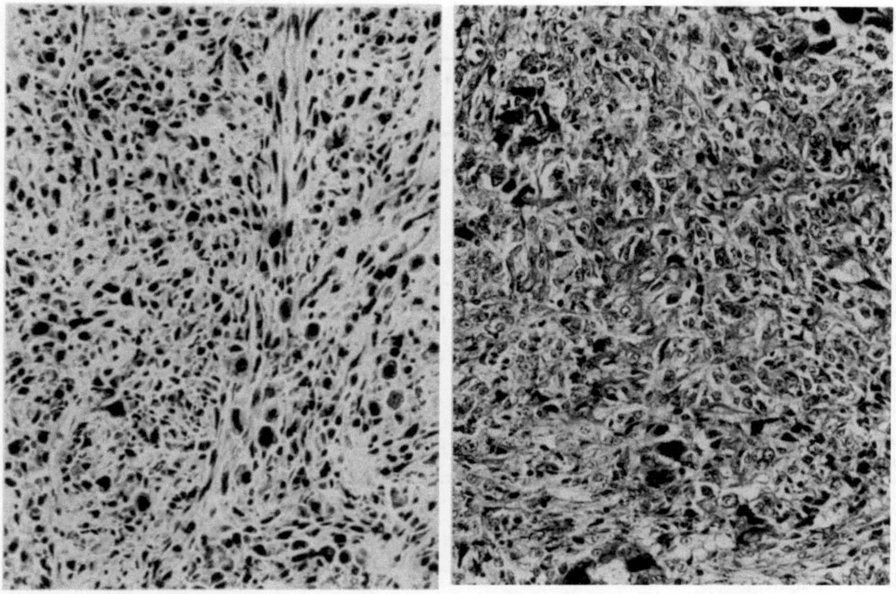 b

Fig. 17. a Anaplastic area of highly malignant anaplastic osteosarcoma with mostly round and some spindly polymorphic tumor cells. No osteoid formation (H & E, × 136). **b** Incipient osteoid formation in anaplastic osteosarcoma with small, osteoid-like collagenous bundles between polymorphic, anaplastic tumor cells (H & E, × 136)

tase and β-glucuronidase activities are higher, both indicating increased bone remodeling activities. Calcification seems to be nearly completed; the calcium content is about 19% (weight per dry mass) and the phosphorus content is also very high. The water content, as well as hexosamine and collagen contents, is lower than in the areas of lower differentiation, reflecting that these more differentiated sites of the rare small cell sclerosing osteosarcoma reach a high density of mineralization with relatively low amounts of incorporated matrix.

The parosteal osteosarcoma seems to be the most homogeneous of the bone-forming tumors investigated in this study. However, in some areas tumor bone growth occurs while in other compartments of the tumor a more mature bone could be recognized. In Table 7 the analytical data of these two different stages are summarized (for the typical morphological pattern, see Fig. 16a, b). In areas of growing tumor bone the alkaline phosphatase and acid phosphatase activity was higher than in the well differentiated tumor bone. In fact, the highest alkaline phosphatase activity of all four osteosarcomas studied here was observed in the growing bone regions of this parosteal osteosarcoma. No proteolytic activity, however, was detectable in these areas. The high amount of extractable protein reveals increased cellular activity. The high contents of collagen and comparatively elevated amounts of hexosamine and isotonically extracted P_0 also reflect an increased matrix formation being prepared for calcification. The parosteal osteosarcoma shows an average content for total hexosamine of 0.27% (weight per dry mass) in those areas of growing tumor bone.

Table 5. Highly malignant osteoblastic osteosarcoma. Topochemical analyses of two different areas of tumor differentiation (cf. Fig. 14)

	Poorly differentiated osteoblastic areas	Areas with mature tumor bone
acPase[a]	61 ± 11 (7)	15 ± 4.9 (8)
APase[a]	275 ± 30 (10)	121 ± 26 (9)
Proteolytic activity[a]	18.6 ± 2.4 (9)	1.8 ± 0.29 (9)
β-Glucuronidase[a]	8.2 ± 2.1 (10)	2.8 ± 0.8 (9)
$Protein_{extr.}$[b]	23.8 ± 4.4 (11)	12.9 ± 3.1 (9)
Hydroxyproline[c]	3.1 ± 0.29 (11)	3.7 ± 1.1 (9)
$Hexosamine_{total}$[c]	1.1 ± 0.17 (10)	0.61 ± 0.12 (9)
$Hexosamine_{extr.}$[c]	0.75 ± 0.17 (10)	0.35 ± 0.07 (9)
P_{total}[c]	4.6 ± 0.6 (11)	5.3 ± 0.48 (9)
$P_{i\ extr.}$[c]	1.1 ± 0.15 (11)	0.46 ± 0.09 (9)
$P_{0\ extr.}$[c]	0.1 ± 0.03 (11)	0.06 ± 0.009 (9)
Water content[d]	80.1 ± 4.1 (7)	72.3 + 3.8 (7)
Collagen[e]	20.8 + 1.5 (11)	27.4 ± 8.1 (9)

[a] Specific activity (mU/mg protein)
[b] µg per mg fresh weight
[c] % dry weight
[d] % fresh weight
[e] Hydroxyproline × 7.41
All data ± s.d.; number of samples in brackets; extr., extracted by buffer, pH 8.0 (see Material and Methods, ALTHOFF et al. 1985b)

Table 6. Small cell sclerosing osteosarcoma. Topochemical analyses of two different stages of tumor differentiation (cf. Fig. 15a, b)

	Areas of lower differentiation	Sclerosing tumor bone
acPase[a]	16.1 ± 3.2 (11)	42.3 ± 5.3 (11)
APase[a]	171 ± 35 (10)	87 ± 28 (11)
Proteolytic activity[a]	12.0 ± 4.1 (11)	0.1 ± 0.05 (11)
β-Glucuronidase[a]	20.3 ± 4.1 (11)	136 ± 39 (11)
$Protein_{extr.}$[b]	20.7 ± 4.4 (11)	9.4 ± 2.1 (11)
Hydroxyproline[c]	2.8 ± 0.20 (11)	2.1 ± 0.24 (11)
$Hexosamine_{total}$[c]	0.83 ± 0.08 (11)	0.31 ± 0.04 (11)
$Hexosamine_{extr.}$[c]	0.61 ± 0.13 (11)	0.07 ± 0.02 (11)
P_{total}[c]	6.1 ± 1.3 (11)	10.2 ± 1.2 (11)
$P_{i\ extr.}$[c]	0.37 ± 0.05 (11)	0.21 ± 0.01 (11)
$P_{0\ extr.}$[c]	<0.01 (11)	<0.01 (11)
Water content[d]	48.2 ± 6.3 (7)	39.1 ± 5.8 (7)
Collagen[e]	22.9 ± 2.1 (11)	15.6 ± 1.8 (11)

[a] Specific activity (mU per mg protein)
[b] µg per mg fresh weight
[c] % dry weight
[d] % fresh weight
[e] Hydroxyproline × 7.41
All data ± s.d.; number of samples in brackets; extr., extracted by buffer, pH 8.0 (see Material and Methods, ALTHOFF et al. 1985b)

Table 7. Parosteal osteosarcoma. Topochemical analyses of two different stages of tumor differentiation (cf. Fig. 16a, b)

	Areas of growing tumor bone		Areas of mature tumor bone	
acPase[a]	22 ± 2.8	(13)	3.1 ± 0.68	(15)
APase[a]	510 ± 178	(14)	265 ± 61	(15)
Proteolytic activity[a]	0.00	(14)	0.00	(15)
$Protein_{extr.}$[b]	49.9 ± 5.1	(14)	14.4 ± 2.1	(15)
Hydroxyproline[c]	5.4 ± 0.9	(13)	2.6 ± 0.32	(14)
$Hexosamine_{total}$[c]	0.27 ± 0.06	(12)	0.12 ± 0.019	(13)
$Hexosamine_{extr.}$[c]	0.04 ± 0.007	(12)	<0.01	(13)
P_{total}[c]	7.1 ± 1.6	(12)	9.9 ± 2.1	(13)
$P_{i\ extr.}$[c]	0.27 ± 0.037	(12)	0.37 ± 0.028	(13)
$P_{O\ extr.}$[c]	0.1 ± 0.02	(12)	0.02 ± 0.004	(13)
Water content[s]	38.1 ± 7.1	(7)	26.3 ± 4.1	(7)
Collagen[e]	40.0 ± 6.7	(13)	19.3 ± 2.4	(14)

[a] Specific activity (mU per mg protein)
[b] µg per mg fresh weight
[c] % dry weight
[d] % fresh weight
[e] Hydroxyproline × 7.41
All data ± s.d.; number of samples in brackets; extr., extracted by buffer, pH 8.0 (see Material and Methods, Althoff et al. 1985b)

The osteoid-rich tissue of normal, healthy developing bone has hexosamine contents in the range of about 0.6% (Pugliarello et al. 1970). The relatively high amount of total phosphorus indicates that a stage of advanced calcification has been reached.

In the area of mature bone (Fig. 16b, Table 7) the amount of extractable protein is only some 30% of the values found in the less well differentiated areas. The alkaline phosphatase and acid phosphatase activities as well as the hexosamine contents in these mature regions are reduced to 50% or less of those measured in immature tumor bone. The total phosphorus is considerably increased (about 10%), while collagen content per dry mass and the water content are remarkably reduced, reflecting a high degree of calcification. This loss of collagen is not an actual loss. Due to the fact that the water content decreases with progressing mineral deposition the total amount of dry mass increases. Assuming that the absolute collagen content remains constant, its relation to the dry mass would result in an apparent decrease. However, these areas of mature bone still show a high alkaline phosphatase activity and relatively high amount of extractable protein, indicating that bone formation has not been fully completed. This is also confirmed by the calcium content of about 15%. In fully mineralized bone the calcium content is in the range of 22% and phosphorus of about 9%. With regard to the amount of phosphorus the mature bone has reached a bone-like value.

The anaplastic osteosarcoma is a tumor with a mainly undifferentiated matrix. In this tumor, an anaplastic area without a differentiated matrix (Fig. 17a, b, Table 8) was compared with an area showing early stages of differ-

Table 8. Anaplastic osteosarcoma. Topochemical analyses of the undifferentiated areas and the stage of initial differentiation (cf. Fig. 17a, b)

	Anaplastic areas			Osteoid-forming areas		
acPase[a]	<1		(19)	23	± 3	(8)
APase[a]	<1		(21)	180	±61	(8)
Proteolytic activity[a]	<0.1		(19)	<0.01		(8)
$Protein_{extr.}$ [b]	34.2	±3.7	(17)	22.6	± 4.6	(8)
Hydroxyproline[c]	1.3	±0.3	(11)	2.5	± 0.4	(9)
$Hexosamine_{total}$ [c]	1.1	±0.2	(10)	1.1	± 0.15	(9)
$Hexosamine_{extr.}$ [c]	0.71	±0.14	(10)	0.32	± 0.07	(9)
P_{total} [c]	0.95	±0.18	(11)	1.12	± 0.16	(9)
$P_{i\ extr.}$ [c]	0.19	±0.04	(11)	0.25	± 0.06	(9)
$P_{o\ extr.}$ [c]	0.58	±0.10	(11)	0.35	± 0.08	(9)
Water content[d]	81.2	±4.8	(7)	77.4	± 4.2	(7)
Collagen[e]	9.6	±2.2	(11)	18.5	± 2.9	(9)

[a] Specific activity (mU per mg protein)
[b] µg per mg fresh weight
[c] % dry weight
[d] % fresh weight
[e] Hydroxyproline × 7.41
All data ± s.d.; number of samples in brackets; extr., extracted by buffer, pH 8.0 (see Material and Methods, ALTHOFF et al. 1985b)

entiation and the beginning of osteoid formation (Fig. 17b, Table 8). None of the enzymatic activities normally present in bone-forming osteosarcomas could be detected in anaplastic areas without any signs of differentiation The major part of the pooled sections analyzed consisted of this anaplastic tissue. The extracted protein content, and the total and extracted hexosamine content, are high. Unlike nonmineralizing soft tissues, the total phosphorus content is relatively high. Its major part consists of extractable P_0. The collagen content, however, is very low.

In contrast to these anaplastic undifferentiated areas of this tumor, in those small areas that show immature osteoid formation (Fig. 17b, Table 8) alkaline phosphatase and acid phosphatase activities are measurable. Some progressive matrix formation is indicated by an increased collagen content when compared with the values of the anaplastic areas and with the decreased amounts of extractable hexosamine. The slight increase of total phosphorus and of extractable P_i confirms this assumption. Analogous results were found for calcium. On the whole, the gradual differentiation of this osteosarcoma towards hard tissue formation is rather low, at least in this stage of tumor development.

4 Comparison of Hard Tissue Formation in Osteosarcomas with Physiological Bone Formation

In the first study (see Sect. 3) it could be shown that the results of the biochemical analyses of the four different osteosarcoma types agree well with their respective histological picture. Furthermore the data reflect the distinct heterogeneity of different areas in the individual tumor. In view of the large number of samples per tumor, the coefficient of variation was remarkably high. The method of combined histological and biochemical analyses offers the advantage of more accurate quantitative differentiation not only between one bone tumor type and another, but also between several stages of differentiation that may coexist in one osteosarcoma. Therefore the aim of these combined analyses was to collect data regarding the different stages of tumor bone formation occuring in the individual osteosarcoma. In the following the different types of osteosarcoma will be discussed based on the results of the combined analyses.

Case 1. The highly malignant osteoblastic osteosarcoma permitted the identification of two biochemically dissimilar areas of tumor metabolism: rather poorly differentiated osteoblastic areas and areas with more mature bone-like material. In the poorly differentiated osteoblastic areas relatively strong enzymatic activities could be detected. High alkaline phosphatase activity on the one hand and increased activity of acid phosphatase and β-glucuronidase on the other, may reflect enhanced bone remodeling (Reddi 1981). High proteolytic activity in those poorly differentiated osteoblastic osteosarcoma may point at enhanced tumor invasion. Thus, from the biochemical point of view, it may be concluded that at least three different processes are overlapping in these so-called osteoblastic areas: (a) calcification, most probably enchondral calcification, (b) remodeling, and (c) tumor invasion. This interpretation is supported by some other observations. The isotonically extracted protein is about twice as high in the rather poorly differentiated areas as in those of maturer bone, which indicates elevated cellular activities. The amounts of total and of isotonically extracted hexosamine are relatively high, which suggests a large soft tissue compartment, e.g., cartilage-like material. These cartilage-rich areas contain high amounts of proteoglycans (Wuthier 1969). The hydroxyproline content implies that a collagenous matrix at a stage of progressive calcification is developing, which is also reflected by the values of total phosphorus and isotonically extracted P_0, while those of extracted P_i may reflect enhanced bone remodeling. The calcium contents are about three times higher in the more mature tumor bone than in areas of poorly differentiated osteoblastic osteosarcoma.

In areas of maturer tumor bone the enzymatic activities are visibly reduced, compared with those in poorly differentiated osteoblastic areas. The decreases seen in isotonically extracted total protein content and extracted hexosamine, extracted P_i and P_0, and water content, express a differentiation towards hard tissue. The inference is confirmed by increased amounts of total phosphorus and calcium as a sign of advanced biomineralization. However, in comparison with normal bone (Pugliarello et al. 1970, 1973) this "maturer" tumor bone is found to be very soft and of insufficient biochemical properties. This bone is comparable with calcified cartilage and primary spongiosa developing during enchondral calcification. In summary, these biochemical analyses combined with morphology have revealed that indeed this tumor contains cartilaginous foci being formed by the differentiation of invaded mesenchymal cells to chondrocyte-like cells. It can therefore be assumed that this osteoblastic osteosarcoma is an enchondral calcifying bone tumor.

Case 2. This tumor was identified morphologically as a small cell sclerosing osteosarcoma. The difference of chemical data between the two stages of tumor growth are first reflected by their enzymatic activities. In areas of lower differentiation acid phosphatase activity is lower, while alkaline phosphatase activity is higher than in areas of sclerosing tumor bone. It can be assumed that in the latter the remodeling activity is enhanced. This assumption is also supported by the high β-glucuronidase activity, the low levels of isotonically extracted protein, and the high amount of total phosphorus and calcium in the areas of sclerosing tumor bone. Furthermore, the values of total and extracted hexosamine and hydroxyproline as well as the water content in those areas reveal the high degree of calcification attained.

The areas of lower differentiation show increased values for proteolytic activities, isotonically extracted protein, hydroxyproline, total and extracted hexosamine, and water content, indicating that this region of small cell sclerosing osteosarcoma is at an invasive stage accompanied by progressive calcification. Increased alkaline phosphatase activity and high values of isotonically extracted P_i as well as higher water content accompanied by elevated hydroxyproline content could indicate the lower degree of calcification.

Case 3. In this parosteal osteosarcoma it was possible to distinguish an area of growing tumor bone from another area with maturer bone. However, this distinction is not easy, due to the fact that this type of tumor is very similar to normal bone. The data from the biochemical analyses reveal increased acid and alkaline phosphatase activities for those areas containing growing tumor bone compared with areas of maturer bone. The occurrence of these two activities indicates that calcification and bone remodeling are taking place. Elevated levels of isotonically extracted protein, hydroxyproline, total hexosamine, extracted P_o, and water content also point to enhanced calcification. Remodeling in these areas of growing tumor bone may also be expressed by the relatively high amount of extracted P_i and the low level of extracted hexosamine.

In the areas of maturer bone acid and alkaline phosphatase activities are reduced and so are the other variables, except for total phosphorus, calcium, and extracted P_i, which are increased. These findings appropriately illustrate the higher degree of bone formation reached in these areas, probably accompanied by certain remodeling activities.

Case 4. Histologically classified as an anaplastic osteosarcoma, this tumor permitted the distinction of two characteristic regions: (a) anaplastic areas and (b) areas of incipient osteoid formation. As revealed by the chemical data, none of the enzymes typical for hard tissue formation were detectable in the anaplastic areas, which suggests that they probably consist of undifferentiated soft tissue. A low collagen content and a high amount of total as well as isotonically extracted hexosamine reveal that this tissue is not even comparable with connective tissue. High amounts of isotonically extracted protein and P_0 would reflect strong cellular activities and mitotic processes. The extremely high water content also suggests a soft tissue with a low degree of differentiation. In contrast, the areas of incipient osteoid formation did show an increased alkaline phosphatase activity and slightly increased acid phosphatase activity. The hydroxyproline content rose to about 2.5% reflecting the increased collagen content up to about 19%. Although the total hexosamine content remains at 1.1% like in anaplastic areas, the isotonically extracted hexosamine and the extracted protein are reduced, which may point to a higher degree of differentiation. The decreased water content as well as the total phosphorus and calcium accompanied by decreased extracted P_i may also indicate that a more differentiated tissue is on the way to form the matrix for hard tissue formation. Further support for this interpretation is given by the data reported by Quint et al. (1988). Finally, decreased levels of extracted P_0 may reflect the reduced rate of mitotic processes.

Summarizing the data it can be stated that a number of similarities and parallel biochemical parameters exist for the osteosarcoma cases 1, 2, and 3. Although absolute values for alkaline phosphatase activity and hexosamine are not the same in the three cases, these two parameters are generally twice as high in undifferentiated as in better differentiated areas of the tumors. There are, however, also characteristic differences between the two stages of tumor growth in each case. While acid phosphatase activity decreases from the less well differentiated stage to the maturer bone in cases 1 and 3, it increases in case 2. This may indicate that the process of bone remodeling is stronger in the sclerosing tumor than in the stage of lower differentiation.

Similarly, the level of isotonically extractable P_0 measurably decreases from the less well differentiated stage to that of maturer bone in cases 1 and 3, but is very low in case 2, obviously proving the low rate of calcification in this tumor. Proteolytic activities are measurable and decreasing in a similar sequence in cases 1 and 2, but are undetectably low in case 3. The above results may demonstrate that topological analyses combining biochemical with morphological and histological methods permit the comparison not only of undifferentiated and more differentiated areas of the same tumor, but also of correlating areas and stages in several tumors as well as of physiological bone formation. However, the differences documented here will stress the need for correlation of topochemical data with histological control sections, in order to determine whether and to what extent poorly and well differentiated stages of different tumors are actually corresponding and thus comparable.

Case 4, the anaplastic osteosarcoma, distinctly differs from cases 1, 2, and 3. Correlation of histology and analytical biochemistry made possible the differentiation between the more frequent anaplastic areas of the tumor and the areas of incipient osteoid formation that were characterized by a measurable alkaline phosphatase activity and an increased collagen formation as can be deduced from the enhanced hydroxyproline levels.

This method, which was first applied and developed for the analysis of enchondral ossification occurring in the epiphyseal growth plate, offers a new approach for the analysis of osteosarcomas regards the definition and documentation of the heterogeneity of bone tumors, and for establishing a classification by sequential grades of differentiation. Biochemical results revealed characteristic data on calcification activities within bone-forming osteosarcoma.

These observations illustrate the potential usefulness of topological analyses guided by histological control sections. Further studies are needed to obtain detailed information about the biochemical processes in osteosarcomas and their stages of differentiation.

References

Ali SY (1976) Analysis of matrix vesicles and their role in the calcification of epiphyseal cartilage. Fed Proc 35:135–142

Althoff J, Quint P, Höhling HJ (1977) Combined zonal chemical and biochemical analysis on mineralizing turkey tibia tendon. Calcif Tissue Res 22 [Suppl]:470–472

Althoff J, Quint P, Höhling HJ (1978) Activation and specificity of alkaline phosphatase of a mineralizing collagen-rich system. Experientia 34:692–693

Althoff J, Quint P, Krefting E-R, Höhling HJ (1982) Morphological studies on the epiphyseal growth plate combined with biochemical and X-ray microprobe analyses. Histochemistry 74:541–552

Althoff J, Quint P, Höhling HJ, Roessner A, Grundmann E (1985a) Biological characterization of human bone tumors: IV. Combined biochemical and histological analyses of different osteosarcomes. Pathol Res Pract 180:383–391

Althoff J, Quint P, Höhling HJ, Roessner A, Grundmann E (1985b) Biological characterization of human bone tumors: V. Zonal charaterization of osteosarcoma: topological biochemical analysis correlated with morphology. Pathol Pract Res 180:392–399

Althoff J, Quint P, Richter K-D, Jones DB (1988) Osteoblasten und Knochenorgankulturen unter "in vivo"-Bedingungen. Z. Zahnärztl Implantol IV, 282–285

Anderson HC (1967) Electron microscopic studies of induced cartilage development and clacification. J Cell Biol 35:81–101

Blumenthal NC, Betts F, Posner AS (1977): Stabilization of amorphous calcium phosphate by Mg and ATP. Calcif Tissue Res 23:245–250

Bonucci E (1967) Fine structure of early cartilage calcification. J Ultrastruct Res 20:33–50

Boyde A, Shapiro IM (1980) Energy dispersive X-ray elemental analysis of isolated epiphyseal growth plate chondrocyte fragments. Histochemistry 69:85–94

Cone CD Jr (1971) Unified theory on the basic mechanism of normal mitotic control and oncogenesis. J Theor Biol 30:151–181

Dahlin DC (1978) Bone tumors. General aspects and data on 6221 cases, 3rd edn. Charles C. Thomas, Springfield

Dahlin DC, Unni KK (1977) Osteosarcomas of bone and its important recognizable varieties. Am J Surg Pathol 1:61–72

Fleisch H, Neuman WF (1961) Mechanism of calcification: role of collagen, polyphosphates and phosphatase. Am J Physiol 200:1296–1300

Granda JL, Posner AS (1971) Distribution of four hydrolases in the epiphyseal plate. Clin Orthop 74:269–272

Grundmann E, Roessner A, Immenkamp M (1981) Tumor cell types in osteosarcoma as revealed by electronmicroscopy. Implications for histogenesis and subclassification. Virchows Archiv [Cell Pathol] 36:257–273

Höhling HJ, Barckhaus RH, Krefting ER, Schreiber J (1976) Electron microscopic microprobe analysis of mineralized collagen fibrils and extracollagenous regions in turkey leg tendon. Cell Tissue Res 175:345–350

Huvos AG (1979) Bone tumors, diagnosis, treatment and prognosis. W.B. Saunders, Philadelphia

Jones DB, Scholübbers G, Althoff J, Becker M, Doty S (1988) Evidence for more than one type of bone forming cell. In: Heuck HW, Keck E (eds). Fortschritte der Osteologie in Diagnostik und Therapie. Springer, Berlin, Heidelberg, New York, pp 311–324

Kakuta S, Golubb EE, Shapiro IM (1985) Morphometric analysis of phosphorus pools in calcified cartilage. Calcif Tissue Int 37:293–299

Krefting E-R, Lißner G, Höhling HJ (1980) Mixtures of salts as standards for quantitative electron-probe microanalysis of biological material. In: Brederoo P, Cosslett VE (eds) Electron microscopy. VIIth European Congress for Electron Microscopy Foundation, Leiden, vol 3, pp 156–157

Landis WJ (1986) A study of calcification in the leg tendons from the domestic turkey. J Ultrastruct Res 94:217–238

Linde A, Bhown M, Butler WT (1981) Non-collagenous proteins of rat dentin. Evidence that phosphoprotein is not covalently bound to collagen. Biochim Biophys Acta 667:341–350

Lukacs GL, Zs-Nagy I, Lustyik GY, Balazs GY (1983) Microfluorimetric and X-ray microanalytic studies on the DNA-content and Na/K ratios of the cell nuclei in various types of thyroid tumors. J. Cancer Res Clin Oncol 105:280–284

Pugliarello MC, Vittur F, de Bernard B, Bonucci E, Ascenzi A (1970) Chemical modifications in osteones during calcification. Calcif Tissue Res 5:108–114

Pugliarello MC, Vittur F, de Bernard B, Bonucci E, Ascenzi A (1973) Analysis of bone composition at the microscopic level. Calcif Tissue Res 12:209–216

Quint P, Althoff J, Höhling HJ (1977) Topochemical analysis of a mineralizing collagen-rich system. Naturwissenschaften 64:389

Quint P, Althoff J, Höhling HJ, Boyde A, Laabs WA (1980) Characteristic molar ratios of magnesium, carbon dioxide, calcium and phosphorus in the mineralizing fracture callus and predentine. Calcif Tissue Int 32:257–261

Quint P, Althoff J, Roessner A, Grundmann E, Höhling HJ (1988) Kombinierte biochemische und histologische Untersuchungen verschiedener Typen von Osteosarkomen. In: Heuck HW, Keck E (eds) Fortschritte der Osteologie in Diagnostik und Therapie. Springer, Berlin Heidelberg New York, pp 154–160

Rath NC, Hand AR, Reddi AH (1981) Activity and distribution of lysosomal enzymes during collagenous matrix-induced cartilage, bone and bone marrow development. Dev Biol 85:89–98

Reddi AH (1981) Cell biology and biochemistry of endochondral bone development. Collagen Rel Res 1:209–226

Roessner A (1984) Zur Cyto- und Histogenese der malignen und semimalignen Knochentumoren. Veröffentlichungen aus der Pathologie H. 122. Gustav Fischer, Stuttgart

Roessner A, Immenkamp M, Hiddemann W, Althoff J, Miebs T, Grundmann E (1985) Small cell osteosarcoma of the tibia with diffuse metastatic disease. Skeletal Radiol 14:216–225

Rozengurt E (1980) Stimulation of DNA synthesis in quiescent cultured cells: exogenous agents, internal signals, and early events. Curr Top Cell Regul 17:59–88

Schlüter E (1978) Die Ultrastruktur der Knorpelmineralisation am Beispiel der bipolaren proximalen Ulnawachstumsfuge des Hausschweins. Doctoral Thesis, University of Münster

Schmidt A, Rodegerdts U, Buddecke E (1978) Correlation of lysozyme activity with proteoglycan biosynthesis in epiphyseal cartilage. Calcif Tissue Res 26:163–172

Urist MR, DeLange RJ, Fineman GAM (1983) Bone cell differentiation and growth factors. Science 220:680–686

Wuthier RE (1969) A zonal analysis of inorganic and organic constituents of epiphysis during enchondral calcification. Calcif Tissue Res 4:20–38

Zs-Nagy I, Toth L, Szallasi Z, Lampe I (1987) On the possible role of intracellular sodium in mitogenesis: X-ray microanalytic measurements of the sodium to potassium ratio in human laryngeal tumors. J Cancer Res Clin Oncol 113:197–202

The Proliferation Behavior of Bone Tumors Investigated with the Monoclonal Antibody Ki-67

E. VOLLMER, A. ROESSNER, P. WUISMAN, A. HÄRLE, and E. GRUNDMANN

1 Introduction 91
2 Materials and Methods 93
3 Results 95
3.1 Malignant Tumors of Bone 95
3.1.1 Primary Bone Tumors 95
3.1.2 Tumors of Hemopoietic Origin 100
3.1.3 Metastases 102
3.1.4 Soft Tissue Tumors with Secondary Bone Involvement 102
3.2 Giant Cell Tumor of Bone 103
3.3 Benign Tumors and Tumor-like Lesions of Bone 104
3.3.1 Aneurysmal Bone Cyst 104
3.3.2 Solitary Bone Cyst 104
3.3.3 Fibrous Dysplasia 106
3.3.4 Chondroma 107
3.3.5 Aggressive Fibromatosis 107
3.3.6 Benign Fibrous Histiocytoma 107
4 Discussion 108
5 Summary 112
References 112

1 Introduction

Bone tumors are a rare kind of neoplasm. Their varied clinical manifestations, together with their rarity of occurrence, involve the pathologist in considerable difficulties in differentiating benign or merely reactive changes from malignant disease. Correct diagnosis of bone tumors calls for close interdisciplinary cooperation, but even then the difficulties may be grave, and sometimes hardly surmountable in differential diagnosis. Further improvement in the prognosis of malignant osseous neoplasm – beyond the progress seen in recent years – will be achieved only by earlier recognition and greater diagnostic accuracy. Any diagnostic considerations should therefore be centered upon the recognition of the tumor type and its biological behavior.

An essential variable in defining the biology of a neoplasm for diagnostic and therapeutic purposes is the assessment and quantification of the tumor

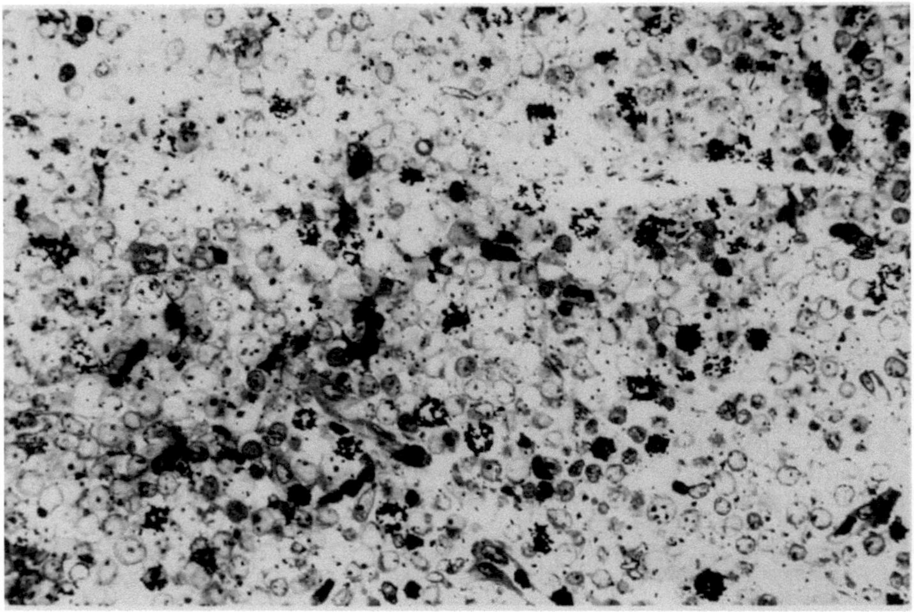

Fig. 1. Ewing's sarcoma: In vitro incubation with ^{3}H-thymidine labeling of many proliferating tumor cells. (The authors are indebted to Dr. D.B. v. Bassewitz for preparing the in vitro incubation.) (Autoradiograph of semithin section, ×330)

cell growth. In the search for a method for correct appraisal, interest has been focused on the "rate of proliferation" as a meaningful criterion for the tumor's biological behavior. Routinely, a quantitative estimate of the mitotic figures is sufficient, but may be difficult in tissues with unusual rates of proliferation reflecting an increased risk of malignancy. Quantitation of proliferating cells in a tissue explant by the assessment of ^{3}H-thymidine incorporation in cell DNA during S-phase by autoradiography (Fig. 1) is rather tedious and time consuming. A somewhat similar method, using bromodeoxyuridine (BrdU), a nonradioactive thymidine analogue, with subsequent immunohistochemical demonstration with a monoclonal anti-BrdU-antibody, is more rapid and less cumbersome. Microscope photometry offers the advantage that cellular foci with different kinetic activities can be studied in histological sections, and directly correlated with standard histological and cytomorphological variables. On the other hand, the cell fraction with DNA of S-phase type can be identified by flow cytometry. However, all these methods take much time and need a lot of mathematical data processing. Moreover, the results of flow cytometry cannot be correlated directly with the tumor's histological picture, which is a major practical disadvantage in routine diagnostics.

The introduction of a new monoclonal antibody, Ki-67, provides another means for rapid and readily reproducible demonstration of the so-called growth fraction in a given cell population (GERDES et al. 1983). This antibody is directed against a nuclear antigen present in all the active phases of the cell cycle (G_1,

S, G_2, M); it can label even those proliferating cells that show no histologically appreciable mitotic configurations. Cells that remain in the postmitotic rest phase (G_0) while differentiating will not express this nuclear antigen Ki-67 (GERDES et al. 1984). As Ki-67 can be applied to frozen sections in conventional immunohistology without additional preparation, its advantages over the other methods are evident (Gerdes 1985).

The proliferative behavior of tumors correlates well with their prognostic outlook (GERDES et al. 1986) and so the application of this antibody Ki-67 appeared to be well suited for the characterization of the biological behavior of bone tumors as a prognostic criterion.

2 Materials and Methods

Using either the double indirect peroxidase method or the monoclonal PAP technique, the nuclei of proliferating cells were labeled in 5-µm frozen sections of bone tumors from the Bone Tumor Registry of Westphalia, which represented a wide variety of malignancy grades (Figs. 2, 3).

To ensure that only freshly excised tissue was subjected to the immunohistological workup, a special messenger service was arranged between the operation room and the Institute of Pathology. Representative areas of the resected tumors were excised and snap-frozen in liquid nitrogen. Separate tissue samples from the same area were preserved for routine histology and for electron microscopy. Frozen sections 5 µm thick were cut with a cryomicrotome 2700 (Reichert/Jung), air-dried for 2 h, and then fixed in acetone for 30 s at 4° C. The sections were then washed in phosphate-buffered saline (PBS) and incubated in 0.4% sodium azide with 0.1% H_2O_2 in PBS for 5 min in order to inactivate endogenous peroxidase. This and the following steps were performed at room temperature. Incubation with monoclonal antibody Ki-67 (Dakopatts, Hamburg) at 1:30 concentration lasted 30 min. Hereafter, the slides were rewashed in PBS, then incubated with rabbit-anti-mouse IgG/M peroxidase-labeled secondary antibodies 1:150 (Dianova, Hamburg), and goat-anti-rabbit IgG/M peroxidase-labeled tertiary antibodies 1:150 (Dianova, Hamburg) for 30 min each. Rewashing in PBS was done between the steps of incubation. Using a monoclonal PAP technique, a rabbit-anti-mouse serum 1:30 (Dakopatts, Hamburg) was applied a secondary, and a mouse PAP complex 1:100 (Dakopatts, Hamburg) as tertiary antibody. After another washing in PBS, the bound peroxidase was developed with 3,3-diaminobenzidine-tetrahydrochloride (DAB, Serva, Heidelberg) at pH 7.4 in TRIS buffer plus 0.02% H_2O_0 for 10 min. Light nuclear counterstaining was performed with acid hemalum. For negative controls, the primary antibody was omitted, or incubation was performed with normal mouse serum. Germinal centers of lymph nodes served as positive controls. The count of Ki-67-positive nuclei was made on ten representative tumor fields, each holding 100 cells, and the proportion of labeled cells was expressed in percent (WEIBEL and ELIAS 1967).

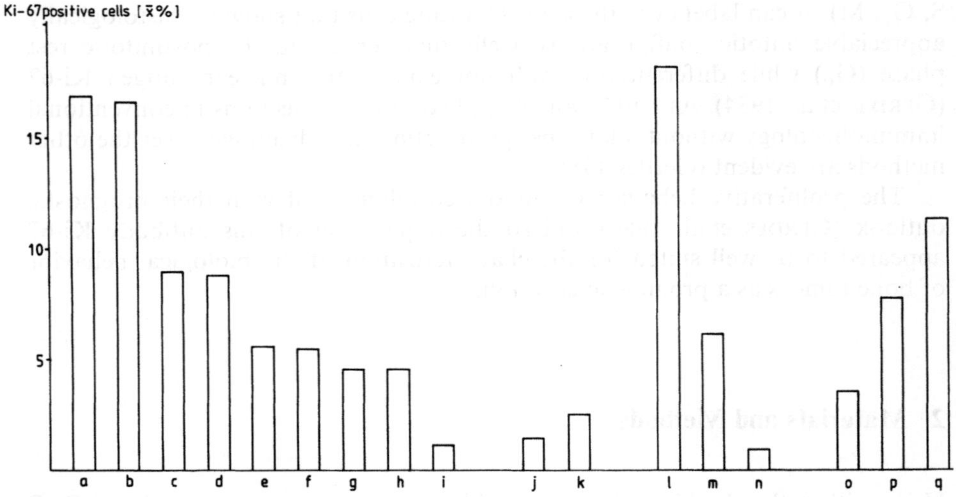

Fig. 2. Determination of growth fractions in different malignant bone tumor entities with the monoclonal antibody Ki-67

	Cases	Range
Primary tumors of bone		
a) Highly malignant osteosarcoma	20	9%–28.8%
b) Malignant giant cell tumor	1	16.6%
c) Malignant fibrous histiocytoma	1	8.9%
d) Ewing's sarcoma	16	5.0%–9.5%
e) Chondrosarcoma	4	2.8%–8.4%
f) Rhabdomyosarcoma	1	5.5%
g) Parosteal osteosarcoma (low-grade)	3	3.4%–5.8%
h) Chordoma	3	4.0%–5.2%
i) Myxoid liposarcoma	1	1.2%
Bone tumors of hemopoietic origin		
j) Plasma cell myeloma	2	0.9%–2.1%
k) Hodgkin's disease	1	2.6%
Bone metastases		
l) From bronchial carcinoma	3	16.2%–19.8%
m) From unidentified primary	1	6.2%
n) From pheochromocytoma	1	1.0%
Soft tissue tumors with secondary bone involvement		
o) Synovial sarcoma	2	5.2%–17.6%
p) Angiosarcoma	1	7.8%
q) Fibrosarcoma	1	11.6%

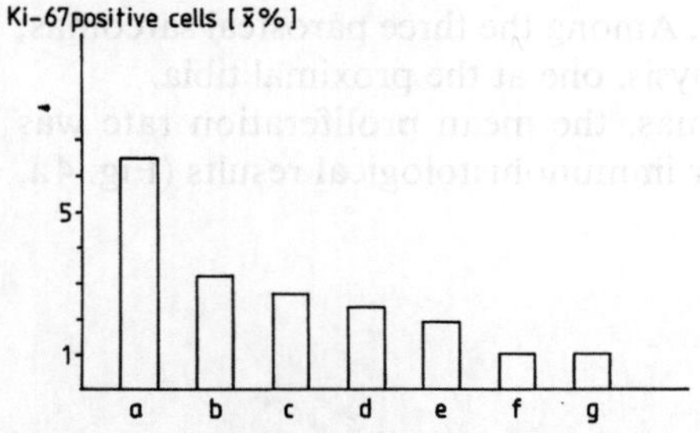

Fig. 3. Determination of growth fractions in different benign bone tumor entities with the monoclonal antibody Ki-67

	Cases	Range
Benign bone tumors		
a) Benign giant cell tumor	7	1.1%–8.9%
b) Aneurysmal bone cyst	6	1.8%–3.6%
c) Aggressive fibromatosis	4	1.2%–4.0%
d) Fibrous dysplasia	8	<1.0%–3.6%
e) Chondroma	4	<1.0%–2.5%
f) Solitary bone cyst	5	<1.0%–4.6%
g) Benign fibrous histiocytoma	1	1%

3 Results

3.1 Malignant Tumors of Bone

3.1.1 Primary Bone tumors

Osteosarcomas are malignant neoplasms characterized by tumor cells directly producing bone and/or osteoid (SCHAJOWICZ et al. 1972; DAHLIN and UNNI 1977). Classification into several subtypes is made according to superficial or central site of origin, and to the respective types of histological differentiation. Unlike the histological subclassification (DAHLIN and UNNI 1986), the site is relevant in prognosis: except for some individual variations (UNNI et al. 1977), central osteosarcomas (some 95% of all) are highly malignant as a rule, in contrast to the superficial lesions.

Our immunohistological studies were performed on 20 highly malignant primary intramedullary osteosarcomas and three parosteal osteosarcomas of low malignancy, in 10 males and in 13 females. The ages ranged from 8 to 48, i.e., four patients in the first, 15 in the second, one in the third, and three in the fifth decade. Among 20 central osteosarcomas, 11 were localized in the distal femur, two in the proximal, two in the distal tibia, and one at the lower leg, at the distal radius, at the os ileum, and at the humerus, respectively. In one case there was a recurrence in the pelvis. Among the three parosteal sarcomas, two were localized near the femoral metaphysis, one at the proximal tibia.

In all 20 highly malignant osteosarcomas, the mean proliferation rate was 16.8% (see Fig. 2, column a). In detail, our immunohistological results (Fig. 4a,

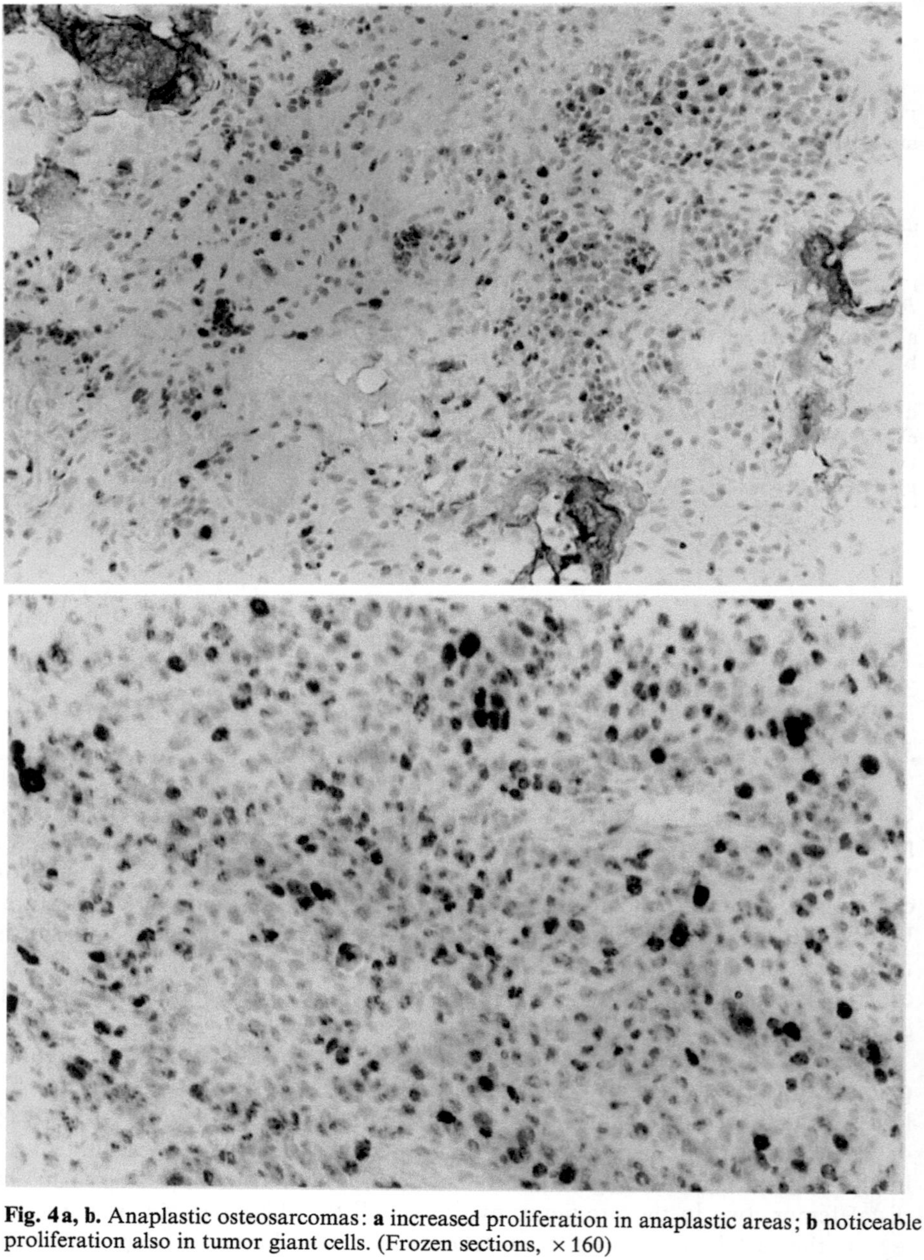

a

b

Fig. 4a, b. Anaplastic osteosarcomas: **a** increased proliferation in anaplastic areas; **b** noticeable proliferation also in tumor giant cells. (Frozen sections, ×160)

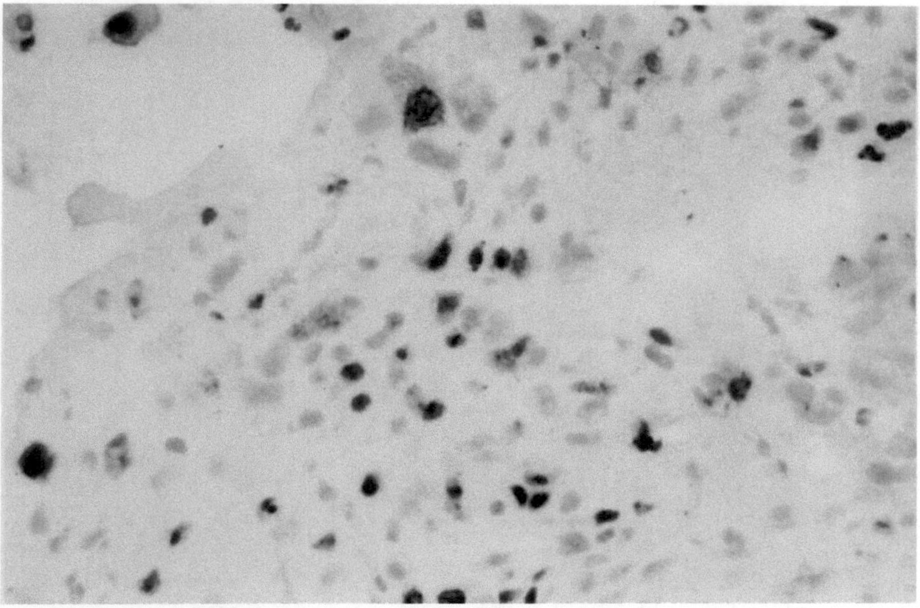

Fig. 5. Telangiectatic osteosarcoma with marked proliferation (frozen section, × 330)

b) showed a wide range of rates in conventional osteosarcomas, between 9% and 28.8%. In this category, the mean value of 16.8% was high, seen against the parosteal osteosarcomas with a mean proliferation rate of 4.6% (see Fig. 2, column g). In one case of recurrent osteosarcoma, we found a proliferation rate of 9% in contrast to the primary, which had shown a rate of 14.8%. In telangiectatic osteosarcoma (Fig. 5), as opposed to conventional osteosarcoma, proliferation rates are rather less variable, ranging only from 12.5% to 17.2% with a mean value of 14.6%. However, a detailed correlation of proliferation rates with certain histological subclassifications such as anaplastic, osteoblastic, chrondroblastic, or fibroblastic osteosarcoma was not possible, due to the small number of cases under observation.

The tumor cells of *chondrosarcoma* produce cartilaginous, but no osseous tissue. Our immunohistological investigation comprised three conventional chondrosarcomas in female patients aged 31, 40, and 61 years. The lesions were all localized in the iliac bone. The fourth case, a boy of 12, had a mesenchymal chondrosarcoma in the scapula. The proliferation rates were 2.8% and 4.4% in two low-grade chondrosarcomas, 6.8% in one high-grade tumor, and 8.4% in the mesenchymal chondrosarcoma. The mean value calculated from all four is 5.6% (see Fig. 2, column e; Fig. 6).

Ewing's sarcoma is one of the round cell sarcomas of more or less similar histological appearance, but with differing prognoses. Lethality rates are particularly high in Ewing's sarcoma (Dahlin and Unni 1986). Adequate pretherapeutic differentiation is important due to the progress in cytostatic therapy (Roessner 1984).

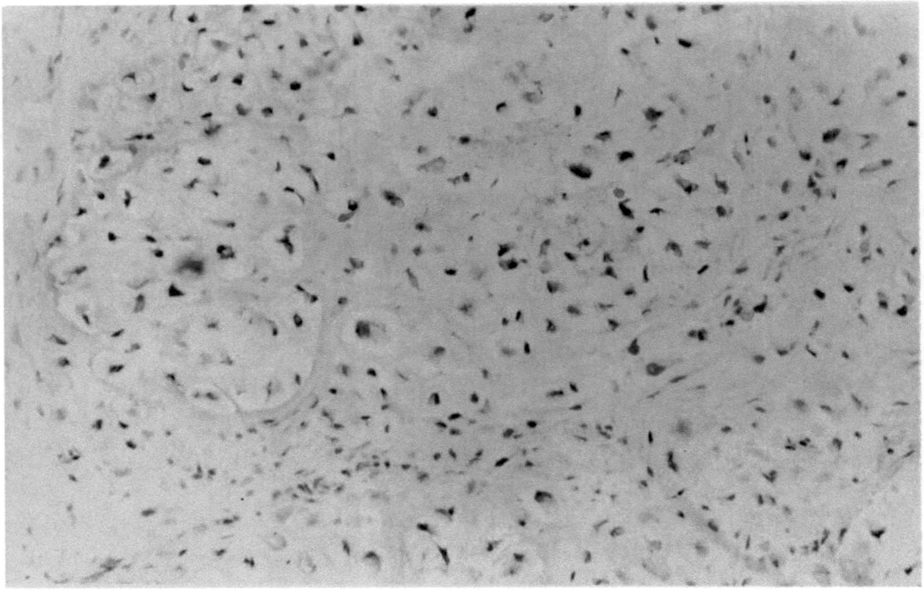

Fig. 6. Chondrosarcoma with marked proliferation (frozen section, ×160)

Histologically, the tumor is characterized by round nuclei without clear cytoplasmic delineation or prominent nucleoli. Fibrous septa often seems to segment the tumor tissue into irregular masses. There is no intercellular network of reticulin fibers such as that characterizing reticulosarcoma (SCHAJOWICZ et al. 1972).

Our immunohistochemical investigations with the monoclonal antibody Ki-67 were performed on fresh material from 16 cases of Ewing's sarcoma (Fig. 7). The patients' age ranged from 7 to 29 years (mean: 16 years). Three were female. Localization was: femur in three cases, humerus in three, tibia in three, fibula in two, scapula in one, and metatarsal bones 3, 4, and 5 plus calcaneus in one. All cases corresponded to the classical type with small cells, much glycogen, and seldom a greater number of mitotic foci; their proliferation rates ranged from 5% to 9.5%, with a mean level of 8.8% (see Fig. 2, column d). The tumors localized in the limbs showed a lower rate (5%–6.2%) than those in the trunk (5.8%–9.5%).

Manifestations of *chordoma* commonly occur between the third and seventh decades (DOMINOK and KNOCH 1982). Originating from residues of the chorda dorsalis, the tumor occurs preferentially in the sacrococcygeal part of the spine and at the base of the skull. Histologically, it is characterized by the presence of physaliferous and stellate cells and an intermediate group of transitional cells. Large vacuolated (physaliferous) cells are mostly found in the central parts of tumor lobules, while stellate cells in a peripheral array show some mitotic activity. The transitional cell type is mostly observed in the periphery of the physaliferous cells. The process of vacuolization itself starts from the

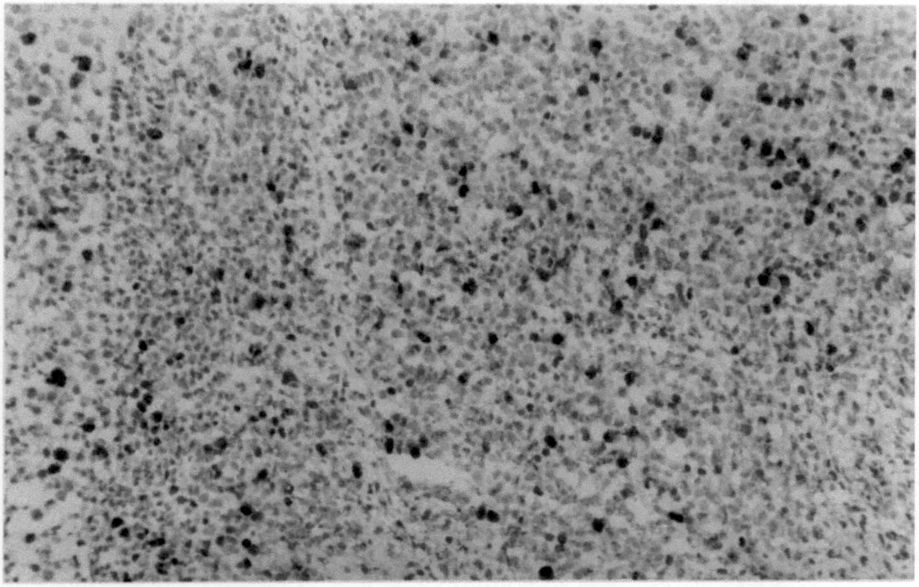

Fig. 7. Ewing's sarcoma with marked proliferation (frozen section, ×160)

stellate cells, implying an enlargement of their endoplasmic reticulum. In addition, we see a kind of pseudovacuolization which, though not clearly defined in light microscopy, can be identified in electron microscopy as an invagination of intracellular space by cytoplasmic protrusions that are interconnected by desmosomes (VOLLMER et al. 1985). Despite its slow growth rate and low metastatic trend, the prognosis of chordoma is poor on account of its infiltrating, destructive growth pattern.

The theoretical notions about the histogenesis of chordoma are controversial, understandably enough in view of the close vicinity of the three germ layers and the very complex transformations during embryogenesis, especially in the chordal region. Several work groups have emphasized the role of a bimodal expression of intermediate filaments in this process (BOUROPOULOU et al. 1987; MIETTINEN et al. 1983; VOLLMER et al. 1985).

Our immunohistological investigations concerned three coccygeal tumors of three male patients aged 62, 65, and 72 years. Proliferation rates (see Fig. 2, column h; Fig. 8) were between 4% and 5.2% (mean value: 4.6%). Of all morphologically distinguishable cells, only the stellate cells could be labeled with the antibody Ki-67. The vacuolated cells and those of intermediate, transitional type were not proliferating.

Malignant fibrous histiocytoma was only recently included in the WHO classification of bone tumors (SCHAJOWICZ 1981). It is currently recognized as the most frequent soft tissue sarcoma of later adult life. The bone variant of malignant fibrious histiocytoma corresponds largely to the soft tissue neoplasm in both light and electron microscopic features (ROESSNER et al. 1979). The tumor

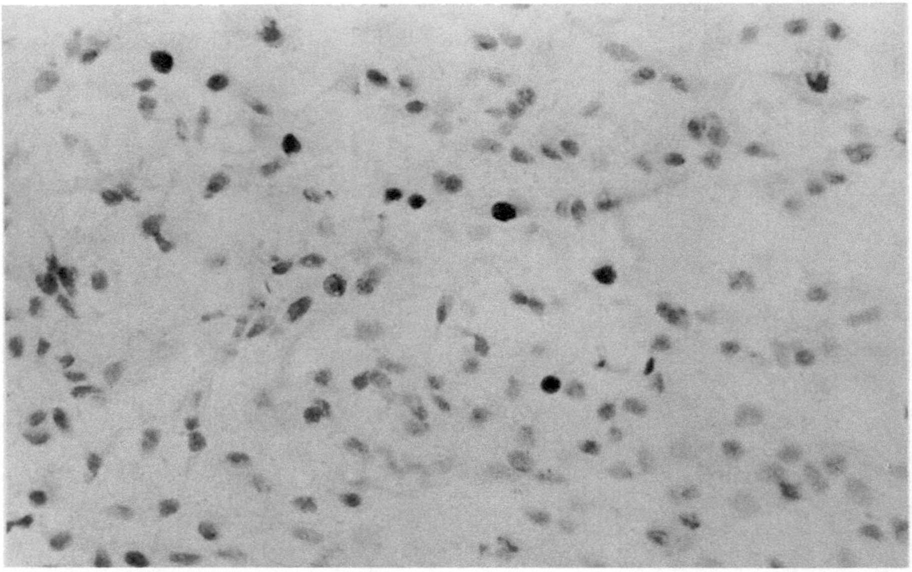

Fig. 8. Chordoma with moderate proliferation only of stellate cells (frozen section, ×330)

is composed of spindle-shaped fibroblastic cells, often arranged in a whorl-like, so-called storiform pattern, without safe evidence of osteoid. Between these fibroblastic cells are seen groups of histiocytic cells which, according to recent investigations, are interpreted as reactive phenomena rather than as an autochthonous tumor compartment (ROESSNER et al. 1984a, 1986). The prognosis is better than that of osteosarcoma (SPANIER 1977). Our immunohistological investigation (see Fig. 2, columne c) focused on representative areas from a large tumor (22 cm) in the minor pelvis of a 52-year-old female patient; revealing a proliferation rate of 8.9%, the positive Ki-67 reaction was found only in the fibroblastic tumor cells (Fig. 9a).

Besides the more common malignant primary tumors of bone discussed above, we were able to investigate two other much less frequent bone tumors with regard to their proliferation behavior: A *rhabdomyosarcoma* in the left upper pubic bone of a 29-year-old male patient had a proliferation rate of 5.5%, and a *myxoid liposarcoma* in the distal femur of a 35-year-old male patient had a rate of 1.2% (see Fig. 2, columns f, i).

3.1.2 Tumors of Hemopoietic Origin

In this category we were able to investigate fresh material from a case of lymphocyte-rich *Hodgkin's disease* of a 36-year-old male patient, manifesting in the 12th thoracic vertebral body with surrounding soft tissue involvement. Its proliferation rate was 2.6% (see Fig. 2, column k).

Another so-called round cell sarcoma of bone of differential diagnostic significance is *plasma cell myeloma*, which is most likely to occur in older patients

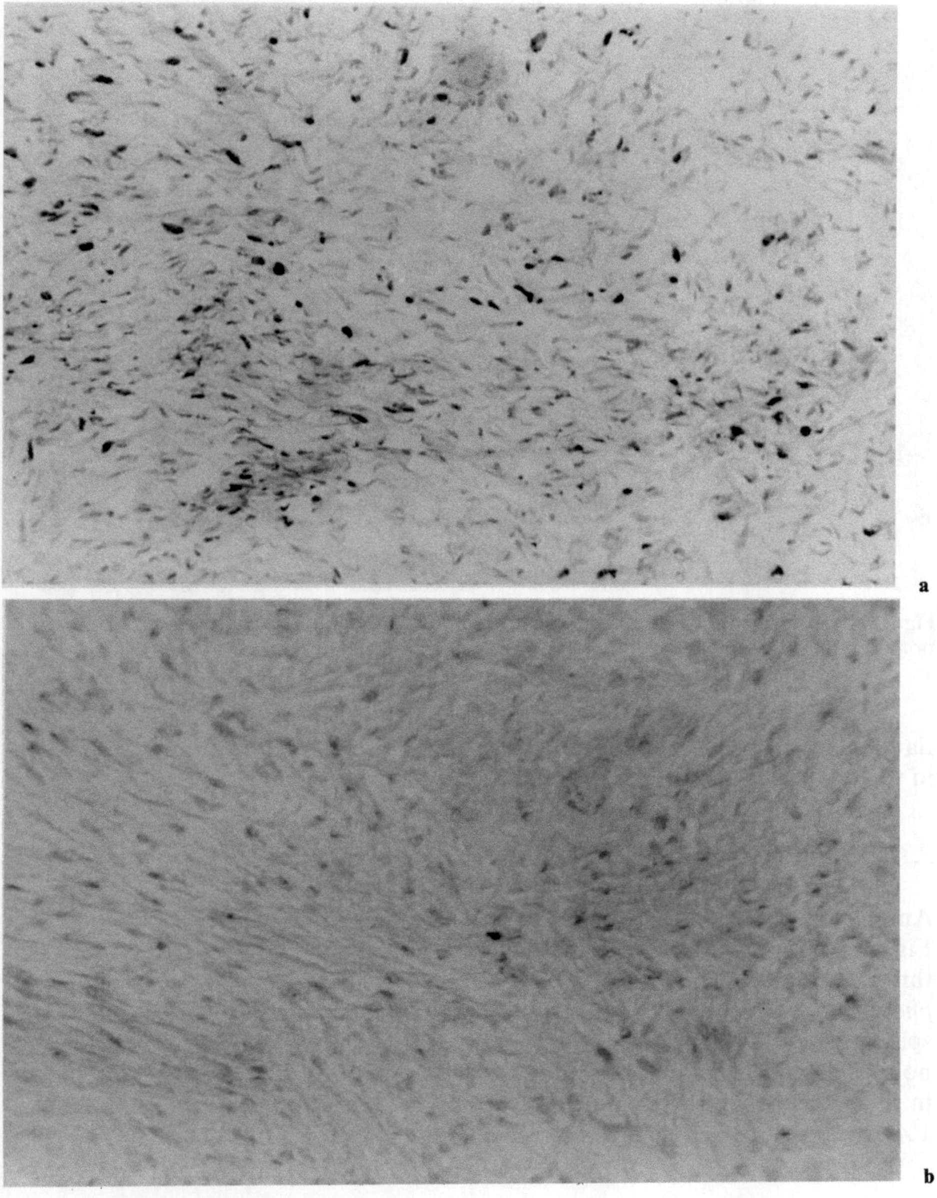

Fig. 9. a Malignant fibrous histiocytoma with marked proliferation. **b** Benign fibrous histiocytoma with little proliferation. (Frozen sections, ×160)

(beyond the sixth decade, (DOMINOK and KNOCH 1982), with an excess in males. The plasmacytomas in our patient group had been recorded in a 31-year-old male and a 53-year-old female patient. They were identified as multiple myeloma, the most frequent type. One was a well-differentiated myeloma with immunohistochemical evidence of IgG; the other was considered as poorly differen-

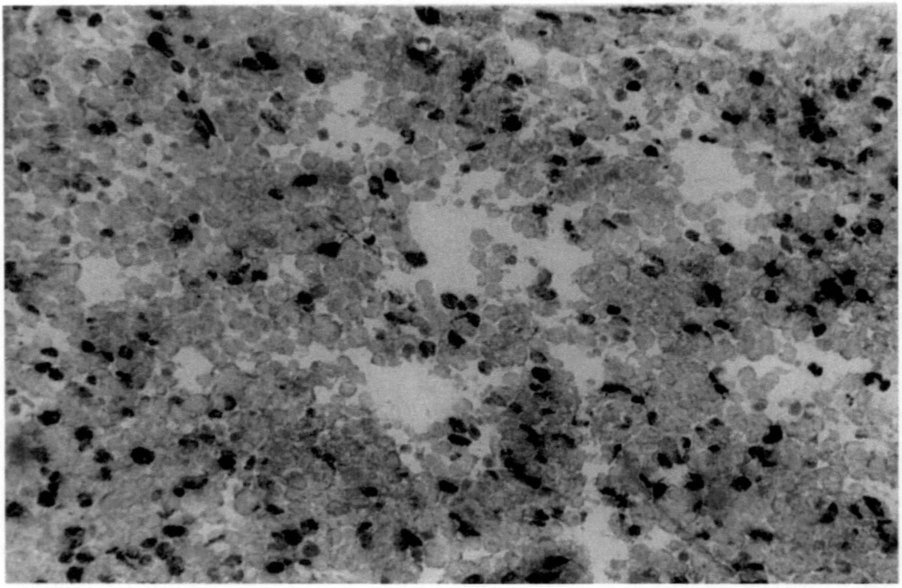

Fig. 10. Osseous metastasis of unidentified carcinoma with moderate proliferation (frozen section, ×160)

tiated according to the criteria of HUVOS (1979). Proliferation rates were 0.9% in the first and 2.1% in the second case (see Fig. 2, column j).

3.1.3 Metastases

Among the five cases included in our immunohistological investigation (see Fig. 2, columns l–n), three were males. Ages ranged from 52 to 67 years. In three cases the primary had been a *bronchogenic carcinoma*, the 4th was a *pheochromocytoma*, the last a carcinomatous metastatic lesion to the thoracic spine with *unknown primary*, and whose nature was unidentifiable even by immunohistochemical methods. Proliferation rates were 16.2%, 18.4%, and 19.8% in the metastases of bronchogenic carcinomas; that of pheochromocytoma was 1%, and that of the unidentified carcinoma, 6.2% (Fig. 10).

3.1.4 Soft Tissue Tumors with Secondary Bone Involvement

The onset of *synovial sarcomas* occurs mostly during the third and fourth decades, seldom earlier (SCHAJOWICZ 1981; LICHTENSTEIN 1977). According to these authors, the male sex is preferentially affected, but the opposite has also been reported (JAFFE 1958). Tumors of this type mostly localized in the limbs, expecially near the joints, which, besides bursae and aponeuroses, are generally the sites of origin. Derivation from synovial tissue, however, has not been fully

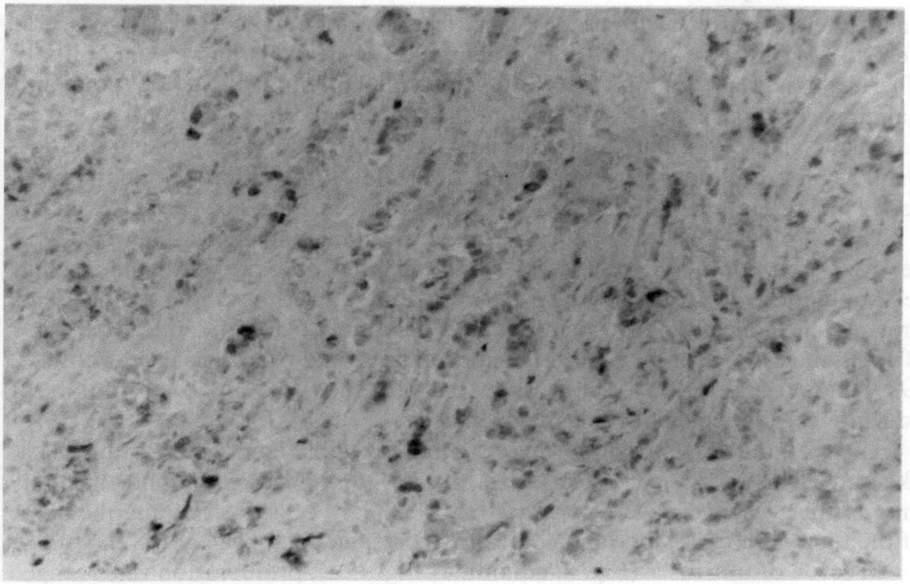

Fig. 11. Synovial sarcoma (biphasic) with marked proliferation (frozen section, ×160)

ascertained (DOMINOK and KNOCH 1982). At an early stage this tumor appears mostly well delineated and encapsulated, but it will show diffuse infiltration into adjacent structures later.

Our immunohistological investigations (see Fig. 2, column o) were performed on fresh material from a monophasic synovial sarcoma in the left calcaneus of a 34-year-old female patient, and on preserved tumor tissue from the right iliac bone of a 54-year-old woman (Fig. 11) with a biphasic synovial sarcoma. The monophasic tumor had a proliferation rate of 5.2%, the biphasic tumor one of 17.6% (mean value: 11.4%).

A rare case of *angiosarcoma*, originating from the paravertebral musculature and eroding the lumbar vertebra of a 42-year-old female patient, is presented under this category. Its proliferation rate was 7.8% (see Fig. 2, column p). The was also a case of well-differentiated mesenterial *fibrosarcoma* infiltrating the iliac wing in a male patient of 60; our immunohistological investigation yielded a proliferation rate of 11.6% (see Fig. 2, column q).

3.2 Giant Cell Tumor of Bone

Giant cell tumors of bone may occur in any age group, but a peak is observed in the third decade. JAFFE et al. (1940), who were the first to describe this entity, proposed a grading of giant cell tumors according to histological findings, ranking benign tumors as grade 1, doubtful lesions as grade 2, and evidently malignant neoplasms as grade 3. However, certain giant cell tumors whose histology placed them obviously with grade 1 were found, rarely, to develop early visceral metastases (DAHLIN et al. 1970). Differential diagnostic alternatives are not only other benign bone lesions, but also giant cell-containing osteosarcoma and malignant fibrous histiocytoma of bone.

In our group of eight cases, the sites of localization were proximal femur, distal femur, proximal tibia, proximal fibula, os ilium, shoulder joint, pubic bone, and os sacrum. The patients' ages ranged from 18 to 60 years.

The histological characteristics of giant cell tumors include vascularized connective tissue composed of mostly spindle-shaped or oval cells, and a giant cell population of osteoclast type evenly distributed over the whole tumor tissue. Previous histochemical investigations had demonstrated the identical behavior of multinucleated cells in giant cell tumor and normal osteoclasts (SCHAJOWICZ 1981; SPJUT et al. (1971). From more recent results, the giant cell tumors of bone are recognized as fibroblastic neoplasms.

The mononuclear stroma of these tumors is mainly composed of fibroblast-like and of histiocytic cells (ROESSNER et al. 1986), and it was found that only the fibroblast-like cells were proliferating. The giant cells determining the name of the tumor were, in fact, nonneoplastic (ROESSNER et al. 1984b, 1987).

In seven of our cases (Fig. 3, column a; Fig. 12a), proliferation rates ranged from 1.1% to 8.9% (mean value: 6.5%); only one had a rate of 16.6% (see Fig. 2, column b; Fig. 12b). According to the documentation in the bone Tumor Registry, the latter case had developed multiple metastases in lung, kidney, thyroid, and myocardium 4 months after the second tumor recurrence, and ultimatively caused the death of the female patient at the age of 60.

3.3 Benign Tumors and Tumor-like Lesions of Bone

3.3.1 Aneurysmal Bone Cyst

Aneurysmal bone cysts are most frequent in the first three decades (DOMINOK and KNOCH 1982). Of our six cases, two patients were in the first, and four in the second decade. Aneurysmal bone cysts may arise in all kinds of bone (JAFFE 1958; DAHLIN and UNNI 1986; LICHTENSTEIN 1977), but they are most frequent in the lower extremities. Spine and upper extremities follow. The aneurysmal bone cyst is an expanding osteolytic lesion with blood-filled spaces of varying size, separated by connective tissue septa, and containing osteoclastic giant cells. Despite current contradictory theories, it is unlikely that the aneurysmal bone cyst originates from the vascular system (VOLLMER et al. 1987).

The growth behavior of such a cyst in unpredictable: Some lesions may continually increase in size over months or years, others may rest for several years (SPJUT et al. 1971). Their prognosis is generally favorable (DOMINOK and KNOCH 1982). The proliferation rates measured in our group were between 1.8% and 3.6% (Fig. 13), with a mean value of 3.2% (see Fig. 3, column b).

3.3.2 Solitary Bone Cyst

These lesions may affect all age groups, with a certain predilection for the first and second decades (JAFFE 1958; SCHAJOWICZ 1981; DOMINOK and KNOCH

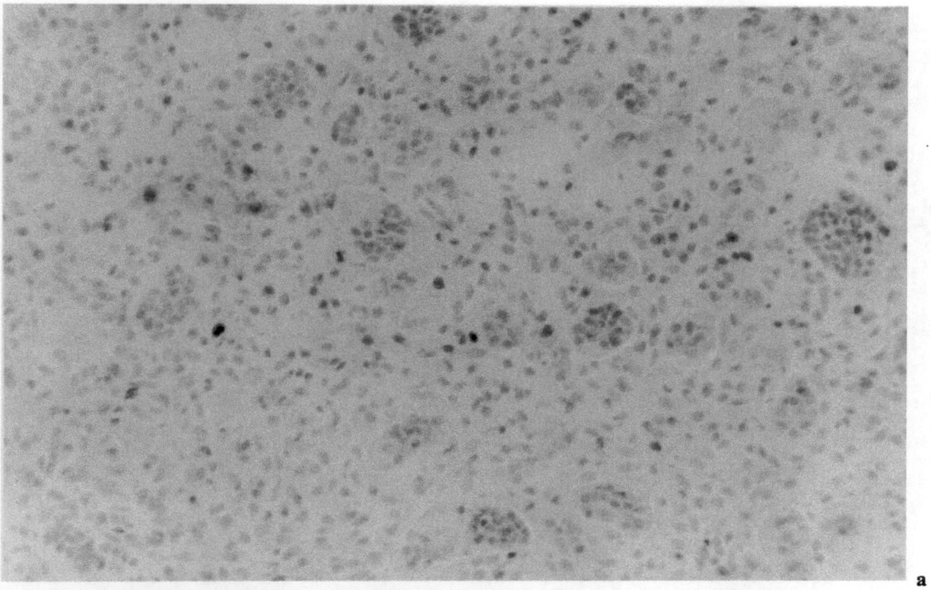

a

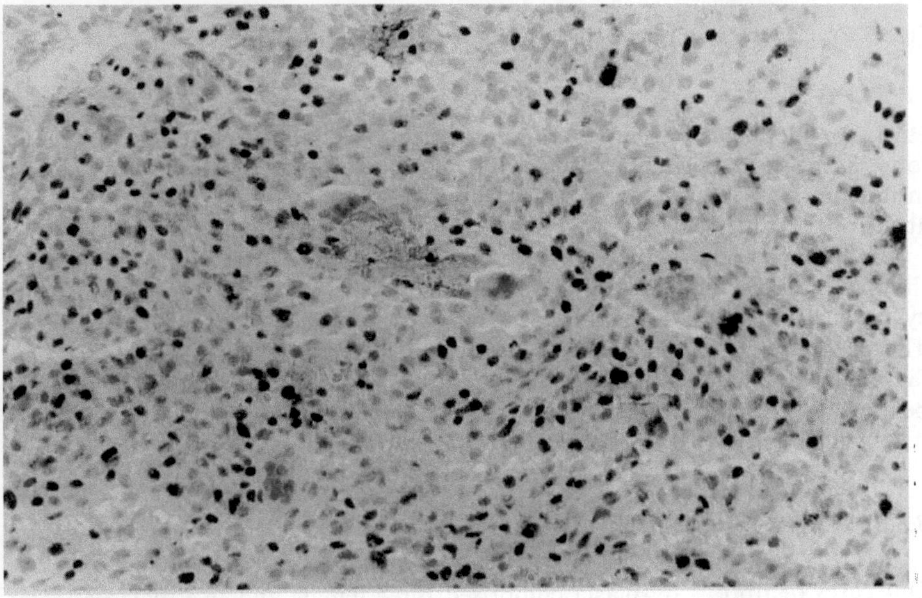

b

Fig. 12. a Benign giant cell tumor with little proliferation. **b** Rare case of malignant giant cell tumor with marked proliferation. (Frozen sections, ×160)

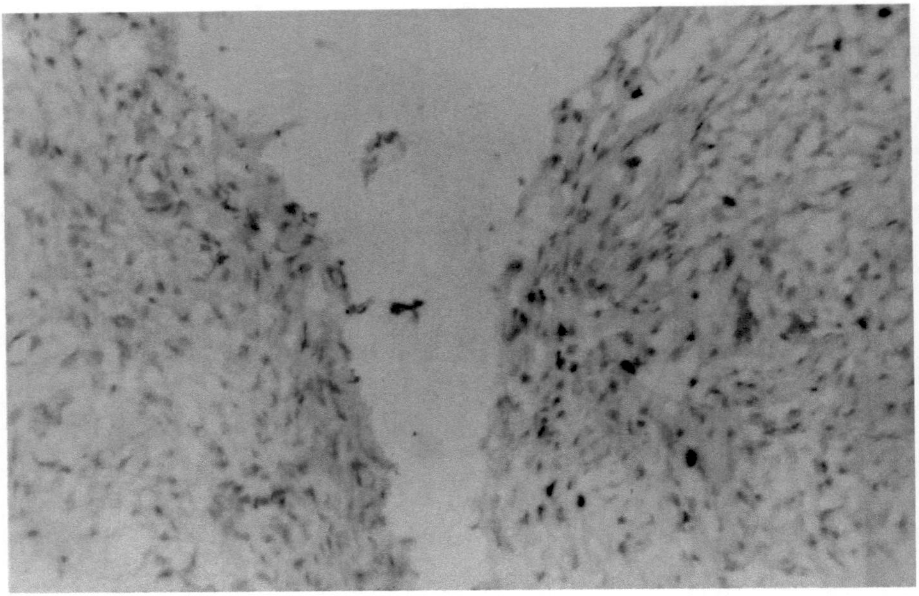

Fig. 13. Proliferating aneurysmal bone cyst (frozen section, × 160)

1982). In fact, of the five cases investigated here, one was in the first, and four in the second decade. Generally, these solitary cysts occur most often in the humerus, and this was the localization of our five, two of them typically at the proximal end.

In solitary bone cysts we may distinguish an active from an inactive type, the first situated near the epiphyseal plate in a state of growing. The inactive cyst is situated at some distance at a state of rest (DOMINOK and KNOCH 1982). The prognosis of this benign cystic, unicameral fluid-filled lesion is generally favorable. In our five cases, proliferation rates (see Fig. 3, column f) were from below 1% to 4.6%, with a mean value of only 1%. The one case with 4.6% reflected an active cyst fractured at the time of diagnosis.

3.3.3 Fibrous Dysplasia

Our cases of fibrous dysplasia comprised three female and five male patients; however, the data on sex ratios in the literature are partly controversial (DOMINOK and KNOCH 1982; SCHAJOWICZ (1981). Immunohistological investigations covered four cases in the second decade, three in the third, and one in the fifth.

Fibrous dysplasia may affect one or more bones at a time, and occur in all kinds of osseous tissue. For monostotic fibrous dysplasia, the main localizations are head, femur, tibia, and ribs; in polyostotic lesions a large number of bones may be involved. In our cases, fibrous dysplasia was localized in the tibia (3), in the femoral region (3), in the humerus (1), and iliac bone (1).

Fibrous dysplasia is characterized as a benign lesion by the presence of fibrious connective tissue with a typical spiral pattern containing trabeculae of immature, nonlamellated bone.

The results with regard to proliferation rates in our cases ranged from below 1% to 3.6% with a mean value of 2.7% (see Fig. 3, column d). No correlation could be established between proliferation rates and patients' ages.

3.3.4 Chondroma

This benign lesion, characterized by the formation of mature cartilaginous tissue, commonly occurs at a later age. Although it starts during the period of growth, its clinical manifestation will not happen before the third or fourth decade, and it is rare in children under the age of 10. The mean age of patients is 35 years. Of our four enchondromas one was situated in the pelvic region, the other three in the feet (two males, two females). Chondromas of the hands and feet show nearly no trend to malignant transformation (1% risk) and will seldom recur (3% risk). In other skeletal localizations, the risk of malignant transformation is higher, i.e., 20%–50% (Dominok and Knoch 1982). In our group of two enchondromas and two enchondromatoses, the proliferation rates were from below 1% up to 2.5%, with a mean value of 1.9% (see Fig. 3, column e).

3.3.5 Aggressive Fibromatosis

These tumors are found predominantly in multiparous women between the third and fifth decades. In our patient group, the cases were aged 13 and 14 (males), and 32 and 40 (females). Microscopically, aggressive fibromatosis resembles hyperplastic scar tissue with spindle-shaped cells and abundant collagenous fibers. The tumors tend to grow infiltrating muscular and fatty tissue and may even cause bone erosion. There are no metastases and spontaneous regression is possible. The etiology is unknown; pathogenetically, an abnormal proliferation of myofibroblasts is considered the main factor.

Aggressive fibromatous lesions in our group were localized at the distal ulna, distal lower arm, and pelvis (two cases). Proliferation rates were 4% (Fig. 14), 3.4%, 2%, and 1.2%, respectively, with a mean value of 2.7% (see Fig. 3, column c).

3.3.6 Benign Fibrous Histiocytoma

This tumor will only very rarely manifest as a primary bone lesion, and clinical data will decide about its differential diagnostic distinction from nonossifying fibroma (Roessner et al. 1981). The histological picture very much resembles that of benign fibrous histiocytoma of soft tissues (Auböck 1975). Our study

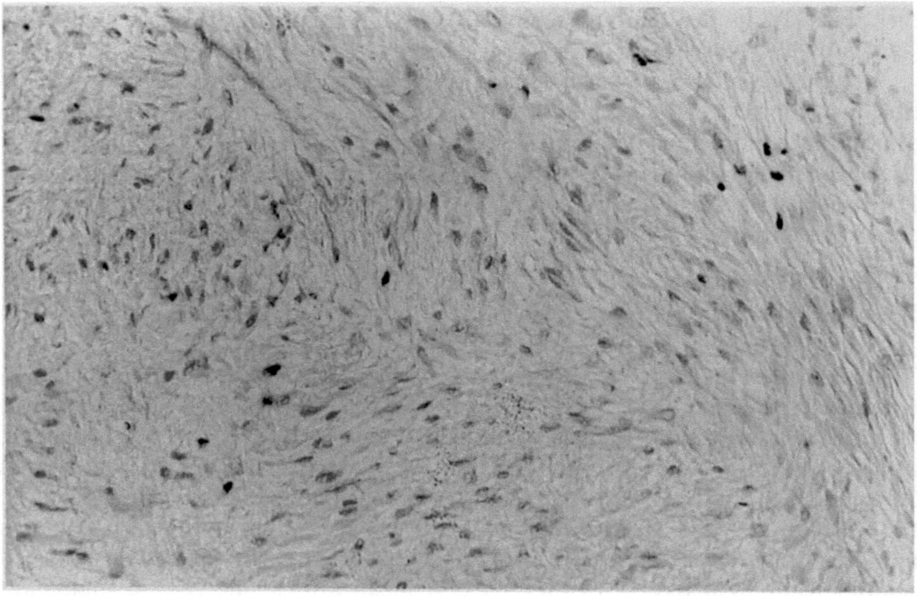

Fig. 14. Aggressive fibromatosis with moderate proliferation (frozen section, ×160)

included such a lesion from the femur of a 32-year-old male patient; the immunohistological result was a proliferation rate of 1% (see Fig. 3, column g; Fig. 9b).

4 Discussion

Immunohistological investigations of various bone tumor entities with the antibody Ki-67 gave results which were largely correlated with the prognoses expected. In general, malignant tumors had a distinctly higher proliferation rate than benign lesions (cf. Figs. 2, 3). The grade of malignancy shows correlation with the proliferation data. In highly malignant conventional osteosarcomas (Fig. 4), for instance, proliferation rates range from 9% to 28.8%, and this wide spectrum suggests, in agreement with SCHAJOWICZ (1981) that histological grading alone is of limited value in predicting the severity of malignancy. Even the mean value of 16.8% calculated from the proliferation rates of our conventional osteosarcoma cases appears high enough to be taken as a sure sign of malignancy; this was confirmed by several authors in a comparison with flow cytometric DNA analysis (ROESSNER 1984; UNNI and DAHLIN 1984; GRUNDMANN et al. 1986; KREICBERGS and TRIBUKAT 1984; HELIÖ et al. 1985).

In low-grade parosteal osteosarcoma, proliferation rates oscillate around the low mean value of 4.6%, which agrees with the observations of GRUNDMANN et al. (1986) that the kinetics of parosteal osteosarcoma are distinctly different from those of highly malignant osteosarcoma: The mean S-phase content of low-grade parosteal osteosarcoma, 7.3%, was distinctly below the mean S-phase value of intramedullary osteosarcoma at 18.8%. Moreover, the low-grade tumors showed only unimodal diploid DNA distribution.

A proliferation rate as low as 9% in a recurrent osteosarcoma is quite rare; it corresponded with a better differentiation than seen in the primary, but it is uncertain in this particular case whether this correlates with a more favorable prognosis as stated by GRUNDMANN (1976). In most cases, the recurrences of bone primaries will show the same histological structure and cytology as the first tumor, although their differentiation may be occassionally poorer, and their prognosis is nearly always less favorable.

Among the chondroblastic tumors, increasing malignancy seemed to be paralleled by increasing proliferation rates, from a conventional low-grade chondrosarcoma with a rate of 2.8%, to a mesenchymal chondrosarcoma with 8.4%. This corresponds to the practice of histological grading and the current knowledge about the clinical course and prognosis of this tumor type: They are generally liable to develop local recurrences and even metastases, often several years after therapy (HUVOS 1979; SPJUT et al. 1971).

Although in our particular case the monoclonal antibody technique was found useful for chondrosarcoma grading, we have to emphasize that chondroblastic bone tumors have to be seen as clinicopathological entities, and that comparison is permitted only between bone tumors in corresponding regions of the skeleton.

The progress of chemotherapy has enhanced the necessity for exact differentiation of round cell tumors. Ewing's sarcoma is a distinctive, small round cell sarcoma which is one of the most highly malignant bone tumors. It has been known for some time, however, that their mitotic rate is not very high (DAHLIN and UNNI 1986). The results of our immunohistological studies confirm this experience: with a mean proliferation rate of 8.8%, Ewing's sarcoma ranks only fourth among the malignant bone primaries (see Fig. 2, column d).

Ewing's sarcoma in the limbs has a lower proliferation rate (5%) than those in the trunk (9.5%) (Fig. 7). This agrees with the observations of SCHAJOWICZ (1981) on the potential prognostic significance of localization in Ewing's tumor. In comparison with Ewing's sarcomas, plasma cell myelomas had a considerably lower proliferation rate (0.9% and 2.1%), adequately correlated with their biological behavior.

The malignant fibrous histiocytoma included in our immunohistochemical study showed a proliferation rate of 8.9%, and was recorded with a diameter of 22 cm at the time of surgery, demonstrating the rapid growth of the lesion. According to histological criteria, the tumor had been classified as high-grade malignant fibrous histiocytoma. In contrast, the very rare benign fibrous histocytoma of bone had a proliferation rate of only 1%, which emphasizes the value of Ki-67 for defining the biological behavior of a tumor and the prognosis (cf. Fig. 9a, b).

The chordomas in our study had a mean proliferation rate of 4.6%, which agrees with the clinical data on these slowly growing tumors. Since it was only the stellate cells that were labeled by positive reaction to the antibody Ki-67

– the same population that shows mitoses in conventional histology – we may assume that these stellate cells are the tumor's stem cells. This is confirmed by ultrastructural findings on the process of vacuolization in the physaliferous cells (VOLLMER et al. 1985).

The labeling results in three cases of metastases from bronchogenic carcinoma, with their high rates of 16.2%–19.8%, reflect the high malignancy of these tumors. However, the low growth rate (1%) documented for a metastasis from malignant pheochromocytoma confirms the fact that neither nuclear polymorphism nor the mitotic count can serve as a reliable criterion for grading the malignancy of this tumor (KERTELGE et al. 1987).

With the exception of giant cell tumors of bone, all benign tumors and tumor-like lesions studied had proliferation rates below 5%, which emphasizes the dubious nature of this entity (cf. Fig. 3). In solitary bone cysts, it is interesting to note that only the active cyst has a slightly increased proliferation rate of 4.6%, in contrast to the inactive one with a rate below 1%. The known benign nature of fibrous dysplasia, chondroma, and aggressive fibromatosis is confirmed by the Ki-67 study yielding mean rates around 2% (see Fig. 3, columns c–e). In the case of fibrous dysplasia it was not possible to correlate the proliferative behavior with the patient's age, presenting no supportive data for the experience that the lesion stops growing at puberty. In view of the small number of cases, our result is hardly representative and a wider series would be needed to study this question.

In giant cell tumors of bone, the results of our immunohistological study with the antibody Ki-67 clearly underline the fibroblastic nature of that neoplasm. None of our eight cases had positive immunohistochemical demonstration of proliferating nuclei in the giant cells for which the tumor is named. Only the mononucleate stroma, composed mainly of fibroblast-like and histiocytic cells, was found to proliferate (Figs. 12, 15a). The well-known observation that no prognosis about a giant cell tumor can be based on its histological pattern alone was substantiated by the immunohistological results. In two cases with markedly atypical stroma cells, the mean proliferation rates were still only 7.2% and 8.9%. In the one case with a growth fraction of 16.6% (Figs. 12b and 15a), multiple metastases developed in the lungs, kidneys, thyroid, and myocardium, which ultimately led to the death of the woman at the age of 60. Subsequent histological examination of these metastases revealed a spindle cell, fibroblastic sarcoma, and so verified the assumed prognosis retrospectively.

In addition to verifying the biological behavior of various tumor entities by observing the expression of the nuclear antigen Ki-67, immunohistological methods may also help in differential diagnosis of giant cell-containing bone tumors. In this context we have to mention that the highest proliferation rates are recorded in the anaplastic giant cell-containing type of osteosarcoma, which can be separated from giant cell tumors (Fig. 15). The Ki-67 technique is also of special interest in telangiectatic osteosarcoma (Fig. 5) with regard to the possible confusion with aneurysmal bone cyst (Fig. 13), the latter showing a considerably lower proliferation.

It may be concluded that the proliferation marker Ki-67 is a handy means to verify, supplement, or correct conventional histological grading. Moreover,

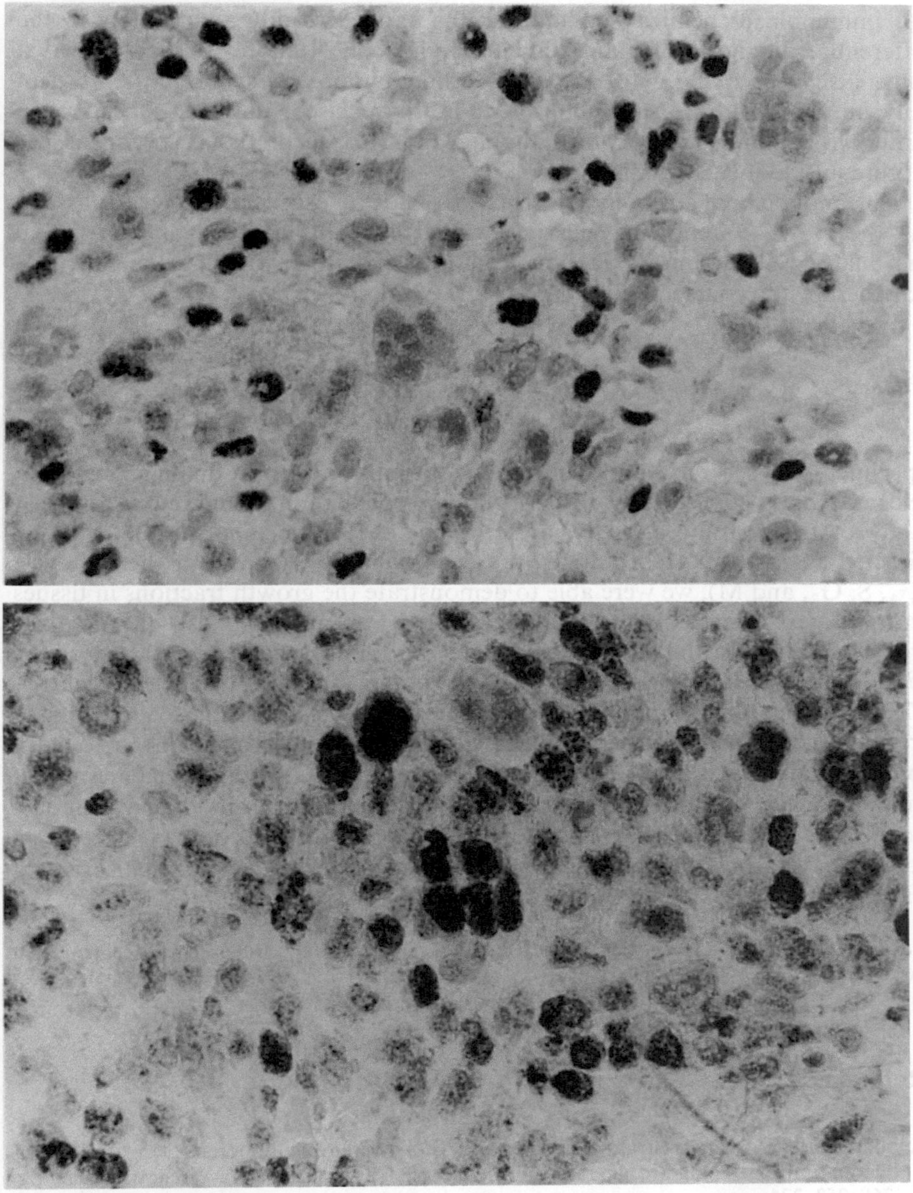

a

b

Fig. 15. a Rare case of malignant giant cell tumor with marked proliferation of mononuclear cells only. **b** Giant cell-containing osteosarcoma with additionally marked proliferation of tumor giant cells. (Frozen sections, ×400)

this immunohistochemical method may be applied readily and reliably in the differential diagnosis of giant cell-containing bone tumors. It even provided some insight into the cytogenesis of certain tumor entities. Since Ki-67 can only be demonstrated satisfactorily in freshly excised, unfixed, shock-frozen material, optimal facilities for sampling and storage of tissue specimens are a prerequisite of such studies.

The monoclonal antibody Ki-67 may provide an excellent marker for assessing the growth fraction of cells in a given tissue. Its practical impact lies in the analysis of a tumor's proliferation rate and in monitoring the pre- and posttherapeutic course of a lesion.

5 Summary

Specimens of several tumor entities at various grades of malignancy were selected from the Bone Tumor Registry of Westphalia for an immunohistological study of their proliferation behavior. Using the monoclonal antibody Ki-67 directed against a nuclear antigen present in all active phases of the cell cycle (G_1, S, G_2, and M), we were able to demonstrate the growth fractions in tissues with an atypical rate of proliferation, implying an increased risk of malignant transformation. In the 97 cases examined we found a good correlation of the biological proliferation behavior with the expression of the nuclear antigen Ki-67. Moreover, our immunohistological results are comparable with the data from the same tumor entities obtained by other methods such as flow cytometry and autoradiogaphy. Thus the monoclonal antibody Ki-67 provides an excellent marker for labeling the growth fraction in a human tissue. Its practical impact lies in the differential diagnostic analysis of the proliferation rate in a given tumor and its possible grading, and in pre- or posttherapeutic monitoring of patients and the establishment of a prognosis.

Acknowledgment. This work was supported by the Deutsche Forschungsgemeinschaft, Grant no. 6481/2.

References

Auböck L (1975) Zur Ultrastruktur fibröser und histiocytärer Hauttumoren (Dermatofibroma, Dermatofibrosarcoma protuberans, Fibroxanthom and Histiocytom). Virchows Archiv [A] 368:253–274

Bouropoulou V, Kontogeorgos G, Papamichales G, Bosse A, Roessner A, Vollmer E (1987) Differential diagnosis of chordoma. Immunohistochemical aspects. Arch Anat Cytol Pathol 35:35–40

Dahlin DC, Unni KK (1986) Bone tumors. General aspects and data on 8542 cases, 3rd edn. Charles C. Thomas, Springfield

Dahlin DC, Cupps RE, Johnson EW Jr (1970) Giant cell tumors: a study of 195 cases. Cancer 25:1061–1070

Dahlin DC, Unni KK (1977) Osteosarcoma of bone and its important recognizable varieties. Am J Surg Pathol 1:61–72

Dominok GW, Knoch HG (1982) Knochengeschwülste und geschwulstähnliche Knochenerkrankungen, 3rd edn. VEB Gustav Fischer, Jena

Gerdes J (1985) An immunohistological method for estimating cell growth fractions in rapid histopathological diagnosis during surgery. Int J Cancer 35:169–171

Gerdes J, Schwab U, Lembke H, Stein H (1983) Production of a mouse monoclonal antibody reactive with a human nuclear antigen associated with cell proliferation. Int J Cancer 31:13–20

Gerdes J, Lembke H, Baisch H, Wacker HH, Schwab U, Stein H (1984) Cell cycle analysis of a cell proliferation-associated human nuclear antigen defined by the monoclonal antibody Ki-67. J Immunol 133:1710–1715

Gerdes J, Pileri S, Bartels H, Stein H (1986) Proliferation marker Ki-67: correlation with histological diagnosis, histological tumor grading, and prognosis. Verh Dtsch Ges Pathol 70:152–158

Grundmann E (ed) (1976) Malignant bone tumors. Springer, Berlin Heidelberg New York (Rec Res Cancer Res, vol 54)

Grundmann E, Mellin W, Roessner A, Bösing Th, Hiddemann W, Vollmer E, Edel G, Lingg G (1986) Zur Klassification und Prognose der Osteosarkome im Erfahrungsgut des Knochengeschwulstregisters Westfalen unter Einbezug proliferationskinetischer Parameter. In: Dietsch P, Keck E, Kruse HP, Kuhlencordt F (eds) Aktuelle Ergebnisse der Osteologie. W. de Gruyter, Berlin, pp 221–226

Heliö H, Karaharju E, Nordling S (1985) Flow cytometric determination of DNA content in malignant and benign bone tumors. Cytometry 6:165–171

Huvos AG (1979) Bone tumors: diagnosis, treatment and prognosis. W.S. Saunders, Philadelphia

Jaffé HL, Lichtenstein L, Portis RB (1940) Giant cell tumor of bone. Its pathologic appearance, grading, supposed variants and treatment. Arch Pathol. 30:993–1031

Jaffé HL (1958) Tumors and tumorous conditions of the bones and joints. Lea & Febiger, Philadelphia

Kertelge E, Roessner A, Vollmer E, Winterberg B, Tenschert W, Vetter H, Hauss J, Buchholz B (1987) Immunohistological evaluation of 36 pheochromocytomas with regard to proteohormone secretion and proliferation. Arch Anat Cytol Pathol 35:155–161

Kreicbergs A, Tribukat B (1984) Flow DNA analysis of primary bone tumors. Relationship between cellular DNA content and histopathologic classification. Cancer 53:129–136

Lichtenstein L (1977) Bone tumors, 4th edn. C.V. Mosby, St. Louis

Matsuno T, Unni KK, McLeod RA, Dahlin DC (1976) Telangiectatic osteogenic sarcoma. Cancer 38:2538–2547

Miettinen M, Letho CP, Virtanen I (1983) Differential diagnosis of chordoma, chondroid, and ependymal tumors as aided by anti-intermediate filament antibody. Am J Pathol 112:160–169

Roessner A (1984) Zur Zyto- und Histogenese der malignen und semimalignen Knochentumoren. Veröffentlichungen aus der Pathologie, H. 122. Gustav Fischer, Stuttgart

Roessner A, Hobik HP, Grundmann E (1979) Malignant fibrous histiocytoma of bone and osteosarcoma. A comparative light and electron microscopy study. Path. Res. Pract. 164:385–401

Roessner A, Immenkamp M, Weidner A, Hobik HP, Grundmann E (1981) Benign fibrous histiocytoma of bone. Light and electron microscopic observation. J Cancer Res Clin Oncol 101:191–202

Roessner A, Mellin W, Hiddemann W, Voss B, Vollmer E, Grundmann E (1984a) New cytomorphologic methods in the diagnosis of bone tumors: possibilities and limitations. Semin Diagn Pathol 1/3:199–214

Roessner A, v. Bassewitz DB, Schlake W, Thorwesten G, Grundmann E (1984b) Biological characterization of human bone tumors. III. Giant cell tumor of bone. Pathol Res Pract 178:431–440

Roessner A, Vollmer E, Sorg C, Grundmann E (1986) Die Rolle der Makrophagen und osteoklastenähnlichen Riesenzellen in Knochentumoren. In: Dietsch P, Keck E, Kruse HP, Kuhlencordt F (eds) Aktuelle Ergebnisse der Osteologie. W. de Gruyter, Berlin, pp 227–232

Roessner A, Vassallo J, Vollmer E, Zwadlo G, Sorg C, Grundmann E (1987) Biological characterization of human bone tumors. X. The proliferation behavior of macrophages as compared to fibroblastic cells in malignant fibrous histiocytoma and giant cell tumor of bone. J Cancer Res Clin Oncol 113:559–562

Rosen G, Caparros B, Huvos AG, Kosloff C, Nierenberg A, Cacavio A, Marcove RC, Labe JM, Metha B, Urban C (1982) Preoperative chemotherapy for osteogenic sarcoma: selection of postoperative adjuvant chemotherapy based on the response of the primary tumor to preoperative chemotherapy. Cancer 49:1221–1230

Schajowicz F (1981) Tumors and tumorlike lesions of the bones and joints. Springer, New York

Schajowicz F, Ackerman LV, Sissons HA, Sobin LH, Torloni H (1972) Histological typing of bone tumours. International Classification of Tumours, vol 6. WHO, Geneva

Spanier SS (1977) Malignant fibrous histiocytoma of bone. Orthop Clin North Am 8:947–961

Spjut HJ, Dorfman HD, Fechner RE, Ackerman LV (1971) Tumors of Bone and Cartilage. AF Atlas of Tumor Pathology II/5 AF Inst of Pathology, Washington/DC

Unni KK, Dahlin DC (1984) Grading of bone tumors. Semin Diagn Pathol 1/3:165–172

Unni KK, Dahlin DC, McLeod RA, Pritchard DJ (1977) Intraosseous well-differentiated osteosarcoma. Cancer 40:1337–1347

Vollmer E, Bouropoulou V, Roessner A, Erwig H, Grundmann E (1985) Immunohistologische und elektronenmikroskopische Untersuchungen an Chordomen. Verh Dtsch Ges Pathol 69:633+

Vollmer E, Roessner A, Lipecki KH, Zwadlo G, Hagemeier HH, Grundmann E (1987) Biologic characterization of human bone tumors. VI. The aneurysmal bone cyst: an enzyme histochemical, electron microscopical, and immunohistological study. Virchows Archiv [Cell Pathol] 53:58–65

Weibel ER, Elias H (1967) Quantitative methods in morphology. Springer, Berlin Heidelberg New York

Flow Cytometric DNA Analysis of Bone Tumors

W. MELLIN, W. DIERSCHAUER, W. HIDDEMANN, A. ROESSNER, G. EDEL, P. WUISMAN, A. HÄRLE, and E. GRUNDMANN

1 Introduction . . . 115
2 DNA Ploidy, Proliferation, and Therapy . . . 116
3 Flow Cytometry, Possibilities, and Special Problems in Bone Tumors . . . 119
4 Bone-Forming Tumors . . . 122
4.1 Osteoblastoma . . . 122
4.2 Osteosarcoma . . . 123
4.3 Conclusion . . . 131
5 Cartilage-Forming Tumors . . . 133
5.1 Chondroma . . . 133
5.2 Chondrosarcoma . . . 133
5.3 Conclusion . . . 134
6 Giant Cell Tumor of Bone . . . 135
7 Malignant Fibrous Histiocytoma . . . 138
8 Fibrosarcoma . . . 139
9 Chordoma . . . 140
10 Ewing's Sarcoma . . . 141
11 Malignant Lymphomas of Bone . . . 143
12 Summary . . . 145
References . . . 148

1 Introduction

It is the foremost objective of every tumor classification to help to determine prognosis. The definition of morphological categories is the generally accepted principle of all current classifications. In bone tumor pathology, the spectrum of morphological criteria has been enlarged by roentgenological features; nevertheless, their classification is often more difficult than that of carcinomatous neoplasms (SCHAJOWICZ et al. 1972; SCHAJOWICZ 1981). This is due not only to the great morphological heterogeneity of bone tumors but also to the close topographical relationship between tumor tissue and the often very similar mesenchymal changes of inflammatory, reactive, or strongly proliferative nature. A major feature is the presence of multinucleated, histiocytic giant cells in bone tumors. Though varying in intensity, the occurrence of giant cells is a typical trait. Differential diagnostic problems are encountered, especially in the morphological distinction of purely reactive alterations from well-differentiated but potentially malignant neoplasms (e.g., parosteal osteosarcoma), and of benign from malignant tumorous lesions (e.g., benign and malignant giant cell tumors).

In addition to purely morphological classification, the evaluation of tumors comprises a growing spectrum of functional properties, including biochemistry, which can be demonstrated by histochemical and immunohistological methods and correlated with the underlying morphological pattern. Examples may be found in enzyme histochemistry and immunohistological demonstration of enzymes, cellular hormone receptors, and other antigenic structures (e.g., cytoskeleton) of significance as tumor markers. Most of these markers give pointers to the histogenetic origin and grade of differentiation of the tumor cells. In bone tumors, however, these tissue markers are less useful. However, the immunohistological demonstration of a proliferation-associated nuclear antigen by means of the monoclonal antibody Ki-67 permits the prognostic evaluation of proliferation patterns within individual bone tumors (VOLLMER et al. 1986).

Further clues to tumor kinetics are provided by DNA cytometry: apart from an estimate of proliferative activity, it can determine DNA ploidy which, in opposition to most other tissue parameters, cannot be estimated even by an experienced pathologist. DNA aneuploidy is known to be a highly specific marker of malignancy, whereas DNA diploid tumors may be either benign or malignant. Thus, the assessment of DNA ploidy provides an additional variable used for estimating the prospective behavior of bone tumors, especially in cases where morphological classification is difficult.

2 DNA Ploidy, Proliferation, and Therapy

In contrast to chromosomal analysis and counting, the assessment of DNA ploidy by cytophotometry consists simply of quantitation of nuclear DNA. The scale for DNA ploidy measuring is the DNA index (DI), set as 1 for the (diploid) $G_{0/1}$ cells in normal lymphocytes as a standard reference (Fig. 1). By definition, a DI of 1 signals diploidy in nonneoplastic tissue or cells. This DI value, however, is observed in benign tumors and a small proportion of malignant neoplasms (10%–30%) where the numerical and structural changes of DNA are reflected in only minimal or nonmeasurable quantitative shifts of DNA. In such cases we speak of DNA diploid, peridiploid, or pseudodiploid neoplasms. Chromosomal abnormalities are, as a rule, less frequent in benign tumors than in malignant, DNA pseudodiploid tumors. Although DNA diploidy as such does not permit a clear verdict on the tumor's biological behavior, overt DNA aneuploidy can be interpreted as a very specific sign of malignancy, according to current experience. Accordingly, the DNA aneuploidies observed so far in melanocytic nevi, dysplastic epithelial lesions of the uterine cervix, the stomach, and the colon, are interpreted as early stages of malignant lesions (STENZINGER et al. 1984; PFITZER 1985; MACARTNEY and CAMPLEJOHN 1986; HAMMARBERG et al. 1984). DNA aneuploidy is attributed, by definition, only to those stemlines that possess neither diploid nor polyploid DIs. These are, as a rule, hyperdiploid, triploid, hypotetraploid, and hypertetraploid DNA values, and DIs below 1 are quite rare. DNA tetraploidy or polyploidy is more

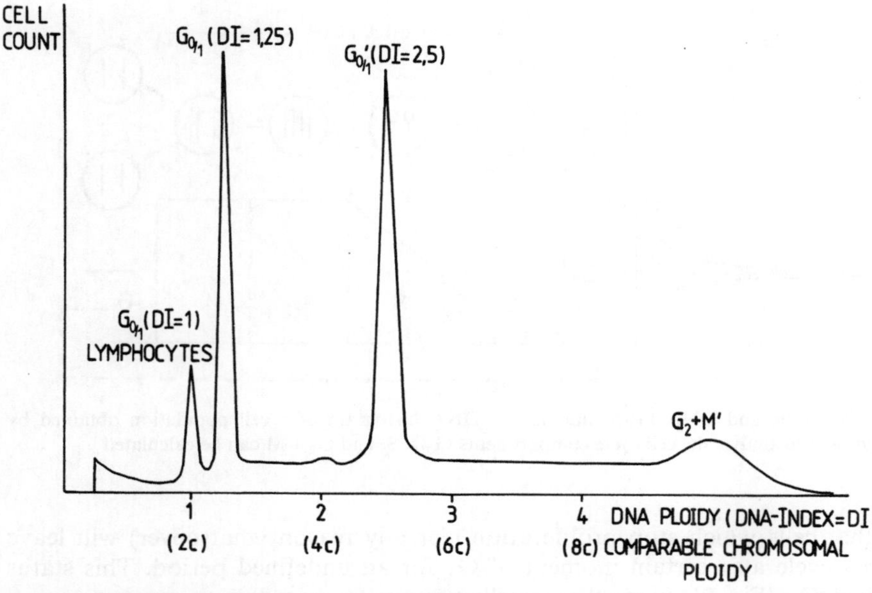

Fig. 1. DNA histogram of a tumor with a DNA diploid $G_{0/1}$ peak of the reactive infiltrate (lymphocytes, DNA index = 1.0) and two aneuploid stemlines (DIs = 1.25 and 2.5)

often associated with malignancy, but may also occur in benign lesions of various organs, where it is mostly associated with enhanced cellular function.

As in DNA pseudodiploid tumors, a certain aneuploid or polyploid DI may reflect a wide variation of structural (oncogenic) or numerical alterations. Except for a few types with characteristic chromosomal aberrations, their prognostic significance is still unknown. Moreover, clear demonstration of chromosomal features in solid tumors is achieved in only 10%–20% of cases (SANDBERG 1980). However, ATKIN et al. (1966) had already shown that the cytometric assessment of DNA content, of what might be called the quasi overall genetic information in tumor cells, is of higher prognostic relevance than variation in the number of chromosomes.

Seen against a background of increasingly differentiated and custom-tailored therapy protocols in oncology, the proliferation kinetics of tumors have also attracted a growing interest. These rates can be largely defined by the distribution of cell cycle phases from flow cytometric DNA measurements.

Within the whole generative cycle of a cell, mitosis occupies a short time. For the major period the cell stays in the interphase, growing in size and doubling its DNA. The four main phases of the cycle are called G_1, S, G_2, and M (mitosis). G_1-phase designates the period between the end of mitosis and the start of DNA synthesis, which occurs exclusively during the S-phase. G_2 then designates the period between the end of DNA replication and the beginning of mitosis. While the periods passed in the S-, G_2-, and M-phases are rather constant for most tissues, the duration of the G_1-phase may vary considerably depending on the varying physiological conditions. This is due to the

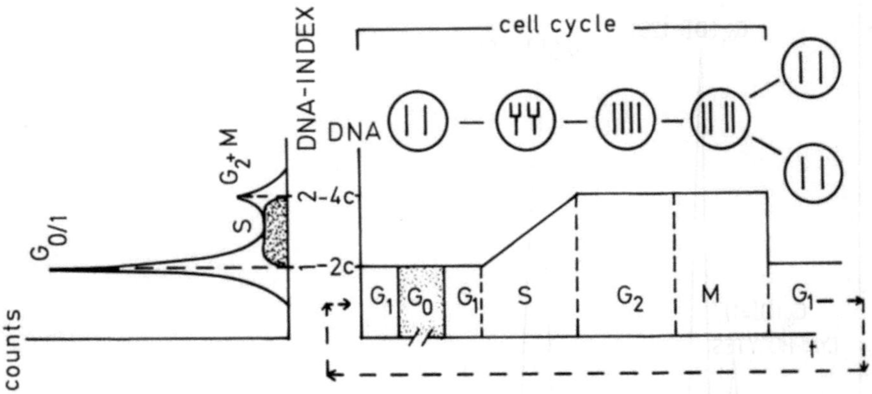

Fig. 2. Cell cycle and DNA histogram: in the DNA histogram of a cell population obtained by flow cytometric analyis the cell cycle compartments $G_{0/1}$, S, and G_2+M can be calculated

fact that cells which stop proliferation (for any reason whatsoever) will leave the cell cycle at a certain moment of G_1 for an undefined period. This status is called G_0 (Fig. 2). Since tumor cells are apt to react less to many external, growth-checking factors than are normal cell populations, they may be expected to possess a much lower portion of G_0 cells.

From DNA histograms obtained by flow cytometry, the distribution of tumor cells in three compartments can be calculated with appreciable accuracy and their percent proportions correlate with the relative duration of the tumor cells in corresponding phases (Fig. 2). Detailed data can be given for the $G_{0/1}$, S, and G_2+M compartments. The S-phase values obtained by flow cytometry correlate well with ^{3}H-thymidine labeling indices obtained by autoradiography in the same tissue, and represent a somewhat gross estimate of its proliferative activity (COSTA et al. 1981). Thus, a high proportion of cells in S-phase will generally reflect a higher proliferation rate, which means rapid and probably malignant growth. The actual growth intensity of a tumor will depend additionally on the overall length of the cell cycle (undefinable by simple DNA flow cytometry) and the cell turnover, i.e., the ratio of cellular replication and cell death.

That malignant neoplasms possess, as a rule, a higher proportion of cells in replication than the corresponding matrix tissue is the basis of radiotherapeutic and most cytostatic tumor therapies. For radiotherapy, the end of the G_1 and the G_2+M phases were found particularly sensitive, with peak sensitivity during mitosis proper (FRINDEL and TUBIANA 1971). The lowest radiosensitivity was found during the S-phase, possibly due to increased enzyme activity and corresponding activation of repair mechanisms in that period.

The effect of different cytostatics on cell cycle phases depends largely on the particular mechanism of action of each drug, and so varies considerably. Exact information about the time course of the cell cycle as well as on the mechanism of action of the drug allows for programming the cytostatic effect in vitro (KRISHAN et al. 1976). Optimal results are obtained only if all tumor cells have entered the cycle, and so it is necessary to accumulate them in a certain phase by synchronization (FRANKE 1972; KRISHAN 1975). This is possible by transitory blocking of tumor cells in a certain phase of the cycle. Defining the (relative) duration of the individual phases with the greatest possible accuracy is another precondition for effective therapy (KRISHAN et al. 1976). In addition to autoradiography and the definition of mitotic indices, this can also be achieved by flow cytometry, which is a most useful tool for the exact analysis of the cell cycle (KRUG 1977). Several methods for synchronization (thermic, mechanical, chemical, irradiation) will mostly achieve a partial effect, mainly because part of the cells is in G_0, and another part blocked in G_2 (GELFANT 1977; DARZYNKIEWICZ 1979). These cells escape synchronization, and are thus less sensitive to cytostatic drugs. Optimal therapeutic results require the combination of several cytostatics with one another, or with radiotherapy.

3 Flow Cytometry, Possibilities, and Special Problems in Bone Tumors

Cytophotometry is a method to assess the relative proportion of certain substances present in cells. Such quantitation is based on the specific and stoichiometrical staining of those substances by certain dyes. While microscope cytophotometry makes use of the proportional relation between extinction (absorption photometry) or intensity of fluorescence (fluorescence photometry) and the amount of measurable substances in the tissue, flow cytometry is best done with fluorescence labeling, which is a more exact method. The absolute prerequisite of all cytometry is a most careful standardization of cell and tissue preparations, staining procedures, and measurements. Only the strictest accuracy in this respect will ensure the comparability of results from different measurements.

The development of a "flow-through cytometer" (DITTRICH and GÖHDE 1969; VAN DILLA et al. 1969) was a true milestone for cytometric techniques. The apparatus allows fluorescence cytometric measurements of cells from a single cell suspension directed through a chamber. On account of the very high rate of flow through (up to 1000 cells per second) the instrument yields histograms with much higher resolution within a few minutes (as a rule, 10000–100000 cells measured) than can be obtained by microscope cytometry (usually 50–300 cells) (BARLOGIE et al. 1983). Thus, it becomes possible to identify even small percentages of DNA-aneuploid tumor cell populations in a given tissue (as low as 2% per sample). The standard reference material for diploid cells in fresh or ethanol-fixed material are normal leukocyte or lymphocyte samples. Beyond the definition of DNA ploidy, flow cytometry (in contrast to microscope cytometry) allows for a statistically reliable analysis of the cell cycle distribution of the tumor cells. Using modern flow cytometers, simultaneous measurements of more than one fluorescence variable are possible (MELLIN et al. 1986a).

The only drawback of flow cytometry is that the value measured for an individual cell cannot be directly correlated with its microscopic picture. In most tumor investigations, however, this fact is irrelevant because cytological or histological evaluation of the tissue is also possible on slides for microscopy, provided the sample is of sufficient size and homogeneity. This is rarely possible in small circumscribed lesions, such as those usually found in precancerous tissue. In such cases microscope cytometry is certainly preferable (MELLIN 1986).

Freshly excised specimens, shock-frozen tissue, and, with qualifications, cells and tissue subjected to various fixation methods and embedded in paraffin are all suitable for cytophotometric investigation. The quality of results will depend mainly on the resistance of the measured substance or antigen structure to the respective preparation procedures. Flow cytometry of antigenic structures of particular sensitivity and low density should be performed only on freshly excised material.

DNA cytophotometry is usually effected on specimens fixed in ethanol or methanol, since the stoichiometric reaction of DNA to diverse specific fluorescence stains is not impaired when compared with fresh material, and the preparations can be investigated years later. Prolonged fixation in unbuffered formol, in contrast, implies increasing and irregular loss of DNA, and even relative quantitation becomes inaccurate. However, HEDLEY et al. (1983, 1985) have shown that flow cytometric analysis of formol-fixed and paraffin-embedded tumor tissue will yield quite satisfactory and reproducible results in a direct comparison with corresponding ethanol-fixed samples (cf. SCHUTTE et al. 1985). The areas suitable for DNA analysis can be selected from the histological slide, which permits a better correlation of histological picture and DNA histogram than would be possible from unfixed or ethanol-fixed tissue. The section taken from the paraffin block is deparaffinized in xylol, rehydrated in graded ethanols, and then prepared in the same way as ethanol-fixed samples.

Optimal preparation of single cell suspensions is achieved by combining enzymatic digestion (0.5% pepsin solution at pH 2) and mechanical mincing, which yields single cells and also naked nuclei. DNA staining is selective using specific fluochromes [such as propidium iodide and 4′-6-diamidino-2-phenylindole (DAPI)]; additional staining of double-stranded RNA can be eliminated by pretreatment with RNAse.

The quality of DNA histograms taken from paraffin-embedded material, like in those from ethanol-fixed tissue, depends principally on the preservation of cell nuclei. During the embedding procedure, the temperature of paraffin certainly plays a decisive role for the preservation and stoichiometric behavior of DNA. If the histological reference slide (H & E stained) shows a marked reduction of nuclear staining, cytophotometric DNA analysis will no longer be possible in the vast majority of cases. Even when nuclear staining is histologically adequate, the quality of DNA histograms is apt to vary considerably.

The flow cytometric DNA analysis of bone tumors is often hampered by the problems of preparing single cell suspensions, especially the collection of sufficient cells. In chondromatous tumors, we found that collecting an adequate amount of well-preserved tumor cells is possible in only a few cases. Histologically, cell density is low, and the majority of cells show regressive changes, and so histology-guided microscope cytometry occasionally may be preferable to flow cytometry for these tumors. In the other types of bone tumors the selection of softer areas for investigation is recommended since they will often show higher cellularity than the more compact osseous structures. Particular difficulties are encountered in well-differentiated osteosarcomas, mostly of the parosteal type, often poorly cellular and rich in bone substance. In such cases we need abundant tumor material that has to be minced and treated with enzyme. In these cases, too, microscope cytometry may sometimes offer a favorable alternative. The use of decalcifying agents induces a loss of measurable nuclear DNA, and so only a few nondecalcified specimens can be suitably worked up for flow cytometry.

In view of these technical problems of cell collection and inadequate tissue pretreatment, flow cytometric DNA analyses of bone tumors are more liable than those of other tumors to yield DNA histograms with less good resolution. The coefficient of variation (CV) of diploid $G_{0/1}$ peaks (=full curve width at half maximum of the peak in channels $\times$ 100/2.35 $\times$ peak channel) is often higher than 5% in such cases, a maximum proposed by many authors. This does not mean, however, that every DNA histogram with a CV above 5% provides unreliable data on DNA ploidy. According to our own experience, clearly DNA aneuploid stemlines with their respective G_2+M peaks can be distinctly separated from the diploid and tetraploid peaks even when the CV is more than 20%. In such cases, the resolution of DNA histograms is often comparable to that achieved in microscope cytometry. Difficulties may be greater when the tumor stemlines are situated near the diploid and tetraploid DNA peaks. We have to be aware that among what is called DNA diploid tumor stemlines, only a few will have an exactly diploid DNA content. Rather, the quantitative deviation of DNA from diploid standard is not yet recognizable even in histograms with a very good resolution. However, a more sophisticated resolution of DNA histograms would enable us to verify the differences between the cell types of normal tissue which are manifested not only in staining variations due to different cellular environment, but especially in the different sizes and structures of nuclei and their functional status (euchromatin, heterochromatin). The very fact that the DNA histogram of a normal lymph node will always have a lower CV than the histogram of gastric mucosa similarly prepared may serve as a convincing example. Consequently, the DNA diploidy of tumor cells must be interpreted as a minor, not clearly discernible deviation of DNA content from normal diploidy. The differentiation between DNA diploidy and DNA aneuploidy must therefore try to identify and distinguish minor from more marked deviations in the DNA content of tumor cells. When we analyze a histogram, the borderline between these two depends largely on the degree of resolution: when the latter was adequate, DNA hyperdiploid stemlines have been distinguished with DIs of less than 1.05 (BÜCHNER et al. 1985).

Reliable comparability of results, however, needs a standardized borderline between DNA diploidy and DNA aneuploidy as well as between DNA polyploidy and DNA aneuploidy, to be accepted and respected in every measurement. In the results of flow cytometric DNA analysis presented in the following sections, deviations of DNA in tumor stemlines from the diploid reference values or from the respective polyploid values were defined as DNA (peri)diploid or (peri)polyploid if below 10%. Deviations of 10% and more were defined as DNA aneuploidy. Unimodal diploid stemlines with a CV up to 10%, and without any recognizable shoulder on the $G_{0/1}$ peak, were called diploid, while diploid tumors with a CV between 10% and 15%, and without a shoulder or definable aneuploid stemline, were called DNA "peri" diploid. Questionable peridiploid tumors with a CV over 15 were not evaluated. Evidence of DNA tetraploidy was taken as confirmed by the presence of a definite G_2+M peak. Since an external standard (reference lymphocytes) cannot be applied to paraffin material on account of differing staining capacities, we selected from the histological block sections that would contain not only tumor cells but also some lymphocytes and other mesenchymal cells, providing a kind of internal standard. Estimating the percent proportions of tumor cells and the reactive infiltrate on the histological slide, and comparison with the histogram, enabled us to identify the diploid peak with sufficient security.

Truly correct cell cycle analysis will be possible only in histograms with a CV up to 5%. In the present study on bone tumors, however, cell cycle analysis has been performed on histograms with a CV up to 10% which, comparing only data with similar CV values, permitted an adequate differentiation of tumors with low proliferation from those with moderate or high proliferation rates. Cell cycle analyses of nonoverlapping populations were made with a computer program based on the mathematical model developed by Dean and Jett (1974). We have to remember that bone tumors usually have significant inflammatory infiltrates and numbers of other reactive mesenchymal cells, which often lead to severe overlapping between tumor cells and reactive mesenchymal cells in their cell cycle distributions. Cell cycle analyses of DNA aneuploid populations were based, as far as possible, on the procedure reported by Baisch et al. (1975).

4 Bone-Forming Tumors

4.1 Osteoblastoma

Osteoblastomas are rare, mostly benign tumors arising preferentially in the spine, and affecting mostly males in the second or third decade. There is a considerable histological likeness to the nidus tissue of osteoid osteomas which, however, are much smaller (up to 1.5 cm) and have a distinctly sclerotic rim. Occasionally, spontaneous tumor regression or cessation of growth has been observed after incomplete removal of the tumor, and has been interpreted as a sign of nonmalignancy. However, there are a few lesions wherein the differential diagnosis between osteoblastoma and certain types of osteosarcoma is particularly difficult. These include:

1. Harmless appearing osteosarcomas of low malignancy in which better differentiated areas may resemble osteoblastoma (Bertoni et al. 1985)
2. Osteoblastomas with degenerative changes and corresponding pseudomalignant pictures
3. Primary conventional osteoblastoma with malignant transformation to osteosarcoma
4. So-called aggressive osteoblastomas (Dorfman 1972) which, according to Dorfman and Weiss (1984), show only locally aggressive growth without metastatic spread.

The nine osteoblastomas in our study, documented in the Bone Tumor Registry of Westphalia, showed no significant deviations in terms of age, sex, and localization. Histologically, they were classified as conventional, obviously nonsuspicious osteoblastomas in seven cases, and as aggressive osteoblastomas in the other two (Fig. 3a, b).

Flow cytometry revealed DNA aneuploidies in three of nine cases. In two DNA aneuploid conventional osteoblastomas the DNA indices were 1.6 and 2.2, but their histological pictures did not differ from those of diploid conventional osteoblastomas (Fig. 3c, d). Of the two aggressive osteoblastomas, one was DNA diploid, the other DNA tetraploid. Cell cycle analysis was possible only in the six DNA diploid tumors: their S-phases ranged from 6.4% to 16.5%, with a mean value of 10.9%. The S-phase of the one diploid aggressive osteoblastoma was also on that medium level (10.3%).

The clinical course was favorable in eight of nine cases. In the case of tetraploid aggressive osteoblastoma, surgery for recurrent tumor was necessary 5 months later, but complete removal was no longer possible. The patient's death was caused by the sequelae of local recurrence, but there was no evidence of metastases. Another recurrence was recorded in one of the DNA diploid conventional osteoblastomas. After successful surgery, performed 7 years ago, this patient remained tumor free (MELLIN et al. 1987a).

4.2 Osteosarcoma

Osteosarcomas (OSs), characterized by a varying production of tumor osteoid and/or bone, arise in at least 90% of cases within the medullary spaces and are hence termed central or medullary OSs. From these have to be separated the juxtacortical OSs, which, in turn, can be subdivided in classical parosteal OSs, periosteal OSs, and highly malignant superficial OSs (MELLIN et al. 1986b). Another extremely rare subtype is the extraskeletal OS.

Medullary OSs are highly malignant, as a rule. The occurrence of central OS of low malignancy is very rare (UNNI et al. 1977). Medullary OSs, which arise preferentially from the long tubular bones, are histologically differentiated into five types: predominantly osteoblastic, chondroblastic, fibroblastic, anaplastic, and telangiectatic. The prognostic relevance of these histological subtypes is rather low (DAHLIN and UNNI 1986). The increasing application of adjuvant chemotherapy in these cases (WINKLER et al. 1983, 1984) may in future enhance the prognostic relevance of the kinetic patterns in these tumors.

The flow cytometric DNA analyses presented in this study have been performed on 21 primary medullary OSs undergoing surgery in the Orthopedic Clinic of Münster University; from each case, either biopsy material or tissue from resection or amputation was at our disposal. All specimens had been taken before any potential radio- or chemotherapy. Histologically, all tumors were classified as highly malignant OSs, that is: six anaplastic, eight osteoblastic, one chondroblastic, three fibroblastic, and three telangiectatic. Nine OSs were divided into several samples (2–16, average 4) for separate investigation in order to assess the distribution and frequency of heterogeneous subpopulations in

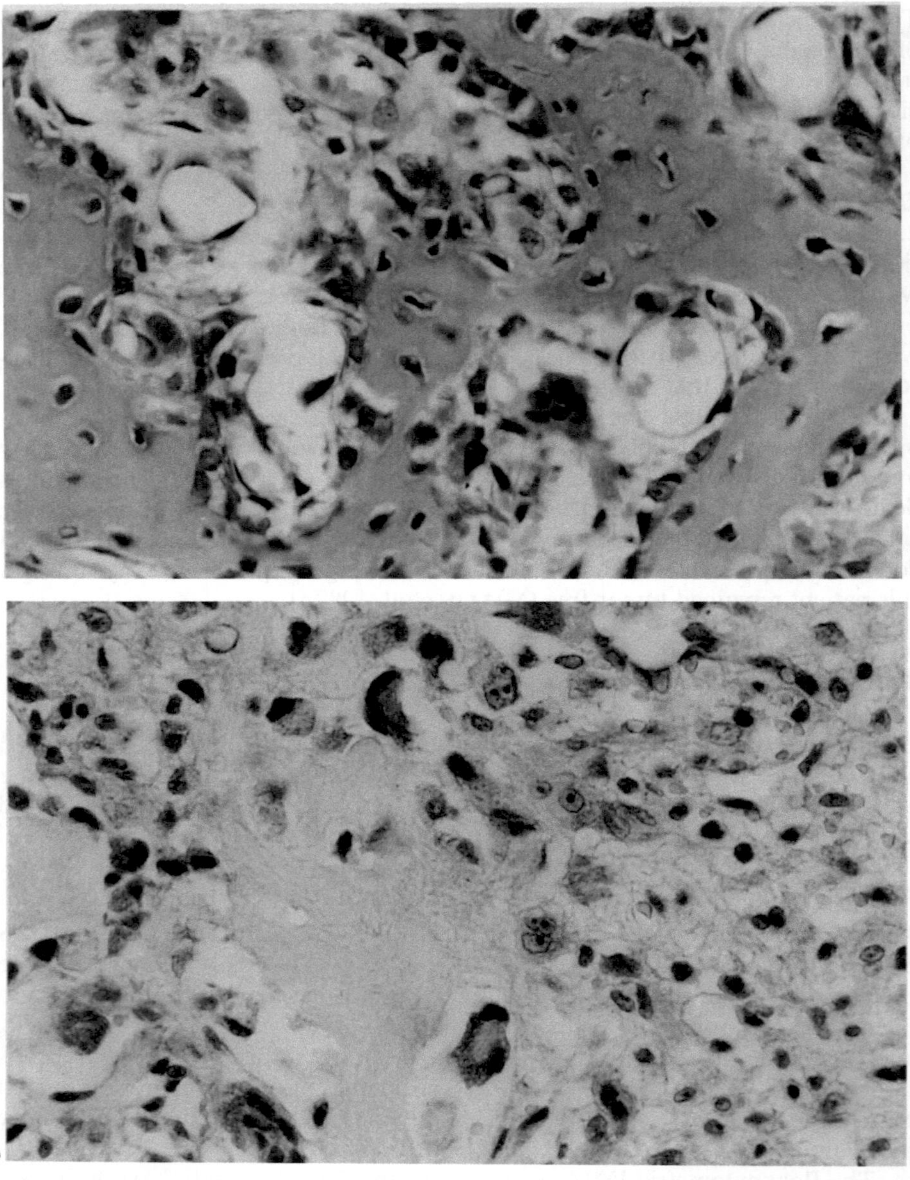

a

b

Fig. 3. **a** Typical histological picture of a conventional osteoblastoma. Bland osteoblasts and osteoclasts form a rim around sharply delineated osteoid trabeculae. Intertrabecular tissue is loose and highly vascular. (H & E, ×435). **b** Aggressive osteoblastoma with enlarged and rounded epithelioid

different areas of the same tumor. For flow cytometric DNA analysis the shock-frozen samples were fixed in 96% ethanol and prepared in routine fashion.

Evidence of DNA aneuploidies was found in 18 of these 21 OSs (86%), with a rather even, noncharacteristic distribution of DNA aneuploidies among

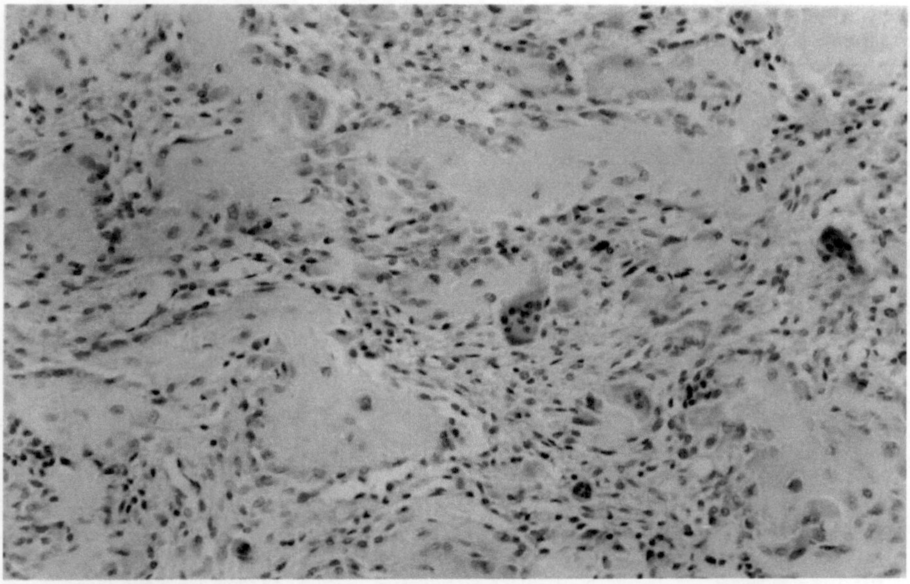

c

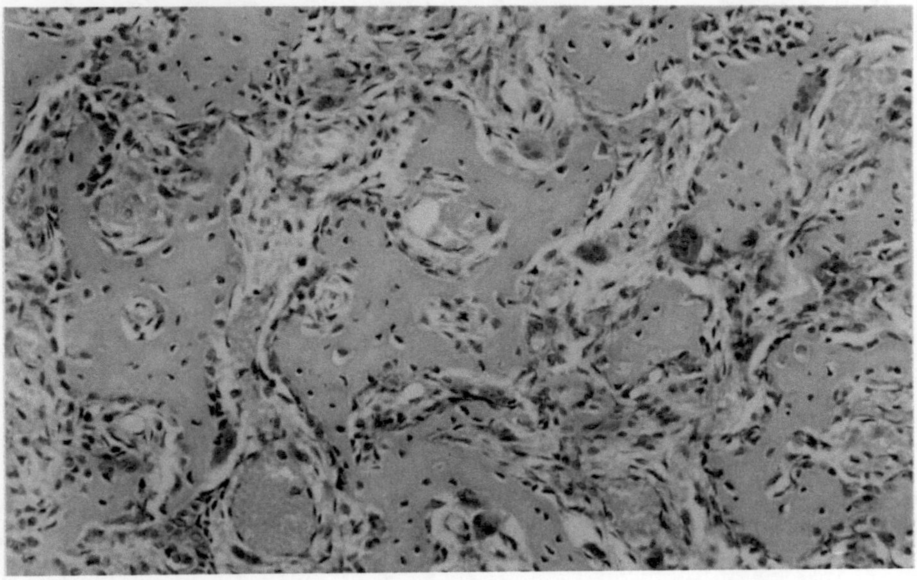

d

osteoblasts which partly show prominent nucleoli (H & E, ×435). **c**, **d** Conventional DNA diploid (**c**) and aneuploid (**d**) osteoblastoma with unsuspicious histiological features in each case (H & E, ×170)

histological subtypes (Table 1). Seven tumors showed only one DNA aneuploid tumor line; in 11 other tumors there was more than one, and in one case even five aneuploid tumor cell populations. Among the total count of 37 aneuploid lines we included two DNA tetraploid stemlines. The DNA indices of

Table 1. Histological subtypes, frequency of DNA aneuploidy and multiple DNA stemlines, percentage of S-phase cells, and DIs in 21 OSs

Highly malignant OS	*n*	DNA aneuploidy	Multiple aneuploid DNA stemlines	% S-phase mean	DI median
Anaplastic OS	6	5	3	23.4	1.66
Osteoblastic OS	8	8	5	17.2	1.74
Chondroblastic OS	1	–	–	6.4	–
Fibroblastic OS	3	3	1	25.6	2.0
Telangiectatic	3	2	1	6.2	1.60

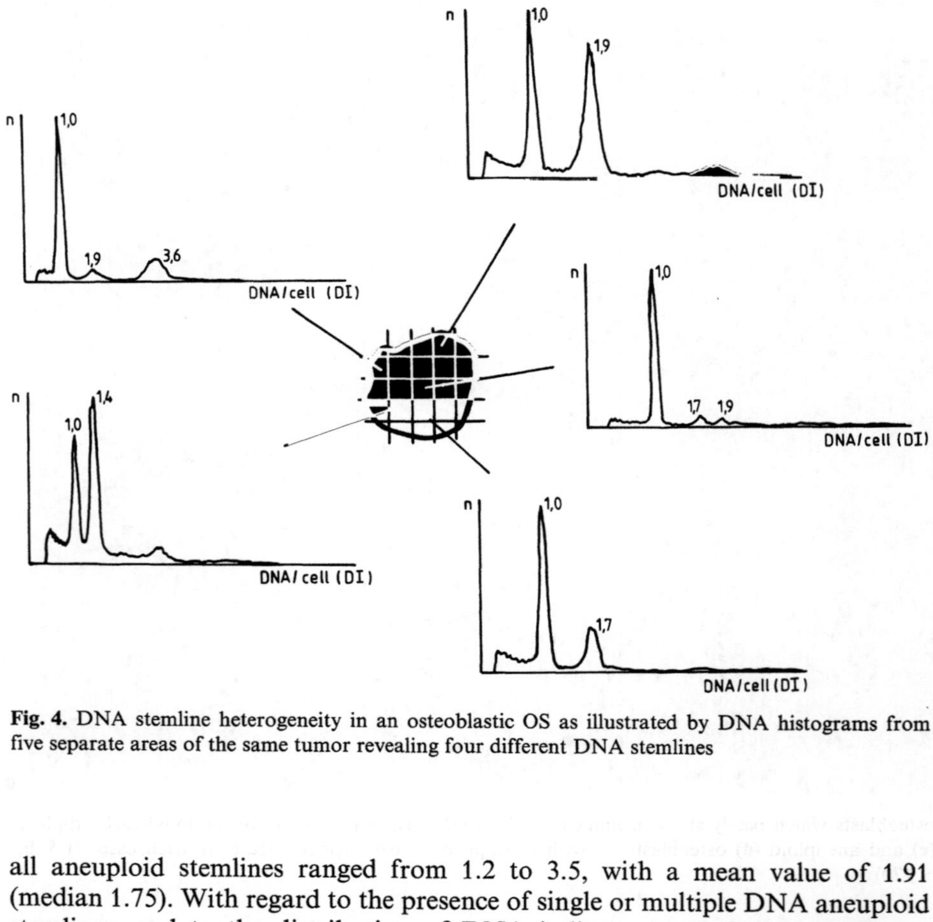

Fig. 4. DNA stemline heterogeneity in an osteoblastic OS as illustrated by DNA histograms from five separate areas of the same tumor revealing four different DNA stemlines

all aneuploid stemlines ranged from 1.2 to 3.5, with a mean value of 1.91 (median 1.75). With regard to the presence of single or multiple DNA aneuploid stemlines, and to the distribution of DNA indices, no particular differences could be ascertained between the histological subtypes of highly malignant (central OS (Table 1). The pattern of stemlines varied considerably from one sample to the other within the same tumor (Table 2, Fig. 4). However, individual DNA stemlines could be reidentified in several areas of one tumor.

Table 2. Distribution of different DNA aneuploidies in 16 separate samples from one highly malignant OS

Sample no.	Tumor DNA indices		
	DI I	DI II	DI III
1	1.40	2.82	
2	1.44	2.84	
3	1.39		
4	1.39		
5	1.39		
6	1.43		
7	1.39		
8	1.36		
9	1.38		
10	1.40		2.34
11	1.39		2.35
12	1.38		
13	1.40		
14			
15			2.37
16			2.42

Cell cycle analysis of individual tumor cell populations was possible in 19 cases. Their S-phase proportion ranged from 6.2% to 38.1%, with a mean value of 18.8%. DNA aneuploid tumor stemlines had higher S-phase percentages (mean 20.6%) than diploid stemlines (12.4%). No characteristic differences, however, could be verified statistically among histological subtypes (HIDDEMANN et al. 1987).

Correlation with clinical courses shows that 9 of 18 patients with DNA aneuploid tumors have died in the meantime, most of them with extensive pulmonary metastases. Three patients with DNA diploid tumors are still living; one of them had to be operated on for recurrence, another for a bone metastasis.

Osteosarcoma After Chemotherapy. Modern therapy protocols involve preoperative chemotherapy of OS, with the objective of reducing tumor mass and preventing metastasis. If there is clear evidence of metastases, palliative chemotherapy follows, as a rule. Initially, chemotherapy is usually partly successful (WINKLER et al. 1983) and this is documented histologically as gradual tumor regression (SALZER-KUNTSCHIK et al. 1983a, b). The distinction of "good responders" from "poor responders" based on histological evidence of tumor regression is also of prognostic significance (WINKLER et al. 1984). With regard to long-term response and cure, however, safe evaluation is still not possible (DAHLIN and UNNI 1986).

The impact of chemotherapy on DNA ploidy and proliferation rates in OSs has not been studied by flow cytometry. Our own investigations were performed on ethanol-fixed material from 20 patients who had been entered in the COSS 80/82 trial, and received preoperative high-dose polychemotherapy (HD-MTX/CF in varying combinations with BCD, cisplatinum, and interferon).

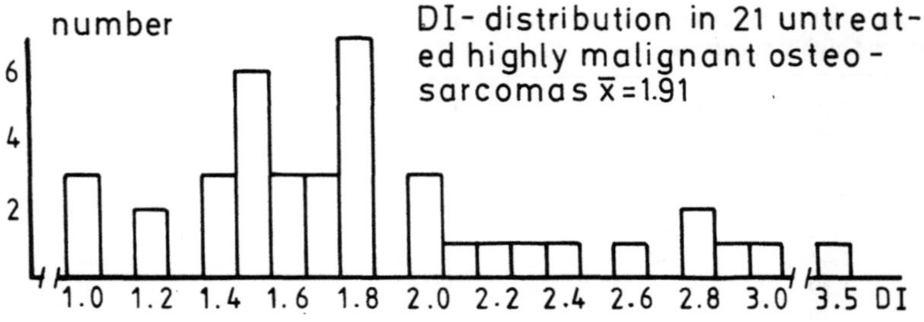

a

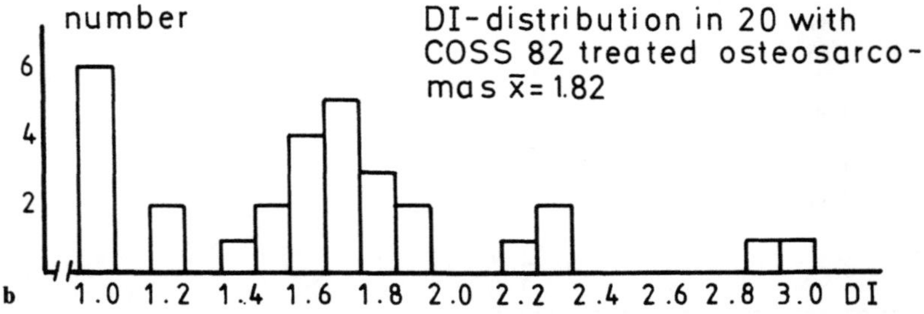

b

Fig. 5. a Distribution of DIs in 21 untreated highly malignant OSs (mean DI = 1.91). **b** DI distribution in 20 OSs treated according to the COSS 82 protocol (mean DI = 1.82)

Table 3. Histological grade of regression in bone tumors after preoperative chemotherapy (SALZER-KUNTSCHIK et al. 1983)

Grade	Morphology
I	No viable tumor cells
II	Isolated viable tumor cells, or a viable islet of tumor cells under 0.5 cm in diameter
III	Less than 10% viable tumor tissue
IV	Between 10% and 50% viable tumor tissue
V	More than 50% viable tumor tissue
VI	No recognizable effect of chemotherapy

Table 4. Grade of regression and DNA ploidy

Grade of regression	No. of cases	Aneuploidies					Mean DI of aneuploidies	Mean S-phase (%)
		0	1	2	3	4		
I	2	2	–	–	–	–	–	11.3
II	3	1	1	1	–	–	1.43	11.9
III	1	–	–	1	–	–	1.71	16.7
IV	6	2	3	1	–	–	1.99	12.8
V	7	1	2	2	1	1	1.87	22.4

Table 5. Flow cytometric data of patients prior to and after high-dose polychemotherapy

Case no.	Histology	Prechemotherapeutic[a]		Postchemotherapeutic[b]		
		DI	S-phase (%)	Grade of regression	DI	S-phase (%)
16	Telangiectatic OS	1.0	6.2	V	1.0	8.6
17	Telangiectatic OS	1.24	–	II	1.0	9.5
		1.78	–			
18	Chondroblastic OS	1.0	6.4	IV	1.0	2.2
19	Fibroblastic OS	1.84	–	V	1.74	25.4
					1.90	–
					2.20	–

[a] Biopsy
[b] Amputate

Following the first cycle, 19 of these patients underwent amputation, and in these cases an average of 14 measurements (range 1–21) from different areas of each tumor were performed. Thus topographical charts of DNA distribution patterns could be related to histology. We also examined three biopsies from patients who subsequently had to undergo ablative surgery. Histological classification (WHO cf. Schajowicz et al. 1972; Schajowicz 1981) verified 1 anaplastic, 11 osteoblastic, 4 chondroblastic, 2 fibroblastic, and 2 telangiectatic OSs. The grades of regression after chemotherapy were evaluated according to the criteria of Salzer-Kuntschik et al. (1983a, b).

Of the 20 pretreated tumors, 14 (70%) revealed DNA aneuploidy with a total of 24 DNA stemlines. Comparing results which those in untreated OSs, the number of tumors without DNA aneuploidy (i.e., with a DI of 1.0) was markedly higher (6 of 20 = 30% in contrast to 3 of 21 = 14%). In pretreated tumors the average DI of aneuploid populations was 1.82 (range: 1.2–3.0, mean 1.67), and in those without chemotherapy, 1.91 (range: 1.2–3.5, median 1.75) (Fig. 5). Seven of 14 (50%) pretreated tumors revealed multiple aneuploid stemlines, as against 11 of 18 (60%) tumors without chemotherapy. The average proportion of cells in S-phase was found to be lower after previous polychemotherapy (16.1%; range 2.2%–33.8%, median 13.9%) than in cases without chemotherapy (19.2%; range 6.2%–38.1%, median 18.8%).

There was a clear correlation of DNA indices and S-phase percentages with the grade of regression (Tables 3, 4): No aneuploid DNA population was found in the responder group I (0/2), whereas aneuploid stemlines could be verified in six of seven cases belonging to responder group V. The only exception was an OS whose clinical course was protracted over 2 years. The two tumors with more than two aneuploid stemlines were also in group V. The five clones with a DI over 2.0 belonged to nonresponder groups IV and V. Here, all DNA aneuploid populations had an S-phase proportion of more than 12%.

Four tumors could be analyzed before and after chemotherapy (Table 5): Two showed normal DNA distributions in the initial biopsy as well as in the postchemotherapeutic amputation specimen (nonresponder patients 16 and 18).

Table 6. Histological classification and DNA ploidy

Histological type	No of cases	Aneuploid stemline	Multiple aneuploid stemlines	Mean DI of aneuploid lines	S-phase (%)
Anaplastic	1	1	–	1.63	–
Osteoblastic	8	6	3	1.88	17.1
Chondroblastic	4	2	1	1.58	11.9
Fibroblastic	2	2	1	1.77	25.4
Telangiectatic	5	3	2	1.90	15.6

In one patient (17), a responder, tumor regression was reflected in the disappearance of a preexisting DNA aneuploidy, while in one nonresponder (19) the DNA aneuploid stemline (DI = 1.84) seen in the pretherapeutic biopsy was again found after chemotherapy, together with two additional subpopulations.

Comparison of tumor histology with DNA histograms in the individual cases failed to yield any significant differences among the histological subtypes of pretreated OSs with respect to either frequency of DNA aneuploidy and occurrence of multiple DNA stemlines distribution of DNA indices and percentage of S-phase cells (Table 6). Chondroblastic OSs alone showed a relatively small number of DNA aneuploid stemlines (two of four) with lower mean DI (1.58) and lower proliferation rates (S-phase 11.9%) than the other histological subtypes. Telangiectatic OSs had the highest mean DI (1.9), and four of five such tumors were nonresponders in group V.

Five patients from this series have died, four with a DNA aneuploid and one with a DNA diploid tumor. Among the eight cases with distant metastases, seven had DNA aneuploid tumors. Recurrence had been noted in one DNA diploid and one DNA aneuploid OS. Since the follow-up periods range from 1 to 7 years, these data are only preliminary (BÖSING et al. 1987).

Osteosarcomas arising at the bone surface are classified as juxtacortical, with subdifferentiation into classical parosteal, periosteal, and highly malignant superficial OSs (UNNI et al. 1976a, b; WOLD et al. 1984). The classical parosteal OSs are typically rather well-differentiated lesions; according to the histological grading systems of AHUJA et al. (1977) and HUVOS (1979) their malignancy is seen as grade I or grade II. Periosteal OSs are characterized by a dominating chondrosarcomatous component and are graded almost exclusively as II or III; accordingly, their prognosis is poorer than that of parosteal OSs. Highly malignant superficial OS corresponds, histologically and with regard to prognosis, to Huvos' grade III, and also to the highly malignant intramedullary OS.

The six juxtacortical OSs of our material were three parosteal, two periosteal, and one highly malignant superficial OSs. One of the parosteal and both periosteal OSs were grade II, two parosteal OS were grade I, and the highly malignant superficial OS was grade III, by definition. The available material was ethanol-fixed tumor tissue of parosteal OS, and formol-fixed, paraffin-embedded tumor tissue of periosteal and superficial OSs.

All three parosteal and two periosteal OSs showed a unimodal, diploid DNA distribution, while the highly malignant superficial OS had an additional, distinctly DNA tetraploid tumor cell population. There was another small hypertetraploid stemline near the base of that tetraploid peak.

Exact cell cycle analysis could only be performed in ethanol-fixed parosteal OSs and the highly malignant superficial OS with a sufficient resolution of the DNA histograms. The S-phase values of parosteal OSs ranged from 6.0% to 11.5% (mean 8.6%), while the DNA tetraploid stemline of the highly malignant superficial OS had a distinctly higher S-phase proportion of 14.3%.

The clinical course to date has been favorable in all cases. Recurrence occurred in one parosteal and in one periosteal OS. No metastases were found even in the case of a highly malignant surface OS of the fibula which had required amputation above the knee joint.

The rare category of *extraskeletal osteosarcoma* occupies maximally 4.6% of all OSs (RAO et al. 1978). It may be defined as an OS that is located in the soft tissue without attachment to the skeleton, as determined by examination of roentgenographs or by inspection during surgery. In contrast to primary OS in bone with an age peak in the 2nd decade, extraskeletal OSs are more frequent after the 5th decade (ALLAN and SOULE 1971). Some cases have been recorded after radiotherapy. The histological spectrum corresponds to that of primary osseous OSs (ENZINGER and WEISS 1983) and no differences were seen on electron microscopy (WILLIAMS et al. 1976). The prognosis does not differ essentially from that of osseous OSs (ENZINGER and WEISS 1983).

From the archives of the Bone Tumor Registry of Westphalia, five extraskeletal OSs were available for flow cytometric DNA analysis in paraffin-embedded specimens, with corresponding undecalcified samples. Histologically, all five tumors were classified as highly malignant osteoblastic OSs.

Flow cytometry identified one aneuploid stemline in each of four cases, and two aneuploid stemlines in one case. DNA indices ranged from 1.2 to 4.0, and in one case an additional peridiploid tumor stemline was safely identified. Exact cell cycle analysis was impossible on account of superposed lines in the DNA histogram, and somewhat limited resolution.

Two of these five patients have died in the meantime from extensive metastases. In two other cases, data about further clinical outcome are incomplete.

4.3 Conclusion

The rarer aggressive osteoblastoma should be distinguished clinically and morphologically from the "conventional" osteoblastoma. The assessment of a DNA tetraploid stemline, as seen in one of our two aggressive osteoblastomas, speaks for malignancy, and so the term "malignant" osteoblastoma used by SCHAJOWICZ and LEMOS appears plausible. The differentiation of such malignant osteoblastomas from well-differentiated OSs of low malignancy is obviously a problem of morphological definition.

Evidence of a DNA aneuploid stemline in two histologically nonsuspicious, normally benign "conventional" osteoblastomas is an unexpected finding, inviting two diverse interpretations: apparently DNA aneuploidy does not reflect malignancy with absolute certainty, and so gives no prognostic clue in these two cases, or DNA aneuploidy might only signal the malignant potential of the lesion before it becomes manifest – as happens in melanoctyic nevi or in dysplasia of various mucosal epithelia (STENZINGER et al. 1984; PFITZER 1985; MACARTNEY 1986; HAMMARBERG et al. 1984). The risk of malignant transformation, noted rarely in conventional osteoblastoma, may speak in favor of the second explanation. Consequently, even conventional osteoblastoma with safely benign histology but a potential DNA aneuploidy would require complete resection of the entire tumor mass.

Among OSs in general, a good 90% of all cases are medullary and, as a rule, highly malignant. The high rate of DNA aneuploid stemlines and the frequency of multiple DNA stemlines are interpreted as criteria of malignancy, and the high proliferation rates observed, particularly in aneuploid stemlines, emphasize the growth potential of these tumors. With regard to the spectrum of histological subtypes as defined by the WHO classification – anaplastic, osteoblastic, chondroblastic, fibroblastic, and telangiectatic OSs – there has been hardly any evidence, so far, of correspondingly significant differences in the pattern of tumor kinetics. This agrees with empirical knowledge on the similar prognosis of all these histological types (DAHLIN and UNNI 1986). However, chondroblastic OSs show a distinctly lower rate of aneuploidy and proliferation than all other OS types, with or without preoperative chemotherapy: 2/5 vs 30/36 DNA aneuploidy, and 10.8% vs 17.6% S-phase. Tumor kinetics of chondroblastic OS correspond to some extent with those of high-grade chondrosarcoma, which also points to a histogenetic relationship.

The preliminary results after preoperative chemotherapy of highly malignant OSs reveal, when compared with the nonpretreated cases, a markedly lower rate of aneuploid stemlines (24/20 vs 37/21), and an even higher proportion of tumors without any evidence of a DNA aneuploid stemline (6/20 vs 3/21). It appears plausible that sensitive stemlines are preferentially destroyed by chemotherapeutic pretreatment. The number of aneuploid stemlines will be lower, of course, in the responder group than in that of nonresponders (5/6 vs 18/13). Apparently the proportion of hypertetraploid stemlines is more strongly restricted after chemotherapy. The reduced proliferation (as reflected in the S-phase content) after chemotherapy (mean value 16.1% vs 18.8%) also illustrates the restricted growth tendency. The above data, however, yield no safe indicators for a better response of certain subtypes to chemotherapy.

Among the juxtacortical OSs, the highly malignant superficial OS has, with regard to histology and prognosis, a marked resemblance to the usually highly malignant medullary OS, for which the presence of hyperdiploid stemlines is but another indicator. The parosteal and periosteal OSs are tumors of better differentiation and lower malignancy, for which absence of DNA aneuploid stemlines and comparably low proliferation, as seen our cases, are valuable signs. The highly malignant extraskeletal OSs of our series did not differ histologically or with regard to other tumor kinetics from the primary osseous OSs of high malignancy.

5 Cartilage-Forming Tumors

5.1 Chondroma

Chondromas are benign tumors composed of mature hyaline cartilage. Most cases present as "enchondroma" arising within bones, which have to be differentiated from the more rare periosteal chondromas. Multiple enchondromas are identified as bone dysplasias characterized by disturbed enchondral ossification. About a third of these cases subsequently develop chondrosarcoma. Unlike chondrosarcoma, about 50% of chondromas arise in the extremities, preferentially in the phalanges of the hand. They are rather rare in the bones of the trunk, which are predominantly affected by chondrosarcoma. The enchondromas of smaller peripheral bones are often highly cellular, but multinucleated chondrocytes with enlarged nuclei are uncommon. A similar histological picture found in a tumor of larger bones would, as a rule, indicate a chondrosarcoma. It is necessary to analyze as many different parts of the lesion as possible in order not to overlook a possible chondrosarcoma; this is especially true in large-sized tumors and those localized in larger bones.

If the tumor is completely removed by curettage or resection, prognosis is favorable. Recurrences with malignant histological features are mostly due to an underlying chondrosarcoma that had not been identified on account of incomplete workup.

Twenty-seven paraffin-embedded solitary chondromas with a largely typical distribution of age, sex, and localization were examined by flow cytometry. In all cases the clinical course followed the typical favorable pattern. Histograms fit for interpretation were obtained in only 17 cases, of which 4 cases were DNA diploid, and 13 DNA peridiploid tumors. No DNA aneuploid stemlines were observed. In view of the generally poor resolution of DNA histograms we did not attempt cell cycle analysis.

5.2 Chondrosarcoma

These tumors are about half as frequent as OSs, arising preferentially in the truncal region. Seventy-six percent of cases are primary chondrosarcomas (CSs), the remaining tumors developing secondarily from or in multiple or solitary osteochondromas or, less often, from enchondromas (Dahlin and Unni 1986). CSs will frequently show regressive changes with occasional calcifications and often marginal zones of ossification. If there is evidence of tumor osteoid, the tumor is by definition a chondroblastic OS, a variety occurring in younger patients with rather less favorable prognosis. About 10% of CSs will subsequently turn into lesions of higher malignancy, such as OS, fibrosarcoma, or malignant fibrous histiocytoma, and are then subsumed under the term "dedifferentiated chondrosarcoma."

Conventional Chondrosarcoma. On account of much lower rates of metastasis, the prognosis of these tumors is much better than that of OSs. Consequently, therapy is focused on complete surgical removal of the lesion, which, however, is often severely hampered by the truncal localization of the tumor. Some 90% of conventional CSs are relatively well differentiated sarcomas of grades I or II, and their histological differentiation from chondroma may be rather difficult. Typical CSs are of comparably low cellularity with marked regressive changes affecting even the nuclei.

Flow cytometric analysis was performed on paraffin-embedded material stored in the Bone Tumor Registry of Westphalia. Only 9 of our 21 CSs had a resolution of DNA histograms sufficient for ploidy assessment, but no adequate cell cycle analysis was possible even in these. DNA aneuploidy was evident in two CSs: one had a peritetraploid stemline, the other had two stemlines with DIs of 1.2 and 2.4. Both tumors were histologically grade III, while the other seven peridiploid tumors showed grades I and II.

Dedifferentiated Chondrosarcoma. These are in fact conventional CSs of varying differentiation and malignancy with an additional component of more malignant sarcomatous tissue. This may be either a spindle cellular dedifferentiation (towards fibrosarcoma or malignant fibrous histiocytoma) or a plain osteosarcomatous transformation. Recently there have been discussions about a rhabdomyosarcomatous component of some dedifferentiated CSs (ASTORINO and TESLUK 1985; NIEZABITOWSKI et al. 1987).

Paraffin-embedded material of 14 dedifferentiated CSs from 1976 to 1985 was available for flow cytometric analysis; six of the tumors had turned towards osteosarcomatous, eight towards spindle cell transformation. The distribution of age, sex and localization was largely similar to that of conventional CSs. Dedifferentiated CSs differed from OS by their occurrence in older patients, and by a more central localization. This is also a distinguishing feature from fibrosarcoma and malignant fibrous histiocytoma, both of which are more common in peripheral bones, especially in the knee region.

DNA aneuploidy was found in 9 of 14 cases, with DIs between 1.2 and 3.3. Five of them had two aneuploid stemlines. The nine aneuploid tumors showed osteosarcomatous dedifferentiation in four cases, and spindle cell transformation in five. The remaining five cases showed unimodal, peridiploid DNA distribution. Aneuploidy rates did not differ significantly in the two types of dedifferentiated CS (spindle cell type = 5/8; osteosarcomatous type = 4/6). Superposition of stemlines and partly reduced resolution of DNA histograms prevented any correct cell cycle analysis. Complete historical data were obtained from ten patients. Eight of them had DNA aneuploid tumors; recurrences were recorded in three patients, metastases in eight. These ten patients have died of their tumors.

5.3 Conclusion

Among all bone tumors studied, chondromas and conventional CSs were the least suitable for flow cytometric DNA analysis, probably due to their poor cellularity and marked regressive changes. In paraffin-embedded material from the registry archives, a potential longer fixation in formol and the frequent use of decalcifiers may also play an important role, but this applies to any retrospective investigation of bone tumors. As reported in previous microscopic photometric studies (CUVELIER and ROELS 1979; KREICBERGS et al. 1980, 1982), the rate of DNA aneuploidy recorded by flow cytometry was low and correlated with the grade of malignancy (ALHO et al. 1983; KREICBERGS et al. 1984), whereas chondromas showed the expected diploid DNA distribution.

As expected, the aneuploidy rates of dedifferentiated CSs (9 of 14=64%) were between those of malignant fibrous histiocytoma 2/10=20%) and those of fibrosarcomas (14/16=87.5%) and highly malignant OSs (18/21=86%), while conventional CSs manifested the typical lower rate of aneuploidies (2/9=22%). There seems to be a close correlation between low aneuploidy rates and comparatively favorable prognosis in conventional CSs. However, the rate of aneuploidy in dedifferentiated CS is found to be lower than that of highly malignant OSs despite its rather poor prognosis. This must be due to the central localization and low operability of dedifferentiated CS, with their additional influence on prognosis.

6 Giant Cell Tumor of Bone

Giant cell tumors of bone are benign in about 90% of cases, but they have a marked trend to recurrence. Histologically they are characterized by an increased occurrence of osteoclast-like giant cells which are interpreted as a reactive phenomenon, arising from the fusion of mononuclear histiocytic forms (ROESSNER 1984). The genuine tumor cells of these lesions are poorly differentiated cells, mostly of spindly shape, existing in diffuse mixture with the histiocytes, giant cells, and round cells that are always present in a tumor. Differential diagnosis has to consider not only benign bone lesions (such as nonossifying fibroma, aneurysmal bone cyst, solitary bone cyst, giant cell reparative granuloma, and fibrous osteoclasia in hyperparathyroidism) but also giant cell-containing OS and malignant fibrous histiocytoma.

Giant cell tumors of bone are far from uniform with regard to their biological behavior, and no general clinical or morphological critera are at hand for its definite assessment in the early individual lesion. Even the system of histological grading in terms of stromal atypia proposed by JAFFÉ et al. (1940) seems of limited and uncertain value (DAHLIN et al. 1970; GOLDENBERG et al. 1970; MNAYMNEH et al. 1964), although only these mononuclear cells of the stroma were identified as true tumor cells. The prognostic value of roentgenological classification is equally uncertain (EDEIKEN and HODES 1973; GEE and PUGH 1958). In fact, the problem of adequate prognostic evaluation is of major importance for the main group of histologically "benign" giant cell tumors, since they are known to become malignant in quite a number of cases. Moreover, the phenomenon of so-called benign, but metastasizing giant cell tumors of bone (GRESEN et al. 1973; ROCK et al. 1984) has never been explained satisfactorily with the aid of conventional morphological methods. So far, flow cytometric analysis has been performed in only isolated tumors of this type (KREICBERGS

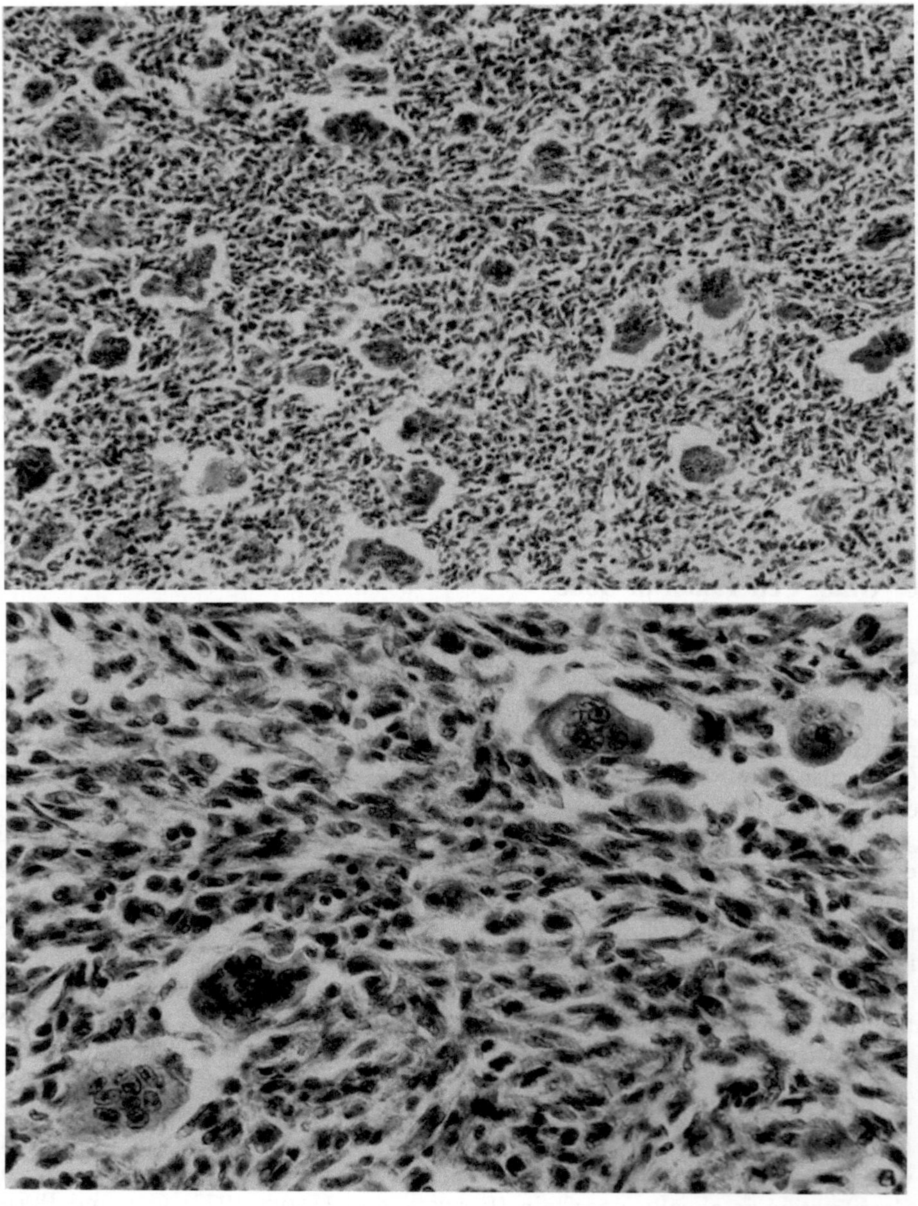

a

b

Fig. 6 a, b. Proliferating DNA diploid giant cell tumor. **a** Multinucleated giant cell in a highly cellular mononuclear stroma (H & E, ×136). **b** Compared with giant cells, mononuclear cells show more chromatin dense nuclei, and generally marked proliferation (H & E, ×330)

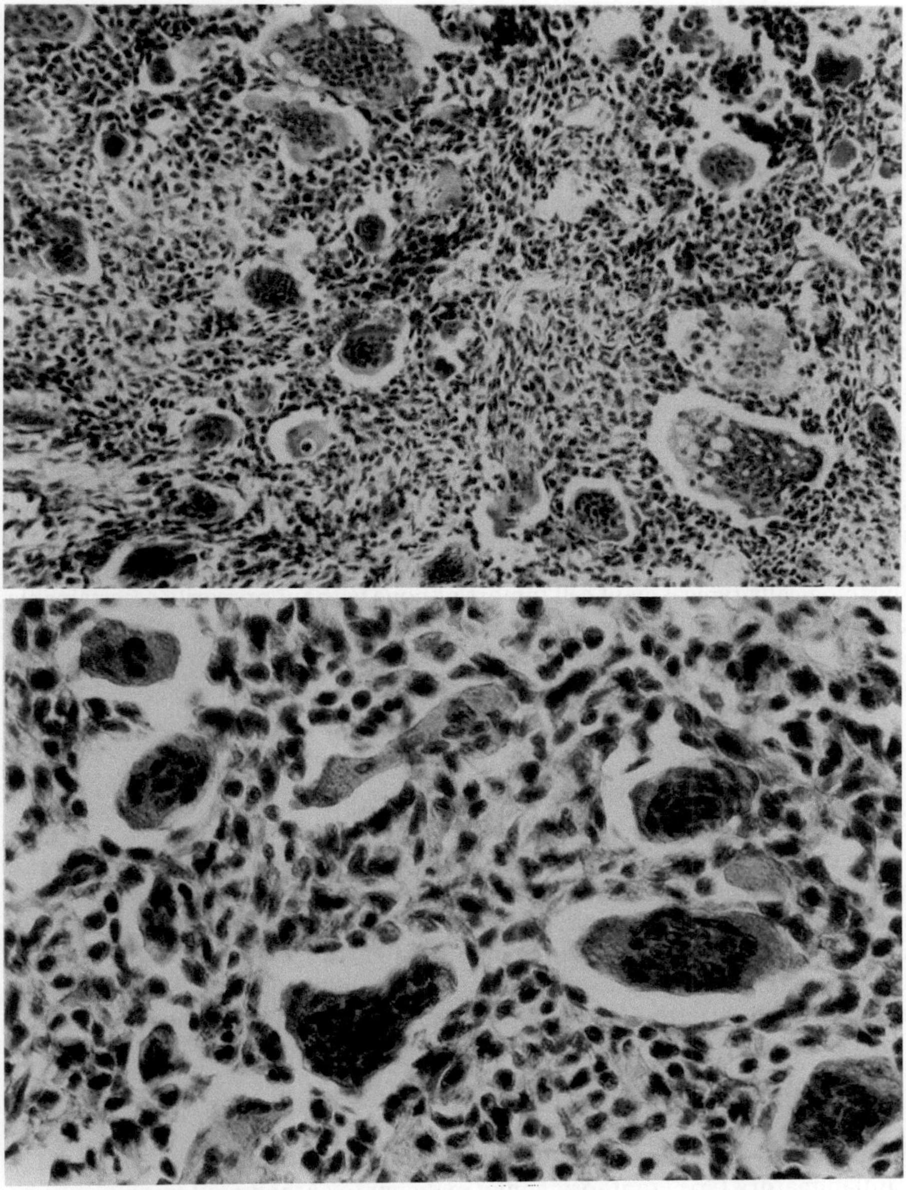

a

b

Fig. 7a, b. Metastasizing DNA aneuploid giant cell tumor of bone. **a** Numerous multinucleated giant cells in diffuse distribution in a cell-rich stroma (H & E, ×136). **b** Relatively uniform stroma cells with chromatin dense nuclei. No remarkable cellular or nuclear atypias in an overall increased proliferation. (H & E, ×330)

et al. 1984; HELIÖ et al. 1985; MANKIN et al. 1985), all of which seemed to belong to the group of clinically benign giant cell tumors.

Our 18 cases (paraffin-embedded material) were identified histologically as typical partly proliferating giant cell tumors of bone (Figs. 6, 7). None of the primaries showed any histological or roentgenological indicators of malignancy; distributions of age, sex, and localization were also largely typical.

Flow cytometry of 14 cases revealed a unimodal diploid pattern in eight cases and peridiploid patterns in six. The other four tumors had DNA aneuploid stemlines whose DI ranged from 1.2 to 2.4. One case examined in several samples revealed three aneuploid stemlines. No cell cycle analysis could be performed as the resolution of DNA histograms was mostly inadequate; moreover, the superpositions of DNA distributions of tumor cells and reactive infiltrates can hardly be calculated in giant cell tumors.

Recurrences have been observed in 5 of our 18 cases; in the case with three DNA aneuploid stemlines, histology of the recurring tumor showed its sarcomatous nature. This patient died 4 years later of extensive metastases. Among the other three tumors with one aneuploid stemline each, only one has had a recurrence; no metastases have occurred as yet.

We may gather from these results that DNA aneuploidy may occur even in histologically typical giant cell tumors of bone without primarily ascertainable malignancy. They have to be interpreted as a sign of probably malignant transformation, and will provide valuable prognostic hints for the physician in charge (MELLIN et al. 1984, 1985a).

7 Malignant Fibrous Histiocytoma

Malignant fibrous histiocytoma (MFH) was first defined as a separate entity among soft tissue tumors by OZZELLO et al. in 1963. Today, MFH is registered as the most frequent soft tissue tumor in late adult age. It has been recognized as a rare primarily osseous sarcoma since 1972 by FELDMAN and NORMAN. There are no histological or electron microscopic differences between the osseous and the soft tissue form, for which ENZINGER (1977) proposed the classification of five subtypes:

1. Storiform pleomorphic type
2. Myxoid type (myxofibrosarcoma)
3. Giant cell type (malignant giant cell tumor of soft tissue)
4. Inflammatory type (xanthosarcoma, malignant xanthogranuloma)
5. Angiomatoid type

All these subtypes show an at least partly storiform array of spindle-shaped tumor cells, interspersed with pleomorphic tumor cells in varying frequency. Occasionally, there is also a fascicular structure. Electron microscopy distinguishes histiocytic cells, fibroblastic cells, xanthomatous cells, tumor giant cells, and reactive histiocytic giant cells (ROESSNER 1984).

The following flow cytometric DNA analyses were performed on formol-fixed, paraffin-embedded material taken from ten primary osseous MFHs, all of the storiform polymorphic type. The cases were documented in the archives of the Bone Tumor Registry between 1977 and 1985. Clinically, uncharacteristic symptoms of pain and swelling were dominant. The age at incidence varied considerably (which is typical), males were more often affected (7/3), and the localizations corresponded to the pattern known from the literature (DAHLIN and UNNI 1986). No diagnostic roentgenological criteria beyond general indicators of malignancy were found, but none have been claimed in the literature (FELDMAN and LATTES 1977).

Flow cytometric DNA analysis yielded an additional hyperdiploid stemline in two of ten MFHs (DI = 2.0 and 2.2, respectively). The other eight MFHs showed unimodal diploid DNA distributions. S-phase values ranged from 5.2% to 14.1% (mean 8.8%). Complete follow-up was available for eight patients. Four of them died of their tumors, of which one was peritetraploid, and three diploid. Among the four surviving patients, recurrence was found in one case and metastases in two. The last patient, operated on in 1984, has been free of tumor since then.

Like the data from light and electron microscopy, the prognosis of MFH in bone corresponds largely to that in soft tissues (INADA et al. 1976; JOHNSON et al. 1978; ROESSNER et al. 1979; KATENKAMP and STILLER 1981; MARTINEZ-TELLO et al. 1981). Although data about 5-year survival rates vary greatly in different reports (HUVOS 1976; FELDMAN and LATTES 1977; SPANIER 1977; DAHLIN and UNNI 1986), the average of 50% is certainly higher than the rates given for highly malignant OS or fibrosarcoma (DAHLIN and UNNI 1986). The generally poor prognosis, reflected in a 5-year survival rate of 20% of highly malignant OSs after surgery alone, is also illustrated by the high rate of aneuploidy (90% mean rate in different reports) and by a high mean S-phase percentage of more than 14% (KREICBERGS et al. 1984; HELIÖ et al. 1985; MANKIN et al. 1985; GRUNDMANN et al. 1985). In the rarer MFH of bone, only recently differentiated from highly malignant OS and fibrosarcoma, such tumor kinetic data are not available.

The kinetic parameters documented in our study suggest a markedly better prognosis than in malignant OS. When we compare our data gathered in ethanol-fixed highly malignant OSs (aneuploidy rate 18/21, mean S-phase content 18.8%) with those of the MFH series (two hyperdiploid tumors in ten, mean S-phase content 8.8%), the lower level is evident. However, plausible prognostic evaluation of tumor kinetic data is not yet possible on account of the low number of cases, the short follow-up, and the diversity of localizations, stages, and therapies. Our own flow cytometric analyses of soft tissue MFH with evidence of DNA aneuploid stemlines in 9 of 19 cases suggest that the rate of DNA aneuploidies in MFH of bone might be expected to be somewhat higher than the current results have shown (MELLIN et al. 1986c).

8 Fibrosarcoma

Fibrosarcomas (FSs) of bone are six times less frequent than OSs, but like these, are predominantly localized in the long tubular bones. In opposition to OS, the age distribution is rather even, starting with the second decade.

The sex ratio is equally balanced. Prognosis is only slightly better than that of OS, and the fibroblastic variant of OS presents the greatest differential diagnostic difficulty. It is only the lack of tumor osteoid that distinguishes FS from fibroblastic OS. Histologically, the grades of differentiation vary greatly, but a kind of herringbone pattern prevails. Decreasing differentiation is paralleled by decreasing production of collagen fibers. Well-differentiated FS has to be distinguished from benign fibrous bone lesions, poorly differentiated or anaplastic FS, and MFH. In the event of myxoid structures, differential diagnosis must also consider liposarcoma. In about 25% of all FSs, the lesion is a secondary one, arising mainly after irradiation, or much less often without irradiation in preexisting bone lesions (DAHLIN and UNNI 1986).

The 16 paraffin-embedded FS specimens from the Bone Tumor Registry were all moderately or poorly differentiated, presenting no differential diagnostic problems, nor did the distribution of age, sex, and localization deviate from normal. Eleven cases were primary lesions while five were secondary; one had been preceded by a primary giant cell tumor, another by a bone infarction. The remaining three occurred after radiotherapy for another tumor.

Flow cytometry revealed aneuploid stemlines in 14 of 16 FSs. Five of these had one DNA tetraploid stemline, two hyperdiploid stemlines were found in only one case, and two tumors showed unimodal diploid DNA distribution. Cell cycle analysis was possible in only four cases, and here the S-phase proportions were between 14.8% and 24.2% (mean value 19.6%). As these were FSs of moderate to poor differentiation, the proliferation levels are certainly above average.

Considering prognosis, the high rates of aneuploidy and proliferation found by flow cytometry could be expected. They are on the same level as in the highly malignant OSs whose prognosis is only slightly worse. There were no significant differences between primary and secondary FSs.

9 Chordoma

This is a rare neoplasm of destructive growth type, arising from remnants of the primordial notochord (chorda dorsalis). The tumor is localized in or near the spine, generally in the sacrococcygeal or sphenooccipital region. In view of the close relations between chorda dorsalis and skeleton, and on account of its clinical and roentgenological features, chordoma is always classified among bone tumors.

Roentgenologically, more than 90% of all cases will display visibly destructive bone involvement (irregular osteolysis) or a soft tissue mass. Macroscopically, the tumor has a softish structure; it is lobated, gray, and semitranslucent. Outside the bone it is commonly encapsulated, resembling a chondrosarcoma or mucinous adenocarcinoma. Histologically, chordomas show a typical lobated array. Electron microscopy distinguishes stellate cells and physaliferous cells, and also intermediate cell types (ERLANDSON et al. 1968). According to the results of several authors (FRIEDMAN et al. 1962; SPJUT and LUSE 1964; PENA et al. 1970; MURAD and MURTY 1970; MIKUZ and MYDLA 1974), the cells of physaliferous type are transformed from the stellate cells via the intermediate type by way of an insidious dilatation of cysterns in the granular endoplasmic reticulum producing and storing acid mucopolysaccharides. According the studies of MIKUZ et al. (1977), stellate cells represent the tumor compartment still capable of proliferation, whereas physaliferous cells are degenerated forms of the tumor cells.

The prognosis of chordoma is dominated by the high rate of recurrence, which remains as high as 28% even after intact and complete removal of the tumor. In case of intraoperative incision into the tumor mass, the rate will rise to 64%. Metastasis or transformation into CS, OS, or FS is very rare. Radiotherapy will achieve varying rates of success which are as yet unpredictable in the individual case (DAHLIN and UNNI 1986).

Paraffin-embedded material from 17 chordomas was available for flow cytometric analysis. Most of them were localized at the caudal spine, with typical distribution of age and sex. Histological pictures were typical, too; four cases showed distinct foci of cellular and nuclear polymorphism. Six of 17 chordomas had a distinctly aneuploid stemline with DIs between 1.3 and 2.0. As the resolution of DNA histograms was often impaired either by extended formol fixation or by a high proportion of regressive, physaliferous tumor cells (four peridiploid tumors), only seven DNA diploid tumors were available for cell cycle analysis. They revealed a wide spectrum of S-phase levels from 2.6% to 16.3% (mean 9.3%). These high levels are somewhat qualified by the fact that measurements were performed predominantly in tumor areas of high cellularity and obvious proliferative activity. Proliferation being rather heterogeneous within the individual chordoma, flow cytometric assessments of proliferation rates has its problems even in fresh samples of a tumor. With the help of comparative immunohistological studies of a proliferation-associated nuclear antigen using the monoclonal antibody Ki-67, this rate can be adequately estimated in routine histology considering cellularity and the amount of regressive changes (MELLIN et al. 1987b).

No correlation could be established between tumor kinetic data and histological pictures or clinical course. Recurrences had occurred in 6 of 17 chordomas, identified as DNA diploid tumors in four cases and as DNA aneuploid tumors in two. Five patients have died of their tumors. Liver metastases were found in one of the four diploid tumors, while further spinal metastases had occurred in the aneuploid tumor. Whether DNA ploidy and proliferation rates in chordoma are of any prognostic significance or relevance to therapy will become clear only if larger case numbers can be evaluated; in this particular tumor, prognosis depends to an exceptional degree on the mass and localization of the primary and hence its operability.

10 Ewing's Sarcoma

Classified among round cell sarcomas, Ewing's sarcoma stands out among bone tumors for its very high lethality. Its histogenesis is not undisputed, the origin being assumed to be from a stem cell belonging to either the hemopoietic or the mesenchymal structural system of the bone marrow (ROESSNER 1984). Typical histological pictures show a highly anaplastic small cell tumor with roundish or oval cells bearing the clinical and roentgenological marks of primary bone neoplasia. Intracytoplasmic glycogen storage is evident in most cases. In addition to the common small cell form of Ewing's sarcoma, a rare variant is known with somewhat larger cells and even worse prognosis. Differential diagnosis has to consider malignant lymphoma, mesenchymal CS, small cell OS, and the metastases of neuroblastoma and small cell carcinomas (DAHLIN and UNNI 1986).

Besides irradiation and surgical resection of the primary, modern therapeutic schedules generally involve polychemotherapy, whereby 5-year survival rates have been improved from a mere 10% to about 40% (JÜRGENS 1981; JÜRGENS et al. 1985; DAHLIN and UNNI 1986). Studies on the tumor kinetics of Ewing's sarcoma, which might be interesting in this context, have only been published on isolated cases (WILLNOW 1982; KREICBERGS et al. 1984; MANKIN et al. 1985), and no safe data are available on DNA ploidy and proliferation in this tumor, nor on their relevance for chemotherapy.

Our analyses concerned 24 Ewing's sarcomas from the archives of the Bone Tumor Registry. The specimens were stored in paraffin blocks which could be prepared for flow cytometry. Histologically, all cases presented the classical glycogen-rich, small cell type. Suspicion of Ewing's sarcoma had already been based on clinical and roentgenological findings. Distribution of age, sex, and localization followed the typical pattern of Ewing's sarcoma.

Flow cytometric DNA analysis revealed at least one hyperdiploid stemline in 14 of 24 cases (58%). The presence of two hyperdiploid tumor cell populations was recorded in three cases (Fig. 8). The DI of hyperdiploid stemlines ranged from 1.1 to 3.2. Tetraploidy was found in three cases. The other ten tumors showed either unimodal, diploid (seven cases), or peridiploid (four cases) DNA distributions.

Correct evaluation of S-phase levels in individual tumor cell populations was possible in 16 of 24 Ewing's sarcomas. These levels ranged from 2.2% to 15% (mean: 7.5%). There was no statistically significant correlation between proliferative activity (as expressed in the S-phase proportion) and DNA ploidy, although the mean value of ten hyperdiploid tumors (8.4%) was clearly higher than the mean value of seven diploid tumors (6.2%).

Complete follow-up was available for 20 patients. Only five of them survived; three of their tumors were diploid, two aneuploid. Extensive metastases were found in all fatal cases but one, which had been caused by local tumor spread in the spine.

The tumor kinetics of Ewing's sarcoma differ markedly from those of OS (MELLIN et al. 1985b). Although prognosis for both tumors is similar, the percentage of DNA aneuploid tumors in our series of Ewing's sarcomas (58%) is markedly lower than in our group of OSs (90%). Stemline heterogeneity, too, is less strong in Ewing's sarcoma than in OS. This may reflect favorable conditions for a better response to radio- or chemotherapy, since the potential of therapy-resistant tumor lines will increase with the number of preexistent aneuploid stemlines (MELLIN and GRUNDMANN 1989). However, the distinctly

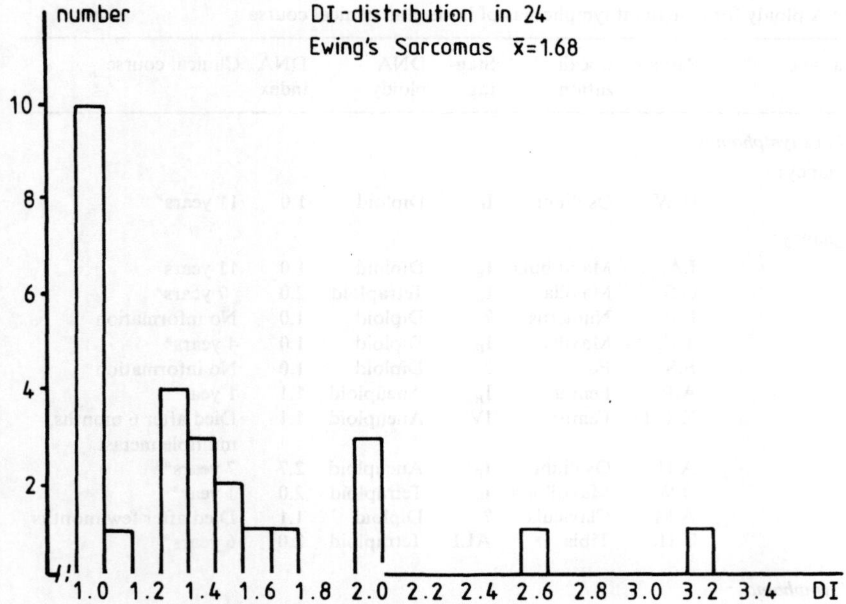

Fig. 8. Distribution of DIs in 24 Ewing's sarcomas (mean DI = 1.68)

lower proliferation rates (as expressed in the S-phase proportion) of Ewing's sarcomas is suggestive of a poorer response to radio- or chemotherapy, which can exert their damaging influence mainly on proliferating cells (FRINDEL and TUBIANA 1971; SINCLAIR 1972; TOBEY 1972). These inferences, however, would contradict the general empirical observation of radiosensitivity in Ewing's sarcoma, and of the success of polychemotherapy in raising the rates of 5-year survival over the past decades (ROSEN et al. 1981). We have to conclude that obviously no close correlation exists between the investigated tumor kinetics and the biological behavior of Ewing's sarcoma.

11 Malignant Lymphomas of Bone

A primary manifestation of malignant lymphomas in the skeletal system is very rare and the classification and histogenesis have been matters of controversy. Particular problems are encountered in the differential diagnosis of those lesions which were originally called reticulum cell sarcomas (LLOMBART-BOSCH et al. 1982). The rather varied group of tumor entities covered by this term is classified today, with few exceptions, as non-Hodgkin's lymphoma. This classification was often possible only with the aid of immunohistological investigations, a method which has hardly been used in the study of malignant lymphomas with primary bone manifestation (Dumont and Mazabraud 1979). Our own histological and immunohistological studies of these tumors have demon-

Table 7. DNA ploidy for malignant lymphomas of bone, and clinical course

Lymphoma type	Patient	Localization	Staging	DNA ploidy	DNA index	Clinical course
Non-Hodgkin's lymphomas						
Low malignancy:						
CB/CC	H.W.	Os ilium	I_E	Diploid	1.0	11 years[a]
High malignancy:						
CB	J.A.	Mandibula	I_E	Diploid	1.0	11 years[a]
CB	O.S.	Maxilla	I_E	Tetraploid	2.0	7 years[a]
CB	F.B.	Numerus	?	Diploid	1.0	No information
CB	T.E.	Maxilla	I_E	Diploid	1.0	4 years[a]
CB	F.S.	Foot	?	Diploid	1.0	No information
CB	A.P.	Femur	I_E	Aneuploid	1.1	1 year[a]
CB	K.H.G.	Femur	IV	Aneuploid	1.1	Died after 6 months, multiple metast.
IB	A.H.	Os ilium	I_E	Aneuploid	2.7	7 years[a]
IB	B.W.	Mandibula	I_E	Tetraploid	2.0	1 year[a]
LB	A.M.	Clavicula	?	Diploid	1.1	Died after few months
LB	T.H.	Tibia	ALL	Tetraploid	2.0	6 years[a]
Hodgkin's lymphomas:						
Nodular sclerosing type	E.H.	Vertebra	?	Diploid	1.1	Died after few months
Mixed cell type	K.S.	Multifocal	IV	Diploid	1.0	Died after few months
Mixed cell type	H.P.	Clavicula	?	Diploid	1.0	No information
Mixed cell type	H.T.	Femur	IV	Diploid	1.0	Too short follow-up[a]
Lymphocytic depleted	H.K.	Vertebra	?	Tetraploid	2.0	Died after few months

[a] Patient living.
CB/CC, centroblastic/centrocytic; CB, centroblastic; IB, immunoblastic; LB, lymphoblastic; ALL, acute lymphoid leukemia

strated that the bone manifestations do not differ from nodal lymphomas with regard to their spectrum of histological subtypes (VASSALLO et al. 1987a). The patterns of DNA ploidy, however, have not yet been ascertained in bone lymphomas.

Flow cytometric DNA analysis was performed in paraffin-embedded tissue samples from 17 malignant lymphomas of bone documented in the Bone Tumor Registry of Westphalia. In none of these cases had there been a clinical suspicion of malignant lymphoma. Five cases were classified as Hodgkin's lymphomas, the remaining 12 as non-Hodgkin's lymphomas, which were then reclassified according to the Kiel nomenclature.

Histology, localization, staging, DNA ploidy, and the main clinical data are listed in Table 7. The proportion of highly malignant non-Hodgkin's lymphomas with hyperdiploid DNA stemlines was 6 in 11, of which three were tetraploid. One non-Hodgkin's lymphoma of lesser malignancy (CB/CC) showed only unimodal diploid DNA distribution. Of five Hodgkin's lymphomas, only the case of lymphocyte-depleted type had a tetraploid stemline; the other four were all DNA diploid (VASALLO et al. 1987b).

This DNA ploidy pattern of bone lymphomas corresponds well with the results from similar studies of nodal lymphomas. Here, too, the Hodgkin's lymphomas were DNA diploid, with few exceptions (Barlogie et al. 1980; Shackney et al. 1980; Hagemeister et al. 1981; Diamond et al. 1982). We have to remember, however, that in cases of Hodgkin's lymphoma the amount of tumor cells in the sample studied may be rather small, which implies the risk of overlooking DNA aneuploid stemlines. In such cases microscope photometry is certainly more suitable.

According to data in the literature, non-Hodgkin's lymphomas show a rising rate of aneuploidy in parallel with increasing histological malignancy (Barlogie et al. 1977, 1980; Braylan et al. 1978; Diamond and Braylan 1980; Diamond et al. 1982; Hagemeister et al. 1981; Sandritter and Grimm 1977; Shackney and Skramstadt 1979; Shackney et al. 1980, 1984; Silvestrini et al. 1977). This in turn corresponds with the clinical course of lymphoma subtypes (Brittinger 1981). In our series of 12 non-Hodgkin's lymphomas we observed a similar pattern of DNA ploidy, whereas only the occurrence of DNA tetraploid stemlines in three of six hyperdiploid high-grade lymphomas presents a particularity. Of course, the low number of cases studied does not warrant definitive interpretation, but the DNA diploidy of low malignancy non-Hodgkin's lymphomas appears to be typical.

In conclusion we emphasize that, from our results, the more favorable clinical course of malignant lymphomas with primary bone manifestations is due to the generally lower tumor stage. The spectrum of high and low malignancy types, which resembles that of nodal lymphomas, seems to offer no meaningful contribution to prognosis.

12 Summary

Flow cytometric DNA analysis was performed in a total of 203 bone tumors, benign and malignant. In more than 80% of cases the material studied was paraffin-embedded tumor tissue, mainly from the archives of the Bone Tumor Registry of Westphalia in Münster. Compared with ethanol-fixed fresh tumor samples, the variation coefficient in DNA histograms of the stored material was increased by a factor of 1.2–1.5, which means that resolution was decreased and that, in many cases, accurate cell cycle analysis was not feasible. However, the results of cell cycle analysis in bone tumors, even if performed on optimally fixed specimens, have to be evaluated with caution and full reference to the corresponding histological slides, since these histograms are apt to show various superpositions from the inflammatory infiltrate. The assessment of DNA ploidy is unimpaired if, in agreement with most researchers today, deviations smaller than $\pm 10\%$ from the diploid standard are still defined as DNA diploid, peridiploid, or pseudodiploid. The coefficient of variation should be kept as low as possible. If it is between 10% and 15%, the near-diploid stemlines with DNA indices of 0.9 or 1.1 may be hard to delineate. On account of the particularly marked regressive changes, the resolution of DNA histograms was most strongly

Table 8. DNA aneuploidy rates in different bone tumors

Histological classification	DNA aneuploidy Rate (incl. DNAtetraploidy)	
Osteoblastoma		
Conventional osteoblastoma	2/7	
Aggressive osteoblastoma	1/2	
Osteosarcoma		
Medullary osteosarcoma	18/21	(85.7%)
Osteosarcoma after chemotherapy	14/20	(70.0%)
Parosteal osteosarcoma	0/3	
Periosteal osteosarcoma	0/1	
High-grade surface osteosarcoma	1/1	
Extraskeletal osteosarcoma	5/5	
Chondroma	0/17	
Chondrosarcoma		
Conventional chondrosarcoma	2/9	
Dedifferentiated chondrosarcoma	9/14	(64.3%)
a) Spindle cell type	5/8	
b) Osteosarcomatous type	4/6	
Giant cell tumor (osteoclastoma)	4/18	(22.2%)
Malignant fibrous histiocytoma	2/10	(20.0%)
Fibrosarcoma	14/16	(87.5%)
Chordoma	6/17	(35.3%)
Ewing's sarcoma	14/24	(58.3%)
Malignant lymphomas		
Hodgkin's lymphomas	1/5	
Non-Hodgkin's lymphomas	6/12	(50.0%)
Low malignancy	0/1	
High malignancy	6/11	(54.5%)

impaired in chondromatous tumors, whereas it was mostly excellent in highly cellular viable tumor tissue, such as that from Ewing's sarcoma or osteoblastoma.

On the whole, there was a distinct correlation between DNA ploidy and the biological behavior of bone tumors (Table 8). The highest rates of DNA aneuploidy were found in highly malignant OSs (18/21) and FSs (14/16), thus reflecting their poor prognosis. Of six juxtacortical OSs, three well-differentiated parosteal OSs and two periosteal OSs were DNA diploid, whereas one highly malignant surface OS and five highly malignant extraskeletal OSs, all DNA aneuploid, corresponded fully to the medullary OSs. Judging by preliminary results, adjuvant preoperative chemotherapy (COSS 80/82: BÖSING et al. 1987) may reduce the rate of DNA aneuploidy and, consequently, of stem cell heterogeneity in general. A selective destruction of those stemlines that respond particularly to chemotherapy appears probable. In contrast to their high malignancy,

Ewing's sarcomas showed an unexpectedly low proportion of DNA aneuploid stemlines (14/24). The comparatively favorable prognosis of MFH of bone is reflected in a lower rate of aneuploidies (2/10), which is also rather low (probably too low) when compared to our own data from soft tissue MFH (9/19). In agreement with their favorable prognosis, only two of nine CSs with evaluable histograms showed DNA aneuploid stemlines. Both tumors manifested grade III malignancy. The marked increase of DNA aneuploidy among dedifferentiated CSs (9/14) illustrates their increasing malignancy impressively; there was, however, no significant difference between tumors of spindle cell (5/8) and osteosarcomatous (4/6) dedifferentiation. As expected, chondromas were always found to be DNA diploid. The rate of DNA aneuploidy found in recurrence-prone chordomas (6/17) may support the concept of their underlying malignancy despite the low trend to metastasis. Malignant lymphomas with primary bone manifestation showed a close correlation between the grade of malignancy of the different histological subtypes and DNA ploidy. That the bone lymphomas have a comparatively better prognosis than their nodal counterparts with the same histological spectrum may be mainly due to the detection at a lower tumor stage in most cases.

Of particular interest will be the results in osteoblastoma and giant cell tumor of bone, both tumors with occasionally malignant variants. In osteoblastoma we want to distinguish with Dorfman and Weiss (1984) conventional, clinically benign osteoblastoma from an aggressive osteoblastoma growing locally in an aggressive way, but without metastatic spread. One of our two aggressive osteoblastomas was DNA tetraploid, a potential sign of its malignancy; the patient died of his local recurrence. Thus, the term "malignant osteoblastoma" proposed by Schajowicz (1981) for this type appears well justified. Whether and how these malignant osteoblastomas can be differentiated from well-differentiated OSs of low malignancy will be a problem of morphological definition. Among our seven conventional osteoblastomas we found an unexpected DNA aneuploid stemline in two cases. Two explanations appear possible: DNA aneuploidy may not be an absolutely safe marker of malignancy, and so is irrelevant in these cases. However, it appears not unlikely that DNA aneuploidy signals the malignant potential of a lesion – as in malignant nevi of the skin or in the dysplasia of various mucosal epithelia – before it becomes fully manifest. The obvious therapeutic conclusion will be that complete tumor resection is required even in conventional osteoblastomas with apparently benign histology but with potential DNA aneuploidy. In 4 of 18 giant cell tumors, DNA aneuploid stemlines were found within primaries of histologically unsuspicious appearance. Of these four, one patient, after manifest recurrence, has died from extensive metastases; among the remaining three aneuploid tumors, only one has had a recurrence, so far. Although the rates of DNA aneuploidy in our series may be rather too high, the observations made in osteoblastomas and giant cell tumors may illustrate that DNA aneuploidy is a valuable and reliable marker of malignancy, especially in tumors of uncertain status.

Acknowledgment. This work was supported by the Minister für Wissenschaft und Forschung, Nordrhein-Westfalen.

References

Ahuja SC, Villacin AB, Smith J, Bullough PG, Huvos AG (1977) Juxtacortical (parosteal) osteogenic sarcoma. Histological grading and prognosis. J Bone Joint Surg 59A:632–647

Alho A, Connor JF, Mankin HJ, Schiller AL, Crawford JC (1983) Assessment of malignancy of cartilage tumors using flow cytometry. A preliminary report. J Bone Joint Surg 65A:779–785

Allan CJ, Soule EH (1971) Osteogenic sarcoma of the somatic soft tissues. Clinicopathologic study of 26 cases and review of the literature. Cancer 27:1121

Astorino RN, Tesluk H (1985) Dedifferentiated chondrosarcoma with a rhabdomyosarcomatous component. Hum Pathol 16:318–320

Atkin NB, Mattison G, Baker MC (1966) A comparison of the DNA content and chromosome number of fifty human tumors. Br J Cancer 20:87–101

Baisch H, Göhde W, Linden WA (1975) Analysis of PCP data to determine the fraction of cells in the various phases of cell cycle. Radiat Environ Biophys 12:31–39

Barlogie B, Hittelman W, Spitzer G, Trujilla JM, Hart JS, Smallwood L, Drewinko B (1977) Correlation of DNA distribution abnormalities with cytogenetic findings in human adult leukemia and lymphoma. Cancer Res 37:4400–4407

Barlogie B, Latreille J, Freireich EJ, Fu CT, Mellard D, Meistrich M, Andreef M (1980) Characterisation of hematologic malignancies by flow cytometry. Blood Cells 6:719–744

Barlogie B, Raber MN, Schumann J et al. (1983) Flow cytometry in clinical cancer research. Cancer Res 43:3982–3997

Bertoni F, Unni KK, McLeod RA, Dahlin DC (1985) Osteosarcoma resembling osteoblastoma. Cancer 55:416–426

Bösing T, Roessner A, Hiddemann W, Mellin W, Grundmann E (1987) Cytostatic effects in osteosarcomas as detected by flow cytometric DNA analysis after preoperative chemotherapy according to the COSS 80/82 protocol.

Braylan RC, Fowlkes BJ, Jaffé ES, Sanders SK, Berard CW, Herman CJ (1978) Cell volumes and DNA distributions of normal and neoplastic human lymphoid cells. Cancer 41:201–209

Brittinger W (Kiel Lymphoma Study Group) (1981) Principles and present status of a prospective multicenter study on the clinical relevance of the Kiel classification. Blut 43:155–166

Büchner T, Bloomfield CD, Hiddemann W, Hossfeld DK, Schumann J (1985) Tumor aneuploidy. Springer, Berlin Heidelberg New York

Costa A, Mazzini G, Del Bino G, Silvestrini R (1981) DNA content and kinetic characteristics of non-Hodgkin's lymphoma: determined by flow cytometry and autoradiography. Cytometry 2:185–188

Cuvelier CA, Roels HJ (1979) Cytophotometric studies of the nuclear DNA content in cartilaginous tumors. Cancer 4:1363–1374

Dahlin DC, Unni KK (1986) Bone tumors. General aspects and data on 8,542 cases. Charles C. Thomas, Springfield, pp 269–321, 357–366

Dahlin DC, Cupps RE, Johnson EW Jr (1970) Giant cell tumor: a study of 195 cases. Cancer 25:1061–1070

Darzynkiewicz Z, Traganos F, Andreeff M, Sharpless T, Melamed MR (1979) Different sensitivity of chromatin to acid denaturation in quiescent and cycling cells as revealed by flow cytometry. J Histochem Cytochem 27:478

Dean PN, Jett JH (1974) Mathematical analysis of DNA distributions derived from flow microfluorometry. J Cell Biol 60:523–527

Diamond LW, Braylan RC (1980) Flow analysis of DNA content and cell size in non-Hodgkin's lymphoma. Cancer Res 40:703–712

Diamond LW, Nathwani BN, Rappaport H (1982) Flow cytometry in the diagnosis and classification of malignant lymphoma and leukemia. Cancer 50:1122–1135

Dittrich W, Göhde W (1969) Impulsfluorometrie bei Einzelzellen in Suspension. Z Naturforsch 24[B]:360

Dorfman HD (1972) Malignant transformation of benign bone lesions. Seventh National Cancer Conference Proceedings 901–913

Dorfman HD, Weiss SW (1984) Borderline osteoblastic tumors: problems in the differential diagnosis of aggressive osteoblastoma and low-grade osteosarcoma. Semin Diagn Pathol 1:215–234

Dumont J, Mazabraud A (1979) Primary lymphoma of bone: histological review of 75 cases according to the new classification of non-Hodgkin's lymphomas. Biomedicine 31:271–275

Edeiken J, Hodes P (1973) Roentgen diagnosis of diseases of bone, 2nd edn. Williams & Wilkins, Baltimore, pp 998–999

Enzinger FM (1977) Recent developments in the classification of soft tissue sarcomas. In: Management of primary bone and soft tissue sarcomas. Year Book Medical Publishers, Chicago

Enzinger FM, Weiss SW (1983) Soft tissue tumors. C.V. Mosby, St. Louis, pp 166–198

Erlandson RA, Tandler B, Liebermann HP, Higinbotham NL (1968) Ultrastructure of human chordoma. Cancer Res 28:2115–2125

Feldman F, Lattes R (1977) Primary malignant fibrous histiocytoma (fibrous xanthoma) of bone. Skeletal Radiol 1:145–160

Feldman F, Norman D (1972) Intra- and extraosseous malignant histioma (malignant fibrous xanthoma). Radiology 104:497–508

Franke HD (1972) Die Anwendung strahlensensibilisierender Substanzen in der Strahlentherapie. Strahlentherapie 143:296

Friedmann I, Harrison DFN, Bird ES (1962) The fine structure chordoma with particular reference to the physaliferous cell. J Clin Pathol 15:116–125

Frindel E, Tubiana M (1971) Radiobiology and the cell cycle. In: Baserga R (ed) The Cell cycle and cancer. Marcel Dekker, New York, pp 391–447

Gee VR, Pugh DG (1958) Giant cell tumour of bone. Radiology 70:33–41

Gelfant S (1977) A new concept of tissue and tumor cell proliferation. Cancer Res 27:3845

Goldenberg RP, Campbell CJ, Bonfiglio M (1970) Giant cell tumor of bone. An analysis of 218 cases. J Bone Joint Surg 52A:619–664

Gresen AA, Dahlin DC, Peterson CFA, Payne WSP (1973) "Benign" giant cell tumor of bone metastasizing to the lung. Ann Thorac Surg 16:531–535

Grundmann E, Mellin W, Roessner A, Hiddemann W, Vollmer E, Edel G, Lingg G (1985) Zur Klassifikation und Prognose der Osteosarkome im Erfahrungsgut des Knochengeschwulstregisters Westfalen unter Einbezug proliferationskinetischer Parameter. Dtsch Ges Osteol 221–226

Hagemeister FB, Raber M, Barlogie B, Maddox A, Cabanillas F (1981) Flow cytometry analysis in lymphoma: effect of abnormal DNA content. Proc Am Assoc Cancer Res 22:42+

Hammarberg C, Slezak P, Tribukait B (1984) Early detection of malignancy in ulcerative colitis. A flow cytometric study. Cancer 53:291–295

Hedley DW, Friedländer ML, Taylor JW, Rugg CA, Musgrove EA (1983) Method for analysis of cellular DNA content of paraffin-embedded pathological material using flow cytometry. J Histochem Cytochem 31:1333–1335

Hedley DW, Friedländer ML, Taylor IW (1985) Application of DNA flow cytometry to paraffin-embedded archival material for the study of aneuploidy and its clinical significance. Cytometry 6:327–333

Heliö H, Karaharju E, Nordling S (1985) Flow cytometric determination of DNA content in malignant and benign bone tumors. Cytometry 6:165–171

Hiddemann W, Roessner A, Wörmann B et al. (1987) Tumor heterogeneity in osteosarcoma as identified by flow cytometry. Cancer 59:324–328

Huvos AG (1976) Primary malignant fibrous histiocytoma of bone. Clinico-pathologic study of 18 patients. NY State J Med 76:552–559

Huvos AG (1979) Bone tumors: diagnosis, treatment and prognosis. Saunders, Philadelphia, pp 94–106

Inada O, Yumoto T, Furuse K, Tanaka T (1976) Ultrastructural features of malignant fibrous histiocytoma of bone. Acta Pathol Jpn 24:491–501

Jaffé HL, Lichtenstein L, Portis RB (1940) Giant cell tumor of bone. Its pathologic appearance, grading, supposed variants and treatment. Arch Pathol 30:993–1031

Johnson WW, Cobrun TP, Pratt CB, Smith JW, Kumar APM, Dahlin DC (1978) Ultrastructure of MFH arising in the acromion. Hum Pathol 9:199–209

Jürgens H (1981) Ewing-Sarkom bei Kindern und Jugendlichen: Planung einer kooperativen Therapiestudie der Gesellschaft für Pädiatrische Onkologie (CESS 81). Klin Pädiat 193:254–257

Jürgens H, Göbel V, Michaelis J et al. (1985) Die kooperative Ewing-Sarkom Studie CESS 81 der GPO-Analyse nach 4 Jahren. Klin Pädiatr 1978:225–232

Katenkamp D, Stiller D (1981) Malignant fibrous histiocytoma of bone. Light microscopic and electron microscopic examination of four cases. Virchows Arch [A] 391:323–335
Kreicbergs A, Zetterberg A, Söderberg G (1980) The prognostic significance of nuclear DNA content in human chondrosarcoma. Analy Quant Cytol Histol 2:272–279
Kreicbergs A, Boquist L, Borssen B, Larsson S-E (1982) Prognostic factors in chondrosarcoma. A comparative study of cellular DNA content and clinicopathologic features. Cancer 50:57–583
Kreicbergs A, Silfverswärd C, Tribukait B (1984) Flow DNA analysis of primary bone tumors. Relationship between cellular DNA content and histopathologic classification. Cancer 53:129–136
Krishan A (1975) Rapid flow cytophotometric analysis of mammalian cell cycle by propidium iodide staining. J Cell Biol 66:18
Krishan A (1976) Effect of adriamycine on the cell cycle traverse and kinetics of cultured lymphoblasts. Cancer Res 36:143
Krishan A, Palka KD, Frei E (1976) Cell cycle synchronisation of human lymphoid cells in vitro by 2,3-dihydro-1H-imidazo(1,2-b) pyrazole. Cancer Res 38:138
Krug H (1977) Der Wert der Impulszytophotometrie in der klinischen Onkologie. Acta Histochem [Suppl] 19:167–172
Llombart-Bosch A, Blache R, Peydro-Olaya A (1982) Roundcell sarcomas of bone and their differential diagnosis (with particular emphasis on Ewing's sarcoma and reticulosarcoma). Pathol Annu 17(2):113–145
Macartney JC, Camplejohn RS (1986) DNA flow cytometry of histological material from dysplastic lesions of human gastric mucosa. J Pathol 150:113–118
Mankin HJ, Connor JF, Schiller AL, Perlmutter N, Alho A, McGuire M (1985) Grading of bone tumors by analysis of nuclear DNA content using flow cytometry. J Bone Joint Surg 67A:404–413
Martinez-Tello FJ, Navas-Palacios JJ, Calvo-Asensio M, Loizaga Iriondo JM (1981) Malignant fibrous histiocytoma of bone. A clinico-pathological and electron-microscopical study. Pathol Res Pract 173:141–158
Mellin W (1986) Möglichkeiten und Grenzen zytophotometrischer Meßverfahren bei der Untersuchung von Tumoren und Präkanzerosen. MD-GBK: Mitteilungsdienst – Gesellschaft zur Bekämpfung der Krebskrankheiten NRW 49:46–49
Mellin W, Grundmann E (1989) Flow cytometric analysis of stemline heterogeneity. Pathol Res Pract 184:6–10
Mellin W, Roessner A, Wörmann B, Vollmer E, Hiddemann W, Grundmann E (1984) Evaluation of dignity in metastasizing giant cell tumors of bone by flow cytometric DNA analysis. Verh Dtsch Ges Pathol 68:220–223
Mellin W, Wörmann B, Roessner A, Hiddemann W, Immenkamp M, Grundmann E (1985a) Biological characterisation of human bone tumors. VII. Detection of malignancy in a giant cell tumor of bone by flow cytometric DNA analysis. Pathol Res Pract 180:619–625
Mellin W, Roessner A, Ritter J, Sapp H, Grundmann G (1985b) Zur durchflußzytophotometrischen DNA-Analyse des Ewing-Sarkoms. Verh Dtsch Ges Pathol 69:606
Mellin W, Davaris P, Jütte G, Heidl G, Krieg V, Grundmann E (1986a) Comparative flow cytometrical analysis of DNA and CEA in gastric carcinomas. Verh Dtsch Ges Pathol 70:234–237
Mellin W, Roessner A, Immenkamp M, Boeddinghaus D, Grundmann E (1986b) Klassifikation und Differentialdiagnose der juxtakortikalen Osteosarkome. Pathologe 7:94–100
Mellin W, Roessner A, Grundmann E (1986c) Flow cytometric DNA analysis of malignant fibrous histiocytoma of bone. Deutscher Krebskongress 1986. J Cancer Res Clin Oncol [Suppl] 111:149
Mellin W, Roessner A, Pill C, Edel G, Grundmann E (1987a) Durchflußzytophotometrische DNA-Analyse an Osteoblastomen. Verh Dtsch Ges Path (in press)
Mellin W, Roessner A, Schöneich U, Vollmer E, Grundmann E (1987b) Durchflußzytophotometrische DNA-Analyse an Chordomen. Verh Dtsch Ges Pathol (in press)
Mikuz G, Mydla F (1974) Elektronenmikroskopische und zytophotometrische Untersuchungen des Chordoms. Verh Dtsch Ges Pathol 58:447–453
Mikuz G, Mydla F, Gütter W (1977) Chordoma: ultrastructural, biochemical and cytophotometric findings. Beitr Pathol 161:150–165
Mnaymneh WA, Dudley HR, Mnaymneh LG (1964) Giant cell tumor of bone. An analysis and follow-up study of the 41 cases observed at the Massachusetts General Hospital between 1925 and 1960. J Bone Joint Surg 46A:63–79
Murad TM, Murthy MSN (1970) Ultrastructure of chordoma. Cancer 25:1204–1215

Niezabitowski A, Edel G, Roessner A, Timm C, Wuisman P, Grundmann E (1987) Rhabdomyosarcomatous component in dedifferentiated chondrosarcoma. Pathol Res Pract 182:275–279
Ozzello L, Stout AP, Murray MR (1963) Cultural characteristics of malignant histiocytomas and fibrous xanthomas. Cancer 16:331
Pena CE, Horvat BL, Fisher ER (1970) The ultrastructure of a chordoma. Am J Clin Pathol 53:544–551
Pfitzer P (1985) The karyological basis of atypia. Pathol Res Pract 180:675–681
Rao U, Cheng A, Didolkar MS (1978) Extraosseous osteogenic sarcoma. Cancer 41:1488
Rock MG, Pritchard DJ, Unni KK (1984) Metastases from histologically benign giant cell tumor of bone. J Bone Joint Surg 66A:263–273
Roessner A (1984) Zur Zyto- und Histogenese der malignen und semimalignen Knochentumoren. Gustav-Fischer, Stuttgart New York
Roessner A, Hobik HP, Grundmann E (1979) Malignant fibrous histiocytoma of bone and osteosarcoma. A comparative light and electron microscopic study. Pathol Res Pract 164:385–401
Rosen G, Caparros B, Nirenberg A et al. (1981) Ewing's sarcoma: ten-year experience with adjuvant chemotherapy. Cancer 47:2204–2213
Salzer-Kuntschik M, Brand G, Delling G (1983a) Bestimmung des morphologischen Regressionsgrades nach Chemotherapie bei malignen Knochentumoren. Pathologe 4:135–141
Salzer-Kuntschik M, Delling G, Beron G, Sigmund R (1983b) Morphological grades of regression in osteosarcoma after polychemotherapy – study COSS 80. J Cancer Res Clin Oncol [Suppl] 106:2124
Sandberg AA (1980) The chromosomes in human cancer and leukemia. Elsevier/North Holland, New York
Sandritter W, Grimm H (1977) DNA in non-Hodgkin's lymphoma – a cytophotometric study. Beitr Pathol 160:213–230
Schajowicz F (1981) Tumors and tumorlike lesions of bone and joints. Springer, Berlin Heidelberg New York
Schajowicz F, Lemos C (1976) Malignant osteoblastoma. J Bone Joint Surg 588:202–211
Schajowicz F, Ackermann LV, Sissons HA (1972) Histological typing of bone tumours. Int histol classif of tumours No. 6, WHO, Geneva
Schutte B, Reynders MMJ, Bosman FT, Blijham GH (1985) Flow cytometric determination of DNA ploidy level in nuclei isolated from paraffin-embedded tissue. Cytometry 6:26–30
Shackney SE, Skramstadt KS (1979) A dynamic interpretation of multiparameter studies in human lymphomas. Am J Clin Pathol 72:756–764
Shackney SE, Skramstadt KS, Cunningham RE, Dugas DJ, Lincoln TL, Lukes RJ (1980) Dual parameter flow cytometry studies in human lymphomas. J Clin Invest 66:1281–1294
Shackney SE, Levine AM, Fisher RI et al. (1984) The biology of tumor growth in the non-Hodgkin's lymphomas. A dual parameter flow cytometry study of 220 cases. J Clin Invest 73:1201–1214
Silvestrini R, Piazza R, Riccardi A, Rilke F (1977) Correlation of cell kinetic findings with morphology of non-Hodgkin's malignant lymphomas. J Natl Cancer Inst 58:499–504
Sinclair W (1972) Cell cycle dependence of the lethal radiatic response in mammalian cells. Curr Top Radiation Res 7:264
Spanier SS (1977) Malignant fibrous histiocytoma of bone. Orthop Clin North Am 8:947–961
Spjut H, Luse SA (1964) Chordoma: an electron microscopic study. Cancer 17:643–656
Stenzinger W, Suter I, Schumann J (1984) DNA aneuploidy in congenital melanocytic nevi: suggestive evidence for premalignant changes. J Invest Dermatol 82:569–572
Tobey RA, Crissmann HA (1972) Use of flow microfluorometry in detailed analysis of effects of chemical agents on cell cycle progression. Cancer Res 32:2726–2732
Unni KK, Dahlin DC, Beabout JW (1976a) Periosteal osteogenic sarcoma. Cancer 37:2476–2485
Unni KK, Dahlin DC, Beabout JW, Ivins JC (1976b) Parosteal osteogenic sarcoma. Cancer 37:2466–2475
Unni KK, Dahlin DC, McLeod RA, Pritchard DJ (1977) Intraosseous well-differentiated osteosarcoma. Cancer 40:1337–1347
Vassallo J, Roessner A, Vollmer E, Grundmann E (1987a) Malignant lymphomas with primary bone manifestation. Pathol Res Pract 182:381–384
Vassallo J, Mellin W, Pill C, Roessner A, Grundmann E (1987b) Flow cytometric DNA analysis of malignant lymphomas with primary bone manifestation. J Cancer Res Clin Oncol 113:249–252

Vollmer E, Roessner A, Gerdes J, Mellin W, Stein H, Chong-Schachel S, Grundmann E (1986) Improved grading of bone tumors with the monoclonal antibody Ki-67. J Cancer Res Clin Oncol 112:281–282

Williams AH, Schwinn CP, Parker JW (1976) The ultrastructure of osteosarcoma – a review of 20 cases. Cancer 37:1293

Willnow U (1982) Autoradiographic in vitro study of the cell kinetics of osteogenic sarcomas and Ewing's sarcomas in children. Arch Geschwulstforsch 52:9–16

Winkler K, Beron G, Kotz R et al. (1983) Adjuvant chemotherapy in osteosarcoma. Effects of Cis-platinum, BCD and fibroblast interferon in sequential combination with DH/MTX and adriamycin. Preliminary results of the COSS-80 study. J Cancer Res Clin Oncol [Suppl] 106:1–7

Winkler K, Beron G, Kotz R et al. (1984) Neoadjuvant chemotherapy for osteogenic sarcoma: results of a cooperative German/Austrian study. J Clin Oncol 2:6

Wold LE, Unni KK, Beabout JW, Pritchard DJ (1984) Highgrade surface osteosarcomas. Am J Surg Pathol 8:181–186

Steroid Receptors and Giant Cell Tumor of Bone

L.E. Wold, T. Spelsberg, N. Jiang, and F. Sim

1 Introduction . . . 153
1.1 Historical Perspectives on Giant Cell Tumor of Bone . . . 153
1.2 Steroid Receptors in Bone and Soft Tissue Tumors . . . 156
1.3 Steroid Receptors in Giant Cell Tumor of Bone . . . 156
1.3.1 Clinical Data Relating to Theoretical Possibility of Steroid Receptors Playing a Role in Giant Cell Tumor . . . 156
1.3.2 Experimental Data: Histochemical Techniques . . . 157
1.3.3 Experimental Data: Immunohistochemical Techniques . . . 157
1.3.4 Experimental Data: Biochemical Techniques . . . 158
2 Analysis of Methods for Determination of Steroid Receptors . . . 159
2.1 Histochemical Techniques . . . 159
2.2 Immunohistochemical Techniques . . . 160
2.3 Biochemical Techniques . . . 161
3 Summary and Conclusion . . . 162
References . . . 162

1 Introduction

1.1 Historical Perspectives on Giant Cell Tumor of Bone

Jaffe and co-workers defined the specific criteria for the diagnosis of giant cell tumor of bone in 1940. Although giant cells are nearly ubiquitous in bone tumors and tumor-like conditions, giant cell tumor of bone is a unique clinical-radiographic-pathological entity (Fig. 1) which is characterized by (1) female predominance, (2) peak incidence in the third and fourth decades of life, and (3) propensity to involve the long bones in the epiphyseal and metaphyseal location. Pathologically, the major diagnostic criteria include the presence of mononuclear stromal cells which are oval or polygonal, containing round or oval vesicular nuclei. Multinucleated giant cells are scattered approximately uniformly throughout the lesion and the nuclei of these multinucleated giant cells are nearly identical morphologically to the mononuclear stromal cells of the tumor. The tumor shows no evidence of matrix production (Fig. 2). Extensive morphometric, cell culture, and histochemical techniques have been employed in an effort to define the relationship of the mononuclear stromal cells to the multinucleated giant cells of this lesion. These techniques have also been used to speculate regarding the cell of origin of the lesion.

Sophisticated cell culture techniques have been extensively employed to study giant cell tumors of bone. In primary cultures of mechanically and enzymatically dispersed giant cell tumors, the multinucleated giant cells quickly become nonvi-

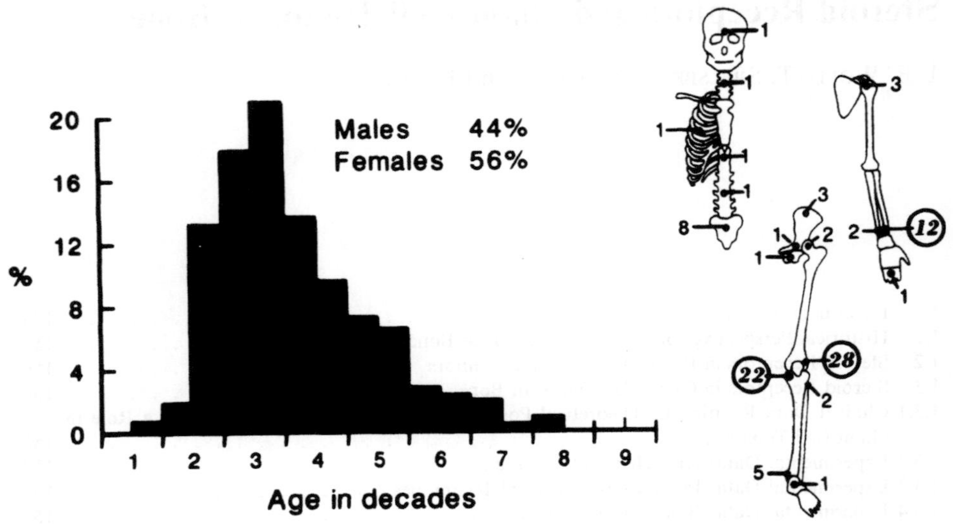

Fig. 1. Skeletal distribution for giant cell tumor

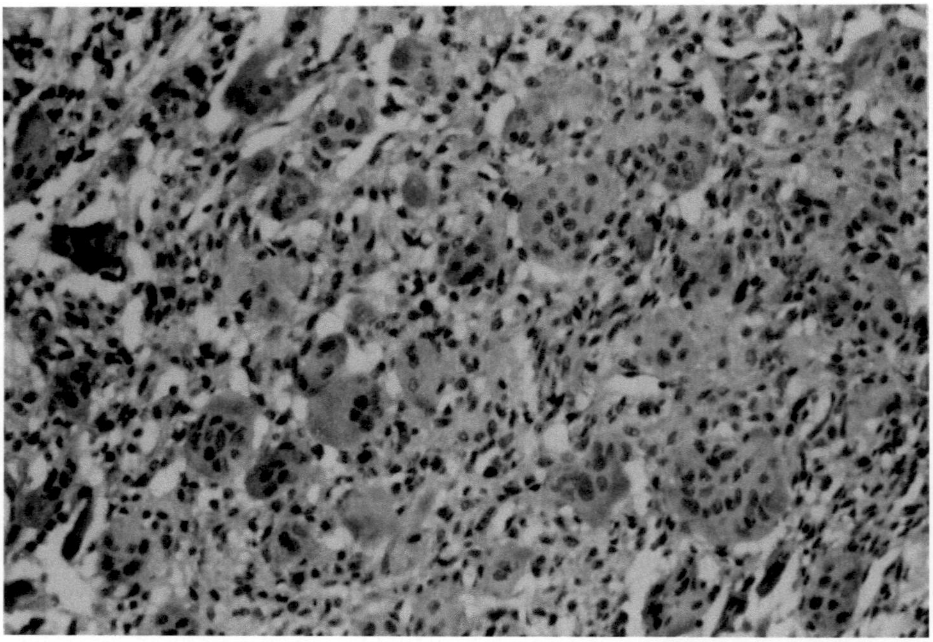

Fig. 2. Photomicrograph of giant cell tumor showing characteristic sea of mononuclear cells within which multinucleated giant cells are identified uniformly scattered through the lesion. No matrix production is identified by the stromal cells

able (GOLDRING et al. 1977, 1978, 1979, 1986; GALLARDO et al. 1970). Although several tumors have been maintained in long-term cultures (GOLDRING et al. 1986), after passage to secondary and subsequent cultures, the multinucleated giant cells have not been identified. BYERS et al. (1975) also failed to detect multinucleated giant cells when mononuclear cells from giant cell tumor were injected into and grown in nude mice. Organ culture techniques, utilizing 2- and 3-mm fragments of tumor (GOLDRING et al. 1986), have demonstrated that the multinucleated giant cells may survive for up to 6–8 weeks. However, their viability was apparently related to the presence of the tissue fragment as removal of the fragment resulted in loss of multinucleated giant cells from the culture. Some investigators have identified the formation of multinucleated giant cells from mononuclear cells, if the appropriate culture medium was used (GALLARDO et al. 1970; WIENTROUB et al. 1982).

Histochemical techniques have also been used to study giant cell tumors. The multinucleated giant cells in giant cell tumor have been noted to be rich in acid phosphatase (APARISI et al. 1977; JEFFREE and PRICE 1965). Lysozyme production has also been demonstrated in cell cultures of giant cell tumor (SCHAJOWICZ 1961; GORDON et al. 1974). These features have suggested a macrophage or monocytic origin for the lesion.

The presence of other macrophage "markers" has also been investigated. Immunohistochemical techniques have been utilized to detect the presence of lysozyme and α_1-antitrypsin in giant cell tumors (LING et al. 1986). The presence of F_c receptors (GOLDRING et al. 1986; UGOLINI et al. 1980; WOOD et al. 1978) and the functional ability of cells to phagocytize India ink particles (GOLDRING et al. 1986) have also been used in an effort to identify macrophage characteristics in giant cell tumor. Although cultured cells and the multinucleated giant cells in giant cell tumor show some similarity to macrophages, they show quantitative differences in these features and are thus distinct from this phagocytic system. Other studies (BYERS et al. 1975; GOLDRING et al. 1984; WOOD et al. 1978) have likewise concluded that macrophage markers are present on the minority of mononuclear cells in giant cell tumor. Although the cell of origin for giant cell tumor remains unknown, more is known about the response of these tumors, or cultures of them, to various hormones.

Reports have demonstrated that cultures of giant cell tumor respond to parathyroid hormone with increased production of cyclic AMP (GOLDRING et al. 1977; GOLDRING et al. 1978). Small increases in cyclic AMP production have also been identified after incubation with calcitonin (GOLDRING et al. 1986). In addition, autoradiographic techniques have been used to demonstrate calcitonin receptors (GOLDRING et al. 1986) on some of the cells. Cultured cells from giant cell tumor, when incubated with PGE_2 (GOLDRING et al. 1986), have also shown an increase in the cyclic AMP content. In spite of this biochemical suggestion that parathyroid hormone, calcitonin, and PGE_2 may bind to "receptors" and giant cell tumor, GOLDRING and co-workers did not note any morphological changes in the cultured cells or increased survivial when cultured cells were exposed to any of these substances (GOLDRING et al. 1986).

Finally, the proliferative effect of estrogen on cell cultures from giant cell tumor has also been studied (GOLDRING et al. 1986). One patient in this study experienced a rapid growth of her tumor during the last trimester of her pregnancy. Observations like this, as well as the female predilection and occurrence in the "child-bearing" years, have suggested to some that giant cell tumors may be hormonally responsive via receptors. Goldring et al. (1986), however, failed to demonstrate any effect of estrogen on "cell growth or replication."

1.2 Steroid Receptors in Bone and Soft Tissue Tumors

Steroid receptors have been identified in a variety of human neoplasms utilizing biochemical techniques. Although the majority of tumors classified as receptor positive have their origin in tissues which are known to be hormonally responsive, some preliminary reports have also suggested that mesenchymal tissues and mesenchymal tumors may also have steroid receptors (Weiss et al. 1986; Bracaglia et al. 1982; Brentoni et al. 1983; Choudhuri et al. 1980, 1981; Walker et al. 1980). Some of these mesenchymal lesions have also shown apparent response to hormonal manipulative therapy (Kinzbrunner et al. 1983; Banner et al. 1981; Gloor et al. 1982; McCarty et al. 1980). However, in general the concentration at which estrogen and progesterone receptors have been identified in mesenchymal lesions has been significantly less than that seen for receptor positive tumors of the breast, endometrium, or ovary. The clinically recognized phenomenon that some soft tissue tumors develop during periods of changing hormonal status (Weiss et al. 1986) has lent further credence to the possibility of mesenchymal lesions being estrogen and progesterone receptor positive. This is particularly true with respect to neurofibromas in von Recklinghausen's disease and aggressive fibromatosis of the desmoid type (McDougall and Garity 1979). Lymphangiomyomatosis occurs almost exclusively in women and has been successfully treated with hormonal manipulation, as has endolymphatic stromal myosis. The largest series in the literature (Weiss et al. 1986; Choudhuri et al. 1980) indicate an overall rate of estrogen receptor positivity of between 18% and 24%.

1.3 Steroid Receptors in Giant Cell Tumor of Bone

1.3.1 Clinical Data Relating to Theoretical Possibility of Steroid Receptors Playing a Role in Giant Cell Tumor

Although the majority of bone tumors and tumor-like conditions are more common in males than in females, giant cell tumor has a marked female predilection (Fig. 1). This tumor also has its peak incidence in the third and fourth decades of life, in the child-bearing years when hormonal changes play a central role in the female's life. Giant cell tumors have been clinically seen to change dramatically during pregnancy as well (Goldring et al. 1986). Response to endocrine manipulative therapy has not been noted. Nor have giant cell tumors been noted to fluctuate in size with the menstrual cycle. However, given these clinical data, some have suggested that giant cell tumors may, in fact, be estrogen and progesterone receptor positive lesions.

1.3.2 Experimental Data: Histochemical Techniques

MALAWER et al. (1984) have utilized commercially available reagents to investigate giant cell tumor for hormone receptors. In their study, five cases of giant cell tumor were analyzed for estrogen and progesterone receptors utilizing commercially availabel reagents (Zeus Scientific Incorporated, Raritan, New Jersey). These histochemical reagents consisted of 17β-estrodial–6-carboxy-methyoxime–bovine serum albumin–fluorescein–isothiocyanate and 11α-hydroxyprogesterone–hemisuccinate–bovine serum albumin–tetramethylrhodamine–isothiocyanate. Three of the five tumors studied showed intense cytoplasmic fluorescence of nearly all stromal cells and the remaining two tumors showed only mild fluorescence with reagents used to investigate the estrogen receptor. In contrast, three of the five patients showed some fluorescence of stromal cells with the reagents utilized to demonstrate progesterone receptor. Both of the tumors in which standard cytosolic assays for estrogen and progesterone receptors were done were negative. These results suggested to MALAWER et al. (1984) the presence of cytoplasmic binding sites for estrogen and progesterone in the stromal cells of giant cell tumors. However, the authors did recognize that the binding may not have been to high affinity type I receptors. In addition, they noted an absence of staining of the multinucleated giant cells with reagents used to demonstrate estrogen receptors. WEISS et al. (1986) subsequently utilized these same histochemical reagents on one case of giant cell tumor in an 11-year-old male and failed to identify convincing positive staining. In addition, they analyzed 32 other soft tissue and bony tumors utilizing these reagents and concluded that the procedure "seems unreliable and was responsible for an unacceptable number of both false positives and false negatives" (WEISS et al. 1986). In our hands, these reagents have only shown cytoplasmic reactivity which was not inhibitable by estrogen or progesterone analogs.

1.3.3 Experimental Data: Immunohistochemical Techniques

Recently, monoclonal antibodies to the estrogen receptor (GREENE et al. 1980) have been developed. A major advantage of the monoclonal antireceptor methodology for estrogen receptor determination is that the method does not require functional preservation of the receptor molecule. Commercially available reagents (Abbott Laboratories, Chicago, Illinois) have been marketed for use with frozen tissues and some studies have been performed utilizing formalin-fixed, paraffin-embedded tissue (SHIMADA et al. 1985; SHINTAKU and SAID 1987). This methodology has, in general, shown a favorable comparison with the biochemical techniques for estrogen receptor determination in a series of breast carcinomas which have been studied. Although early studies utilizing monoclonal antibodies to the estrogen receptor were both cytoplasmic and nuclear staining (GARANCIS et al. 1983), the majority of studies have shown an exclusive nuclear location for the estrogen receptor protein (SHIMADA et al. 1985; PRESS et al. 1985; POUSEN et al. 1985; GREENE et al. 1984). This difference in location of the receptor as determined by histochemical and the immunohistochemical monoclonal antibody techniques emphasizes the difference in these two assays.

WEISS and co-workers, in a study of 33 bone and soft tissue tumors, failed to identify any estrogen receptor positive lesions utilizing the commercially available antiestrogen receptor monoclonal antibody (WEISS et al. 1986). This included the six mesenchymal tumors which were classified as estrogen receptor positive on the basis of dextran-coated charcoal biochemical assays. In that study, the single case of giant cell tumor which was investigated was not positive with the immunohistochemical technique.

1.3.4 Experimental Data: Biochemical Techniques

Three biochemical techniques have been utilized in an effort to determine whether giant cell tumors are steroid receptor positive lesions. These include (1) the enzyme immunoassay on cytosolic extracts using the monoclonal kit marketed by Abbott (Abbott Laboratories, Chicago, Illinois), (2) the standard dextran-coated charcoal assay, and (3) a new biopsy nuclear binding assay developed by SPELSBERG et al. (1984). The enzyme immunoassay utilizes a double monoclonal antibody technique with antibodies directed at the estrogen receptor and an enzymatic indicator system. The dextran-coated charcoal assay utilizes a homogenate of tissue and radiolabeled steroid with a Scatchard plot analysis (Fig. 3). The biopsy nuclear binding assay utilizes a suspension of cells and radiolabeled steroid analog (Fig. 4).

The enzyme immunoassay has been reported on one giant cell tumor studied by WEISS et al. (1986). This tumor was defined as positive utilizing this assay

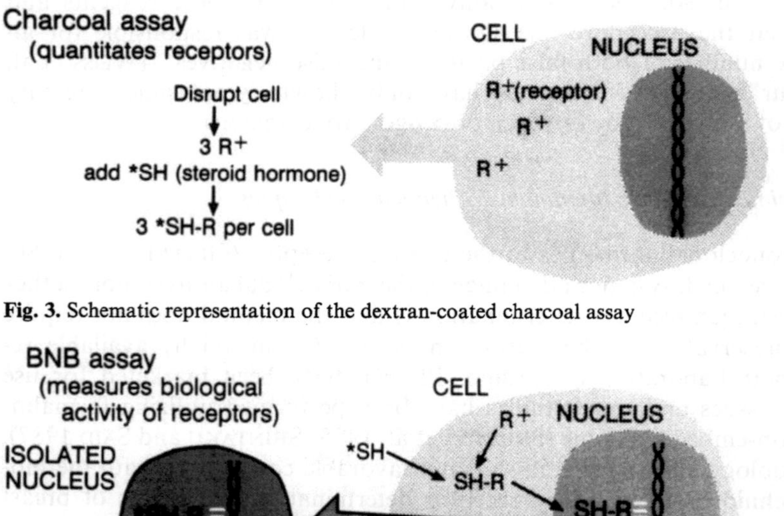

Fig. 3. Schematic representation of the dextran-coated charcoal assay

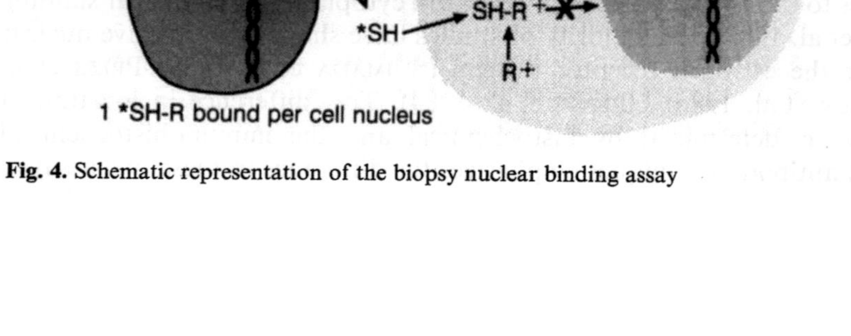

Fig. 4. Schematic representation of the biopsy nuclear binding assay

Table 1. Results of chemical analysis (dextran-coated charcoal assay methodologies) of giant cell tumors for steroid receptors

Patient	References	ER (fmol/mg protein)	PR (fmol/mg protein)
1	Patient 3, 5	–	–
2	Patient 4, 5	–	–
3	Patient 48, 2	–	24.6
4		–	–
5		–	–
6		–	–
7		–	–
8		–	–
9		–	–

ER, estrogen receptor; *PR*, progesterone receptor

with an absolute concentration of 19.4 fmol/mg protein. In addition, this tumor was also progesterone receptor positive by dextran-coated charcoal assay (24.6 fmol/mg protein), but was negative for the estrogen receptor on the basis of the dextran-coated charcoal assay.

In contrast to the single case which has been reported utilizing the enzyme immunoassay, the body of information regarding steroid receptors which has been tabulated utilizing standard dextran-coated charcoal assay methodologies has shown uniform negative results for the estrogen receptor. These results are summarized in Table 1. In only one case reported in the literature (i.e., that mentioned above) has a low level of progesterone receptor been identified in giant cell tumor utilizing dextran-coated charcoal assay.

The biopsy nuclear binding assay for estrogen receptor has been done on 11 samples from eight patients with giant cell tumors (Wold et al. 1986). In only one of the eight tumors were low levels of receptor apparently identified. However, in this tumor it was at the borderline between the definition of negative and positive results. The biopsy nuclear binding assay for progesterone receptor has been done on eight samples of giant cell tumors from six patients. Four of the patients' tumors showed low level of progesterone receptor by this assay. Androgen receptors have been studied in two cases of giant cell tumor (one female and one male patient) and neither tumor was positive.

2 Analysis of Methods for Determination of Steroid Receptors

2.1 Histochemical Techniques

Fluorescently labeled estrogen and progesterone bovine serum albumin conjugates have been employed quite widely in the past for estrogen and progesterone receptor determinations (Penny and Hawkins 1982; Pertschuk et al. 1980; Lee 1978, 1984; Lee and Markland 1979). Although these reagents utilize frozen sections in which the receptor presumably remains functional, consider-

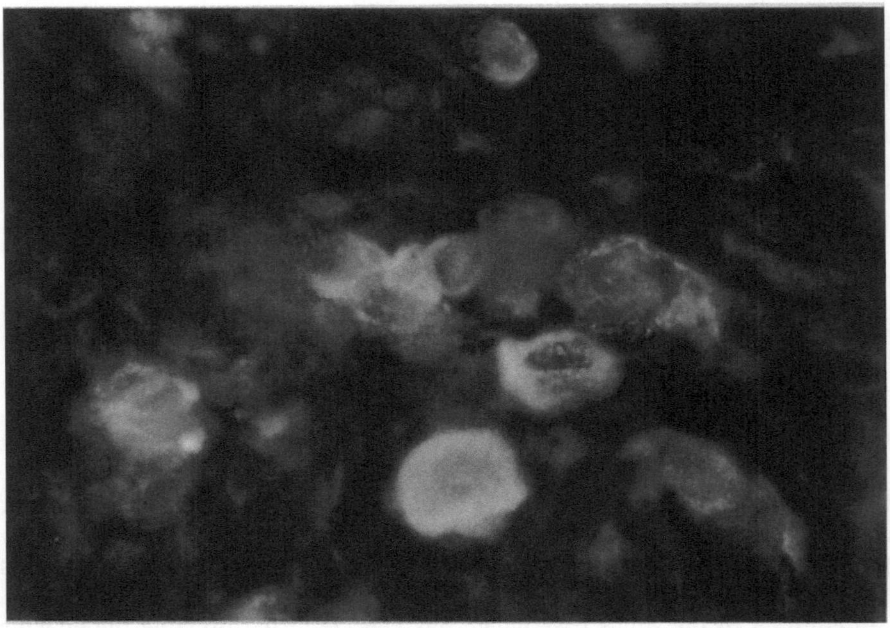

Fig. 5. Although apparent cytoplasmic estrogen and progesterone receptors have been identified with histochemical reagents, inhibition of this staining by estrogen and progesterone has been variable and these reagents probably identify type II receptors rather than high affinity type I receptors (Fluorescent reagents for estrogen receptor, Zeuss Scientific, Raritan, New Jersey)

able controversy exists regarding whether they correlate with standard chemical determinations (PANKO et al. 1982; LEE 1984). Some authors have noted considerable inter- and intraobserver variability with respect to the interpretation of these stains (WEISS et al. 1986). In our experience, although cytoplasmic fluorescence has been identified in tumors known to contain estrogen and progesterone receptors by biochemical techniques (Fig. 5), inhibition of staining has not been possible with estrogen or progesterone analogs.

MCCARTY et al. (1980) have likewise concluded that these reagents probably do not identify type I receptors. The earlier reports by MALAWER et al. (1984) regarding receptor positivity in giant cell tumor should be interpreted in light of this information. As these authors pointed out in their discussion, the apparent cytoplasmic staining with histochemical reagents does not "indicate if these sites are high affinity (type I) estrogen/progesterone receptors...." Such histochemical techniques must, therefore, be considered suspect with respect to the identification of true high affinity, type I receptors in giant cell tumor.

2.2 Immunohistochemical Techniques

The monoclonal antibody assay to the estrogen receptor has been widely used to identify estrogen receptors in fixed frozen tissue (PRESS and GREENE 1984;

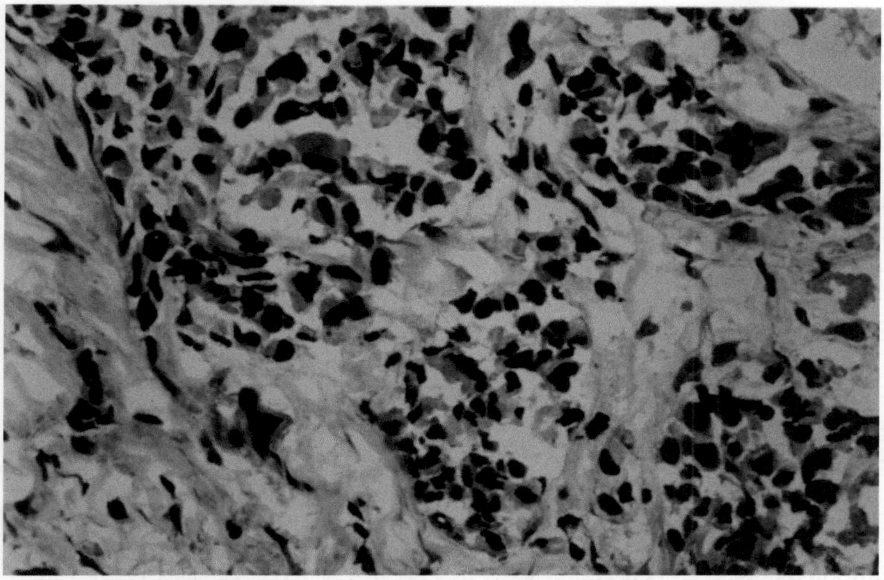

Fig. 6. Immunohistochemical techniques utilizing monoclonal antibodies to the estrogen (estrophilin) can be used with fixed frozen sections and show strong nuclear positivity in tumors known to contain estrogen receptor, as in this case of breast carcinoma. No cases of giant cell tumor have been reported which are estrogen receptor positive utilizing this technique

PRESS et al. 1984), as well as formalin-fixed, paraffin-embedded tissue (SHINTAKU and SAID 1987; SHIMADA et al. 1985). These reagents yield good positive results with tumors known to be receptor positive by biochemical methods (Fig. 6). Few giant cell tumors have been investigated utilizing these techniques, and no positive results have been reported. The excellent qualitative agreement between the immunohistochemical technique and standard chemical assays for the estrogen receptor reported by some authors (SHIMADA et al. 1985; KING et al. 1985; KING and WEIGARD 1986; MCCARTY et al. 1985; DEGEOIJ and BOSMAN 1986; PERTSCHUK et al. 1985) tends to validate that this technique does identify high affinity type I receptors. In addition, favorable agreement between monoclonal immunohistochemical assays and clinical responsiveness to hormonal manipulation has also been reported (MCCLELLAND et al. 1986). Therefore, on the basis of this assay, the weight of the evidence suggests that giant cell tumors are not estrogen receptor positive.

2.3 Biochemical Techniques

The dextran-coated charcoal chemical assay remains the standard by which all other assays for estrogen and progesterone receptors must be measured. The biopsy nuclear binding assay compares favorably with the dextran-coated charcoal assay. Both of these techniques utilize the preparation of tissue which does not allow for the localization of receptor at the histological level. Reports of low and borderline levels of estrogen and progesterone receptor in some mesenchymal tumors may, in fact, be related to "contamination" of the specimen by tissue known to contain receptors. However, the low positive or borderline values which have been observed with either the dextran-coated charcoal assay or biopsy nuclear binding for giant cell tumor of bone lend further support to the argument that these lesions do not contain significant levels of receptor from a clinical perspective.

3 Summary and Conclusion

The cell of origin and giant cell tumor remains unknown, but on the basis of most experimental evidence it is probably a mesenchymal cell showing some macrophage characteristics. The clinical features which have led people to suggest that this tumor may be a steroid receptor positive lesion are tenuous at best. Early histochemical data suggesting a presence of estrogen and progesterone receptors in giant cell tumor have not been substantiated by further studies. Immunohistochemical techniques have not identified estrogen receptors in giant cell tumor. Multiple biochemical techniques have failed to identify clinically significant levels of estrogen or progesterone receptors in giant cell tumor.

References

Aparisi T, Arborgh B, Ericsson JLE (1977) Giant cell tumor of bone: detailed fine structure analysis of different cell component. Virchows Arch [A] 376:273

Banner AS, Carrington CB, Emory WB et al. (1981) Efficacy of oophorectomy in lymphangioleiomyomatosis and benign metastasizing leiomyoma. N Engl J Med 305:204

Bracaglia R, Seccia A, Farallo E, Barile G (1982) Steroid hormone receptors in female breast angiosarcomas. Ann Plast Surg 9:61

Bretoni MM, Pacheco MM, Oshima CTF, Nagai MA, Lemos LB, Goes JCS (1983) Steroid receptors in breast angiosarcoma. Cancer 51:2105

Byers VS, Levin AS, Johnston JO, Hackett AJ (1975) Quantitative immunofluorescence studies of the tumor antigen-bearing cell in giant cell tumor of bone and osteogenic sarcoma. Cancer Res 35:2520

Chaudhuri PK, Walker MJ, Beattie CW, Das Gupta TK (1980) Presence of steroid receptors in human soft tissue sarcomas of diverse histological origin. Cancer Res 40:861

Chaudhuri PK, Walker MJ, Beattie CW, Das Gupta TK (1981) Distribution of steroid hormone receptors in human soft tissue sarcomas. Surgery 90:149

DeGoeij TFPM, Bosman FT (1986) Determination of steroid hormone-dependency of tumours utilizing tissue sections. Survery of histochemical techniques and their application in surgical pathology. J Pathol 149:163–172

Gallardo H, DeLustig ES, Schajowicz F (1970) Growth and maintenance of human giant cell tumors (osteoclastomas) in continuous culture. Oncology 24:146

Garancis JC, Miller LS, Tomita JT, Tiew TM, Clowry LJ Jr (1983) Immunoperoxidase localization of estrogen receptors in human breast carcinoma. Cancer Detect Prev 6:235–239

Gloor E, Schnyder P, Cikes M (1982) Endolymphatic stromal myosis: surgical and hormonal treatment of extensive abdominal recurrence 20 years after hysterectomy. Cancer 50:1888

Goldring SR, Dayer JM, Russell RGG, Mankin HJ, Krane SM (1977) Cells cultured from human giant cell tumors of bone respond to parathyroid hormone. Calcif Tissue Res [Suppl] 22:269

Goldring SR, Dayer JM, Russell RGG, Mankin HJ, Krane SM (1978) Response to hormones of cells cultured from human giant cell tumors of bone. J Clin Endocrinol Metab 46:425

Goldring SR, Dayer JM, Krane SM (1979) Regulation of cells cultured from human giant cell tumors of bone to prostaglandin and parathyroid hormone. In: Copp DH, Talmage RB (eds) Endocrinology of calcium metabolism. Excerpta Medica, Amsterdam, p 362

Goldring SR, Mankin HJ, Roelke M, Amento EP, Bhan AK, Rourke CM, Krane SM (1984) Characterization of cells cultured in human giant cell tumor of bone (GT). Am Soc Bone Mineral Res, Hartford, Connecticut

Goldring SR, Schiller AL, Mankin HJ, Dayer JM, Krane SM (1986) Characterization of cells from human giant cell tumors of bone. Clin Orthop Rel Res 204:59

Gordon S, Todd J, Cohn ZA (1974) In vitro synthesis and secretion of lysozyme by mononuclear phagocytes. J Exp Med 139:1228

Greene GL, Nolan C, Engler JD, Jensen EV (1980) Monoclonal antibodies to human estrogen receptors. Proc Natl Acad Sci USA 77:5115–5119

Greene GL, Sobel NB, King WJ, Jensen EV (1984) Immunochemical studies of estrogen receptors. J Steroid Biochem 20:51–56

Jaffe HL, Lichtenstein L, Portis RB (1940) Giant cell tumor of bone. Arch Pathol Lab Med 30:993–1031

King WJ, Weigand RA (1986) Estrogen receptor detection and measurement using monoclonal antibodies to human estrogen receptor. Pathologist 40:15–19

King WJ, DeSombre ER, Jensen EV, Greene GL (1985) Comparison of immunocytochemical and steroid-binding assays for estrogen receptor in human breast tumors. Cancer Res 45:293

Kinzbrunner B, Ritter S, Domingo J, Rosenthal CJ (1983) Remission of rapidly growing desmoid tumors after tamoxifen therapy. Cancer 52:2201

Lee SH (1978) Cytochemical study of estrogen receptor in human mammary cancer. Am J Clin Pathol 70:197

Lee SH (1984) Validity of a histochemical estrogen-receptor assay supported by the observation of a cellular response to steroid manipulation. J Histochem Cytochem 32:305

Lee YT, Markland FS (1979) Steroid receptors in sarcomatous lesions. J Surg Oncol 11:305

Ling L, Klein MJ, Sissons HA, Steiner GC (1986) Lysozyme and alpha-antitrypsin in giant cell tumor of bone and in other lesions that contain giant cells. Arch Pathol Lab Med 110:713

Malawer M, Bray M, Kass M (1984) Fluorescent histochemical demonstration of estrogen and progesterone binding in giant cell tumors of bone: preliminary observations. J Surg Oncol 25:148

McCarty KS Jr, Woodard BH, Nicholes DE, Wilkinson W, McCarty KS Sr (1980a) Comparison of biochemical and histochemical techniques for estrogen receptor analyses in mammary carcinoma. Cancer 46:2842

McCarty KS Jr, Mossler JA, McLelland R, Sieker HO (1980b) Pulmonary lymphangiomyomatosis responsive to progesterone. N Engl J Med 303:1461

McCarty KS Jr, Miller LS, Cox EB, Konrath J, McCarty KS Sr (1985) Estrogen receptor analysis. Correlation of biochemical an immunohistochemical methods using monoclonal antireceptor antibodies. Arch Pathol Lab Med 109:716–721

McClelland RA, Berger U, Mille LS, Powles JJ, Coombes RC (1986) Immunocytochemical assay for estrogen receptor in patients with breast cancer: relationship to a biochemical assays and the outcome of therapy. J Clin Oncol 4:1171–1176

McDougall A, McGarrity G (1979) Extra-abdominal desmoid tumours. J Bone Joint Surg 61B:373

Panko WB, Mattioli CA, Wheeler TM (1982) Lack of correlation of a histochemical method for estrogen receptor analysis with the biochemical assay results. Cancer 49:2148

Penney GC, Hawkins RA (1982) Histochemical detection of oestrogen receptors: a progress report. Br J Cancer 45:237–246

Pertschuk LP, Tobin EH, Gaetjens E, Carter AC (1980) Histochemical assay of estrogen progesterone receptors in breast cancer: correlation with biochemical assays and patients' response to endocrine therapies. Cancer 46:2896–2901

Pertschuk LP, Eisenberg KB, Carter AC, Feldman JG (1985) Immunohistologic localization of estro-

gen receptors in breast cancer with monoclonal antibodies; correlation with biochemistry and clinical endocrine response. Cancer 55:1513–1518
Pousen HS, Ozello L, King WJ, Greene GL (1985) The use of monoclonal antibodies to estrogen receptors (ER) for immunoperoxidase detection of ER in paraffin sections of human breast cancer tissue. J Histochem Cytochem 33:87–92
Press MF, Greene GL (1984) An immunocytochemical method for demonstrating estrogen receptor in human uterus using monoclonal antibodies to human estrophilin. Lab Invest 50:480
Press MF, Nousek-Goebl N, King WJ (1984) Immunohistochemical assessment of estrogen receptor distribution in the human endometrium throughout the menstrual cycle. Lab Invest 51:495
Press MF, Holt JA, Herbst AL, Greene GL (1985) Immunocytochemical identification of estrogen receptor in ovarian carcinomas. Localization with monoclonal estrophilin antibodies compared with biochemical assays. Lab Invest 53:349–361
Schajowicz F (1961) Giant cell tumors of bone (osteoclastoma). A pathological and histochemical study. J Bone Joint Surg 43A:1
Shimada A, Kimura S, Abe K et al. (1985) Immunocytochemical staining of estrogen receptor in paraffin sections of human breast cancer by use of monoclonal antibody: comparison with that in frozen sections. Proc Natl Acad Sci USA 82:4803–4807
Shintaku IP, Said JW (1987) Detection of estrogen receptors with monoclonal antibodies in routinely processes formalin-fixed paraffin sections of breast carcinoma. Use of DNase pretreatment of enhance sensitivity of the reaction. Am J Clin Pathol 87:161–167
Ugolini V, Nunez G, Smith RG, Stastny P, Capra JD (1980) Initial characterization of monoclonal antibodies against human monocytes. Proc Natl Acad Sci USA 77:6764
Walker MJ, Chaudhuri PK, Beattie CW, Das Gupta TK (1980) Steroid receptors in malignant skeletal tumors. Cancer 45:3004
Weiss SW, Langloss JM, Shnookler BM, Malawer MM, Davis J, Enzinger FM, Stanton R (1986) Estrogen receptor protein in bone and soft tissue tumors. Lab Invest 54:689
Wientroub S, Binderman I, Somjen D, Kletter Y, Salama R, Weissman SL (1982) Response to parathyroid and calcitonin of human giant cell tumor of bone cultured in patients's serum. Clin Orthop 167:277
Wold LE, Sim FH, Riehl EW, Jiang NS, Spelsberg TC (1986) Steroid receptor and giant cell tumors of bone. Lab Invest
Wood GW, Neff JR, Gollahon KA, Gourley WK (1978) Macrophages in giant cell tumors of bone. J Pathol 125:53

Chondroid Chordoma: A Low-Grade Chondrosarcoma and Its Differential Diagnosis

J.J. Brooks, J.Q. Trojanowski, and V.A. LiVolsi

1 Introduction . . . 165
2 Chordoma . . . 165
2.1 Clinical Features and Biological Behavior . . . 165
2.2 Histology . . . 167
2.3 Histogenesis . . . 169
3 Chondrosarcoma . . . 171
3.1 Incidence . . . 171
3.2 Pathology . . . 172
3.3 Prognostic Features . . . 172
4 Chondroid Chordoma . . . 173
4.1 Clinical Description and Behavior . . . 173
4.2 Pathology . . . 174
4.3 Immunohistochemistry in the Differential Diagnosis . . . 176
5 Chondroid Chordoma – a Low-Grade Chondrosarcoma . . . 178
References . . . 179

1 Introduction

Controversy has surrounded chondroid chordoma ever since it was first described as a distinct clinical and pathological entity (Heffelfinger et al. 1973). For, although lesions called chondroid chordoma clearly behave in a far more benign fashion than typical chordoma, the histogenesis of chondroid chordoma has been uncertain. Furthermore, the pathological features distinguishing it from related tumors have been blurred by its supposed bimorphic histology resembling both chordoma and chondrosarcoma. In this chapter, we will review the entities confused with chondroid chordoma from the clinicopathological and histogenetic viewpoints. We will also detail our own immunohistochemical analysis which indicated chondroid chordoma to be a form of low-grade chondrosarcoma.

2 Chordoma

2.1 Clinical Features and Biological Behavior

Chordomas are rare tumors that typically arise within bones of the axial skeleton although they predominantly involve the rostral (i.e., spheno-occipital region) and caudal (i.e., sacrococcygeal region) extremes of the axial skeleton. About

40% arise in the region of the clivus and the remainder occur along the vertebral columns. Chordomas are generally slow growing and produce their symptoms and signs by destruction of bone and by the compression of cranial nerves, spinal nerves, or adjacent neural structures. As discussed below, chordomas resemble notochordal rests in their histology and distribution, and the incidence of such rests in the spheno-occipital region at autopsy is reported to be about 1.5%–2.0% of cases (STEWARD and MORIN 1926). Invasion, as contrasted with compression, of adjacent central nervous system structures is extremely rare, but metastatic dissemination of chordomas is not uncommon and may be seen in over a third of patients with long follow-up (ARIEL and VERDU 1955; BONNEVILLE et al. 1980; BURGER and VOGEL 1982; DAHLIN and MACCARTY 1952; FAUST et al. 1944; GARDNER and TURNER 1941; HEFFELFINGER et al. 1973; HUVOS 1979; JAFFE 1968; LIM 1975; PERZIN and PUSHPARAJ 1986; RICH et al. 1985). Complete surgical removal of chordomas is the treatment of choice, although, because of their location, this is not always feasible. A role for chemotherapy or radiation in the management of these tumors has not been established at this time.

Some of the clinical features of a spheno-occipital chordoma are illustrated in Figs. 1–3 below and the brief clinical synopsis that accompanies the figures. Figure 1 shows the CT scan appearance of a chordoma in the region of the prepontine and supracellular cisterns. The patient was a 68-year-old man who came to medical attention because of difficulty looking to the right and a gait disturbance, both of which were of about 1 year in duration. This patient died of a number of medical problems following attempts to biopsy this lesion. At autopsy, a gelatinous, translucent mass was found to extend from the region of the optic chiasm to the pons (Fig. 2) and it focally compressed these structures (Fig. 3). The tumor appeared to originate from the clivus and there was no evidence of local brain invasion or distant metastasis by this tumor. This case illustrates the low potential of chordomas that arise in this region to invade and metastasize. Nevertheless, because of their location in a relatively inaccessi-

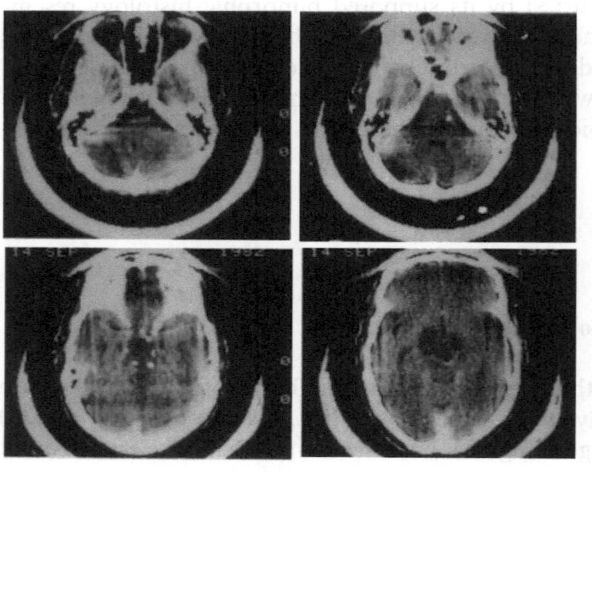

Fig. 1. CT scans without contrast enhancement from a 68-year-old man with a gait disturbance and difficulty seeing to the right. There is a low density mass lesion in the prepontine and supracellar cisterns with focal calcifications that was shown to be a chordoma at autopsy. A resolved cerebellar infarct is also evident

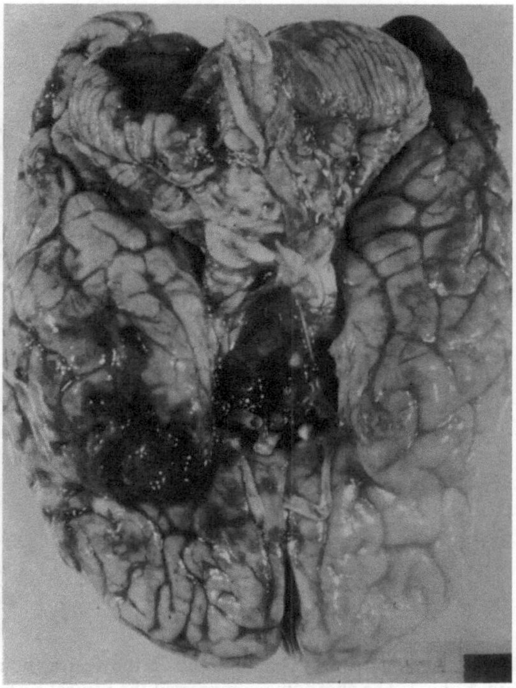

Fig. 2. The ventral surface of the brain from the patient in Fig. 1. There is a soft gelatinous mass, a chordoma, that extends from the optic chiasm to the pons. An old cavitary infarct is present in the cerebellum and a more recent one in the temporal lobe on the same side

ble region that contains many vital central nervous system structures, chordomas that arise in the clivus cannot always be removed surgically, and they may therefore result in serious morbidity and mortality. The median survival of patients with chordomas appears to be about 6 years for spinal chordomas, and about 4 years for those at the base of the skull (Burger and Vogel 1982; Heffelfinger et al. 1973; Sundaresan et al. 1979).

2.2 Histology

The histology of chordomas in routine stains has been extensively characterized by light and electron microscopy, and the distinction between these tumors and other morphologically similar neoplasms (cartilaginous tumors, myxopapillary ependymomas) that arise in the same location has been sharpened recently by reports on the differing immunohistochemical properties of chordomas and other tumors (Burger and Vogel 1982; Brooks et al. 1987; Miettinen et al. 1983). This has served to facilitate the recognition of chordomas as a distinct class of epithelial neoplasms. In particular, these studies have helped resolve the confusion that has existed for a number of years concerning a group of cartilaginous lesions of the spheno-occipital region that have been inappropriately referred to as "chondroid chordomas" (Brooks et al. 1987). The use of antibodies to cell type specific, or relatively cell type specific antigens for the

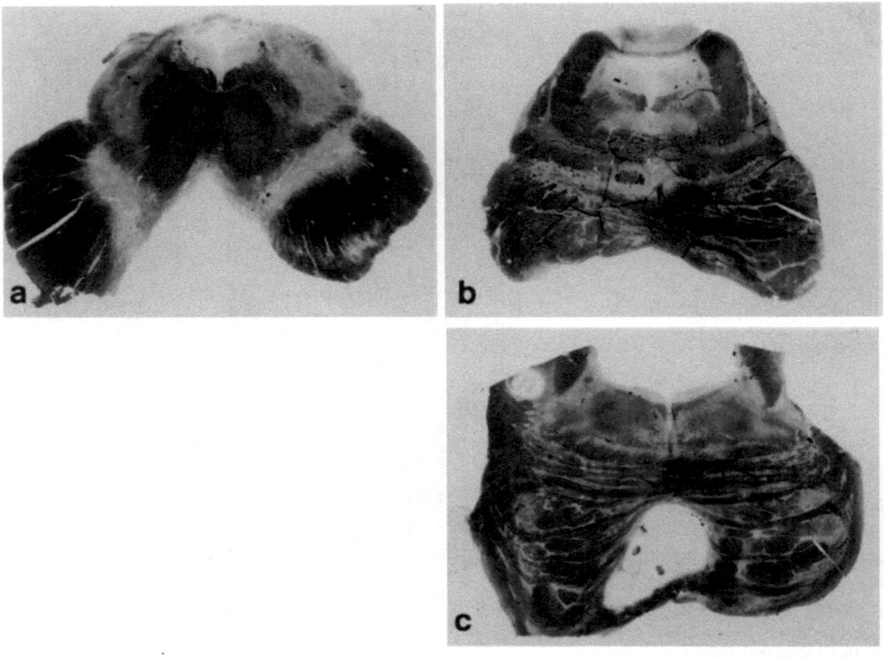

Fig. 3. Sections from **a** the midbrain, **b** the rostral pons, and **c** the mid-pons from the patient in Fig. 1 and 2. The chordoma compressed the ventral surface of these structures. Weil stain

differential diagnosis of chordomas, as compared with so-called chondroid chordomas, is discussed in greater detail later in this chapter.

Chordomas are noted to exhibit a somewhat lobular growth patten that is best seen at low power magnifications by light microscopy. The eosinophilic tumor cells generally are in contact with one another to yield cohesive sheets, nests, strings, and cords of tumor cells within a myxoid ground substance. Linear arrays of tumor cells are generally two or more cells thick but on occasion they may be only one cell thick. The tumor cells may have homogeneous eosinophilic cytoplasm and distinct cell membranes, or they may contain numerous intracytoplasmic vacuoles. The latter may obscure the demarcation between the intracellular and extracellular compartments of the tumor. The highly vacuolated cells are designated "physaliphorous" cells, from the Greek term for bubble ("physallis") bearing ("phoros"). Photomicrographs of the typical appearance of chordomas are shown in Fig. 4. Rarely and particularly after recurrence and/or radiation, chordoma may exhibit unusual morphological patterns simulating either highly aggressive spindle cell sarcoma (MIETTINEN et al. 1987) or malignant fibrous histiocytoma (MIETTINEN et al. 1984; MEIS et al. 1987).

Since some confusion exists about the distinction of chordomas from cartilaginous lesions, especially at the base of the skull, the contrasting histological features of chordomas, chondroid chordomas, and chondrosarcomas are summarized in Table 1, and the immunohistochemical properties of these tumors are summarized in Table 2.

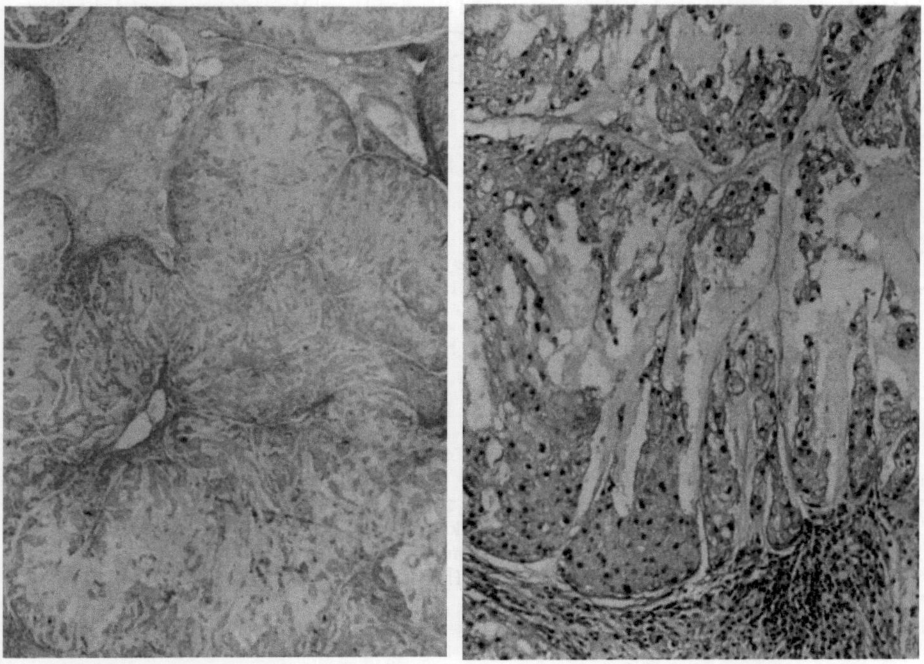

Fig. 4. Photomicrographs illustrating **a** the lobular growth pattern of chordomas and **b** the growth of tumor cells in nests and cords. (BROOKS et al. 1987) H&E

Table 1. Differentiated diagnosis of chondroid chordoma[a]

Feature	Chordoma	Chondroid chordoma	Chondrosarcoma
Sheets	Cohesive	Discohesive	Discohesive
Nests	Present	Absent	Absent
Cords	Present	Absent	Absent
Strings	Rare	Common	Occasional
Eosinophilic cells	Yes	Yes	Yes
Vacuoles	Intracellular	Intracellular + extracellular	Intracellular + extracellular

[a] See text for definitions

2.3 Histogenesis

Because chordomas are similar in histology (see Fig. 5) and distribution to non-neoplastic notochordal rests, chordomas have long been considered to orginate from such rests. To notochord is a cylindrical structure that constitutes the definitive axial skeleton of lower chordates, and, during embryogenesis, it is the primitive axial skeleton of vertebrates (GARDNER and TURNER 1941). In humans, most notochordal tissue disappears during embryogenesis, although

Table 2. Immunohistochemical results on chondroid chordoma, cartilaginous tumors, and chordoma

	S-100	PKER[a]	MKER[b]	AE-1[c]	EMA[d]
Normal tissues					
Fetal notochord	0/2	2/2	2/2	2/2	2/2
Fetal cartilage	2/2	0/2	0/2	0/2	ND
Tumors					
Chondroma	2/2	0/2	0/2	0/2	0/2
Chondrosarcoma					
Typical	6/6	0/6	0/6	0/6	0/6
Myxoid	1/1	0/1	0/1	0/1	0/1
Mesenchymal	1/1	0/1	0/1	ND	ND
Chondroid chordoma	7/7	0/7	0/7	0/7	0/7
Chordoma					
Sacral	12/12	12/12	12/12	12/12	12/12
Base of skull	6/6	6/6	6/6	6/6	6/6

[a] PKER, polyclonal cytokeratin antibody from Dako
[b] MKER, monoclonal antibody to cytokeratin from Dako
[c] AE-1, monoclonal antibody to cytokeratin from Hybriteck
[d] EMA, epithelial membrane antigen
ND, not done

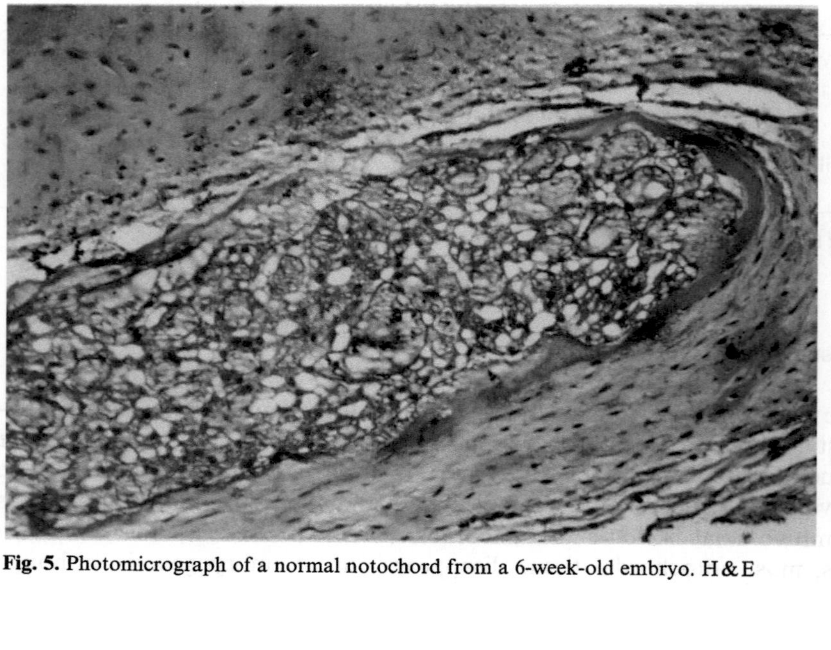

Fig. 5. Photomicrograph of a normal notochord from a 6-week-old embryo. H&E

some residual notochordal tissue does persist in the nucleus pulposus of intervertebral disks or as ectopic rests (HORWITZ 1941; SENSENIG 1956). The latter occur most commonly in the spheno-occipital and sacrococcygeal regions (HORWITZ 1941; SENSENIG 1956). VIRCHOW was the first to identify these rests and he termed them ecchondrosis physaliphora for their presumed origin from cartilage (VIRCHOW 1857). Later, MULLER (1858) suggested that these rests were derived from notochord. The recent demonstration that notochord and chordomas both express epithelial antigens, i.e., keratin polypeptides, unlike cartilage cells, has served to strengthen the notion that chordomas are histogenetically derived from notochordal rests.

3 Chondrosarcoma

Chondrosarcomas of numerous histological subtypes have been described. These lesions can occur both in the bone and in extraosseous soft tissue. Thus, there are reports of dedifferentiated chondrosarcoma, mesenchymal chondrosarcoma, clear cell chondrosarcoma, etc. In considering the differential diagnosis from chordoma, however, the chondrosarcoma which comes to mind is the low-grade myxoid type. This is by far the most common type of chondrosarcoma arising in bone or in the soft tissue.

It is this low-grade myxoid chondrosarcoma and its soft tissue counterpart, dubbed chordoid sarcoma, that resemble chordoma histologically and must be differentiated from it.

3.1 Incidence

True chondrosarcoma of bone comprises approximately 10% of primary malignant bone tumors (DAHLIN 1967). This tumor is primarily a tumor of adulthood, is rarely seen in children, and affects males slightly more than females. Certain conditions predispose the development of chondrosarcoma (i.e., multiple enchondromatosis); in these conditions, sarcoma may be seen as multifocal lesions in many bones and may develop in young individuals.

Most chondrosarcomas arise in the trunk, including the shoulder girdle, in the upper ends of the femurs, the upper humeri, and the iliac and pelvic bones (DAHLIN 1967). However, chondrosarcomas may also arise in the facial bones and it is these lesions which may be confused pathologically with chordoma (FU and PERZIN 1974; COLTRERA et al. 1986).

The symptoms of chondrosarcoma include a local swelling and pain. Since the tumor grows slowly over many years, long intervals occur between initial therapy and recurrences and metastasis (DAHLIN 1967; EVANS et al. 1977; SANERKIN and GALLAGHER 1979).

3.2 Pathology

Grossly, chondrosarcomas are usually large lesions which destroy preexisting bone, producing expansion and thickening of the cortex. Occasionally as the thickened cortex is invaded by tumor pathological fracture may occur.

Histologically chondrosarcomas are characterized by growth in lobules (Dahlin 1967; Fu and Perzin 1974; Coltrera et al. 1986). The center of these lobules can become necrotic, even cystic. Sometimes calcification in these necrotic foci may be seen histologically as well as radiographically. Chondrosarcomas of the myxoid type produce a ground substance that may be firm like hyaline cartilage or may be watery like mucus. The cells are dispersed within lacunae without cell to cell contact. Nuclear pleomorphism is minimal in low-grade lesions; binucleate or multinucleate cells may be seen. The cytoplasm is scanty and occasionally vacuolated.

Differential diagnostic features of chondrosarcoma include those which enable the pathologist to distinguish it from chondroma on the one hand and osteosarcoma on the other. The latter will not be discussed further in this chapter. However, the distinction of chondrosarcoma from chondroma may be extremely problematical for the pathologist. Evidence of malignancy in cartilage tumors includes many cells with plump nuclei, multiple cells with two nuclei, and cells having nuclei with clumped chromatin.

3.3 Prognostic Features

The prognosis for bone chondrosarcomas is that they may occur locally even after 5 years following initial resection. Hence, the use of 5-year survival is not significant in these tumors. In addition, the error of underdiagnosis as chondroma and consequent inadequate therapy shows that the overall long-term survival rate for chondrosarcoma may be less than expected by the low grade of the tumor.

Several studies have enumerated prognostic factors which affect the prognosis of chondrosarcomas: these include site, size, histological grade of the tumor, and initial therapy (Fu and Perzin 1974; Evens et al. 1977; Sanerkin and Gallagher 1979; Marcove et al. 1972; Pritchard et al. 1980). Tumors which involve the axial skeleton are more difficult to cure than those which involve the long bones. Large lesions are more difficult to eradicate and control than smaller ones.

Histological grading of chondrosarcomas has been shown to affect prognosis. Three grades of differentiation are recognized (Evans et al. 1977; Sanerkin and Gallagher 1979; Marcove et al. 1972; Pritchard et al. 1980) based on mitotic rate, cellularity, and nuclear size. Histological grade predicts outcome: hence metastases are found in only 5% of low-grade tumors, but in 75% of high-grade ones (Sanerkin and Gallagher 1979).

Chondrosarcomas of soft tissue origin, although rare, also occur (Angervall et al. 1973). These can be recognized by applying the same histological criteria and can also be graded (Angervall et al. 1973; Dardick et al. 1983; Weiss 1976).

Chondromas and low-grade chondrosarcomas may arise in the head and neck and therefore be confused with chordomas and the so-called chondroid chordoma of the sphenoid region. FU and PERZIN (1974) studied 17 such cartilaginous tumors (seven chondromas and ten chondrosarcomas). Chondromas were usually incidentally found nodules which were treated successfully by local resection. For chondrosarcomas, the location and extent of the lesion, the adequacy of initial surgical therapy, and the degree of differentiation (grade) of the tumor were important in predicting prognosis. Thus, lesions which occur in the region of the head and neck have similar prognostic characteristics to those which occur in other noncranial bones.

The entity of chordoid sarcoma (chordoid tumor, parachordoma) has been reevaluated and recognized as an extraskeletal myxoid chondrosarcoma (ANGERVALL et al. 1973; DARDICK et al. 1983; WEISS 1976). Special stains indicate abundant matrix of sulfated acid mucopolysaccharides interspersed with collagen fibers. These features suggest that the tumor is chondroid rather than chordoid (BUCKWALTER 1983). Ultrastructural evidence of chondroid differentiation has been shown by DARDICK et al. (1983). The ultrastructure of the chordoma is one of cytoplasmic vacuoles whose gradual enlargement leads to the ultimate formation of the physaliphorous cell. Such vacuolization in physaliphorous cells is lacking both at the electron microscopic and light microscopic level in so-called chordoid sarcomas. Benign and neoplastic cartilage, however, does share ultrastructural similarities with so-called chordoid sarcomas. Although there is a superficial light microscopic resemblance of chordoid sarcoma to chordoma, the location of these lesions away from the vertebral and the ultrastructural differences strongly suggest that these lesions are indeed extraskeletal myxoid chondrosarcomas (DARDICK et al. 1983; WEISS 1976).

4 Chondroid Chordoma

4.1 Clinical Description and Behavior

Most chondroid chordomas occur at middle age, with an age peak from 20 to 60 years and an average age of 35 years (HEFFELFINGER et al. 1973). Females slightly outnumber males. Unlike chordomas, the location is almost exclusively limited to the base of the skull. The presenting symptoms and signs are related to the expansion of a mass in this vital area and include diplopia, headache, nasal stuffiness, visual field cuts, and cranial nerve palsies. On occasion these complaints may have been noted for some time (5–10 years) before diagnosis. The surgeon attempting complete removal is faced with a difficult task and only partial excision is effected in many cases. Therefore, the rate of local recurrence is high and patients are often incurable. Despite this, chondroid chordoma characteristically is a nonaggressive tumor with a very indolent course. Metastases do not occur but patients may eventually die of problems relating to local extension. The average survival is nearly 16 years, in sharp contrast to the 4.1 years of the more aggressive chordoma. Likewise, there is a relatively high 10-year survival rate in the chondroid tumor compared to chordoma (47% vs 3%) (HEFFELFINGER et al. 1973).

4.2 Pathology

Chondroid chordoma was originally defined by HEFFELFINGER et al. as a tumor exhibiting histological features common to both chordoma and cartilaginous tumors. Thus, vacuolated cells in "cords" resembling chordoma were described accompanied by foci of cartilage. Interestingly, by their review, practically all previously diagnosed chondrosarcomas were renamed chondroid chordoma (CC). As a result of this pioneering report, very few chondrosarcomas of this region have been diagnosed over the past decade (SUIT et al. 1982). The fundamental difference in the natural history of these lesions accentuated the importance of distinguishing CC from chordoma.

However, examination of our cases together with prior reports showed CCs were distinctly different and demonstrated little relationship to the epithelial-like nesting pattern of chordoma (see Table 1). Unlike classic chordoma, CC cells grew within the matrix either as individual cells or as strings just one cell layer thick (Fig. 6). No thicker cords or cohesive nests were noted. Even when sheets of cells were noted, the individual cells did not directly abut one another. Rather, cells were discohesive and surrounded by ground substance. *Intracytoplasmic* vacuoles mimicking those in physaliphorous chordoma cells were only rarely seen and similar appearing cells can be found in chondrosarcoma (Fig. 7). Vacuoles were commonly observed in an *extracellular* location in the myxoid material (Fig. 8). Clear-cut foci of cartilaginous differentiation were easily identi-

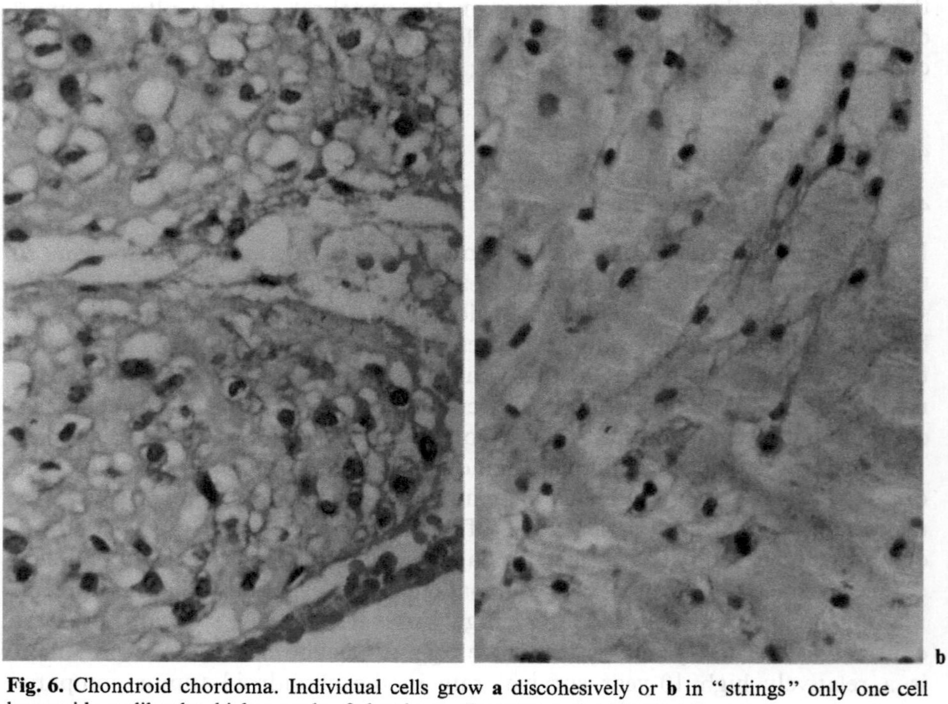

a b

Fig. 6. Chondroid chordoma. Individual cells grow **a** discohesively or **b** in "strings" only one cell layer wide, unlike the thicker cords of chordoma. (BROOKS et al. 1987) H&E

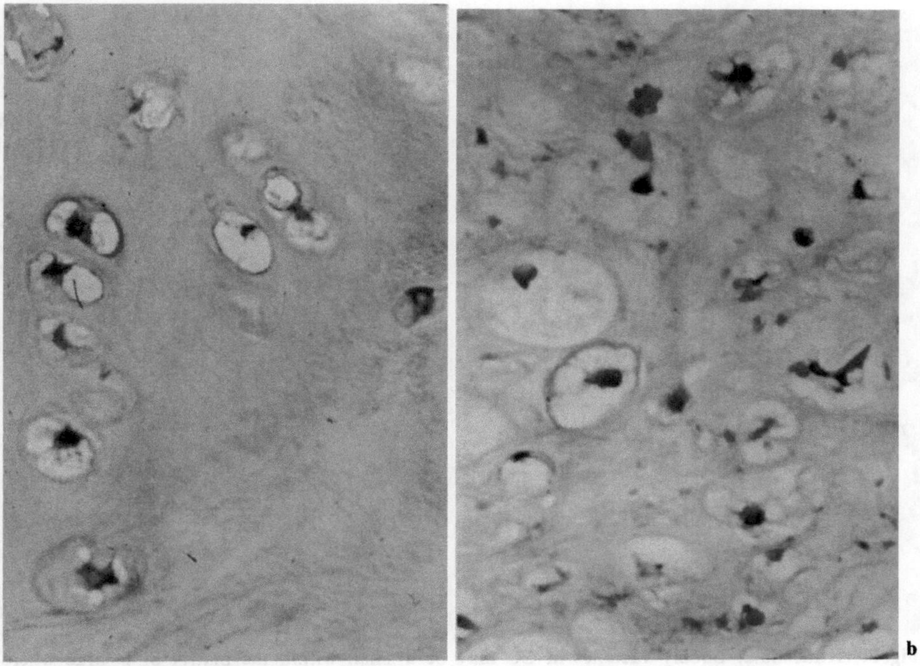

a b

Fig. 7. Intracytoplasmic vacuolization is not specific for chordoma; it occasionally occurs in both **a** benign and **b** malignant cartilaginous tumors. (BROOKS et al. 1987)

fied in every case (Fig. 9). With its thin string-like growth, CC more closely simulated the pattern typically observed in myxoid chondrosarcoma, a variant found in the soft tissues. The combination of this pattern and the site of vacuolization sets CC apart from any chordomatous tumor, and it is also immunohistochemically different from chordoma, as discussed below.

In the literature, CC cases also fail to show the true chordoma pattern. Approximately 48 cases can be found within 14 separate articles on the topic. A large number contained no photographic documentation (CHAMBERS and SCHWINN 1979; HARWICK and MILLER 1979; HASEGAWA et al. 1985; RICH et al. 1985; VOLPE and MAZABRAUD 1983; WOLD and LAWS 1984; PERZIN and PUSHPARAJ 1986). In many, a chondroid component was recognizable, but the thick cords of chordoma were not depicted. Instead, there were either sheets of vacuolated but discohesive cells (VALDERRAMA et al. 1983; RICHTER et al. 1975) or thin strings as found in chondrosarcoma (HEFFELFINGER et al. 1973; SPODEN et al. 1980; RUTHERFOORD and DAVIES 1987). Two reports (HEATON and TURNER 1985; ABENOZA and SIBLEY 1987) illustrated thicker cords consistent with chordoma; however, the chondroid component was not demonstrated convincingly. In short, the classic features of chordoma as redefined above were not identified in reports of CC.

Ultrastructurally, CC does not contain the obvious epithelial markers of chordoma. Desmosomes or simple cell junctions are nonspecific and can be

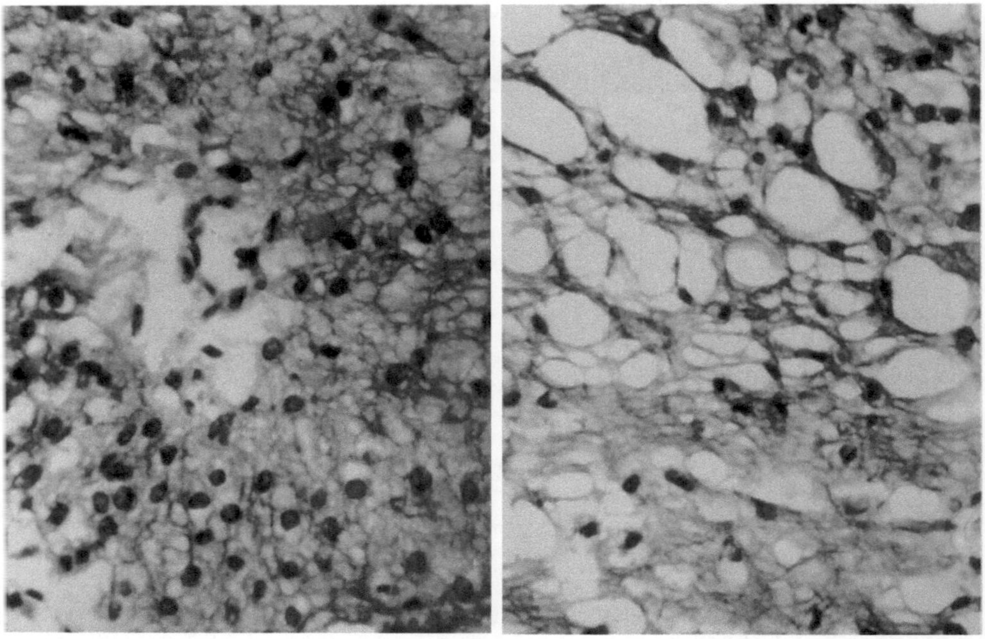

a b

Fig. 8. Extracellular bubbly vacuoles in CC may be **a** small within the matrix or **b** large where they compress the cytoplasm

found in nonepithelial lesions, including chondrosarcoma (WEISS 1976; PARDO-MINDAN et al. 1981; ROBERTSON and HOGG 1980; MARTINEZ-TELLO and NAVAS-PALACIOS 1982). Thus, while well-formed desmosomes have frequently been seen in chordoma (PENA et al. 1970; SPJUT and LUSE 1964; PARDO-MINDAN et al. 1981; KAY and SCHATZKI 1972), and ill-defined ones rarely in CC (VALDERRAMA et al. 1983), they cannot be used as exact documentation of a chordomatous or epithelial feature. Also, the peculiar crystalline tubular structures supposedly unique to CC (VALDERRAMA et al. 1983) had been described in myxoid chondrosarcoma (WETZEL and REUHL 1980). More compelling ultrastructural support of the epithelial nature of chordoma is provided by the findings of true tonofilaments (MIETTINEN 1984) or dense areas of intermediate filaments, neither of which are found in the chondroid tumor (RUTHERFOORD and DAVIES 1987). Although tonofilaments were described by VALDERRAMA et al. in CC, they were short and the illustration appeared to show a thick desmosome.

4.3 Immunohistochemistry in the Differential Diagnosis

Immunohistochemical studies have proven chordoma to be epithelial in nature and easily distinguished from cartilaginous lesions by its antigenic profile. MIETTINEN et al. (1983) first demonstrated the presence of cytokeratin (CK) in six

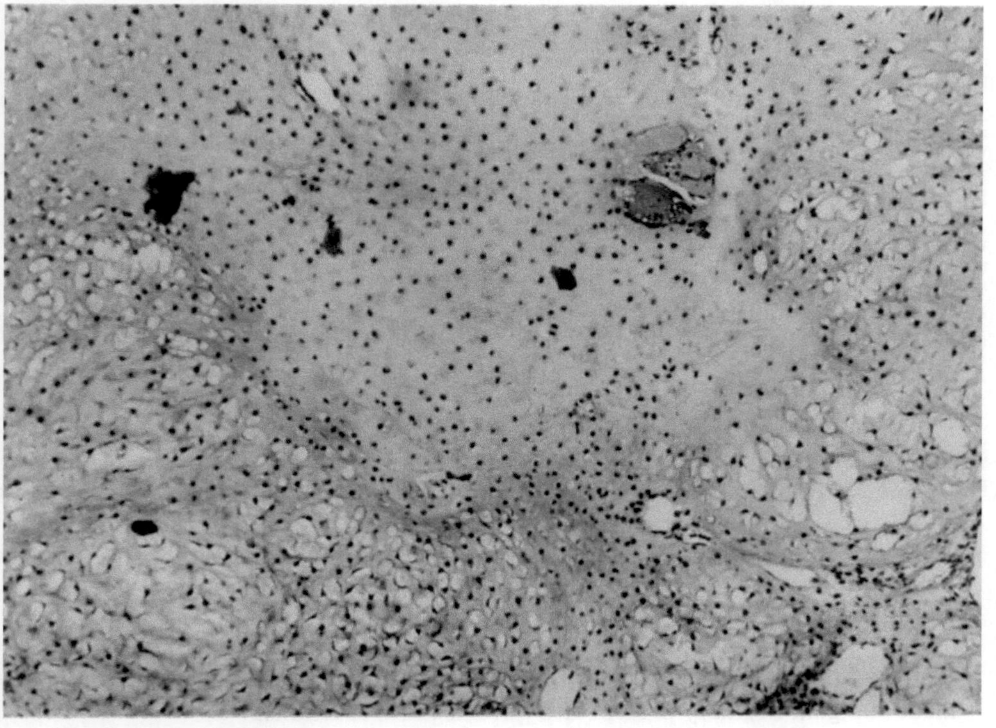

Fig. 9. Cartilaginous regions (*upper middle area*) in CC merge with the discohesive sheets of cells now known to be immunohistochemically chondroid rather than chordoid in nature

chordomas. Later, other authors confirmed the epithelial nature of this lesion (Miettinen 1984; Salisbury and Isaacson 1985; Sibley 1985; Abenoza et al. 1985). In addition to CK, chordomas have been shown to express epithelial membrane antigen (EMA) (Miettinen 1984; Salisbury and Isaacson 1985), carcinoembryonic antigen (CEA) (Sibley 1985; Abenoza et al. 1985), and S-100 protein (Nakamura et al. 1983). In our hands, all chordomas displayed strong and diffuse reactivity with each of three CK reagents and with EMA (Fig. 10), and in this respect resembled normal notochordal tissue (Brooks et al. 1987; Salisbury and Isaacson 1985). The additional expression of S-100 was also noted in chordomas. The results of the immunohistochemical analysis are contained in Table 2.

In contrast, the epithelial markers CK and EMA were negative in chondromas and chondrosarcomas. Only S-100 immunoreactivity was expressed, a reaction pattern identical to fetal cartilage. These results are identical to those in previous reports. Chondrosarcomas have been shown to contain vimentin instead of CK (Miettinen et al. 1983), and to lack EMA (Salisbury and Isaacson 1985; Abenoza et al. 1985) and CEA (Abenzoa et al. 1985).

Chondroid chordomas had the exact same immunohistochemical profile as cartilaginous tumors (S-100+, CK-, EMA-) in each of the seven cases we tested

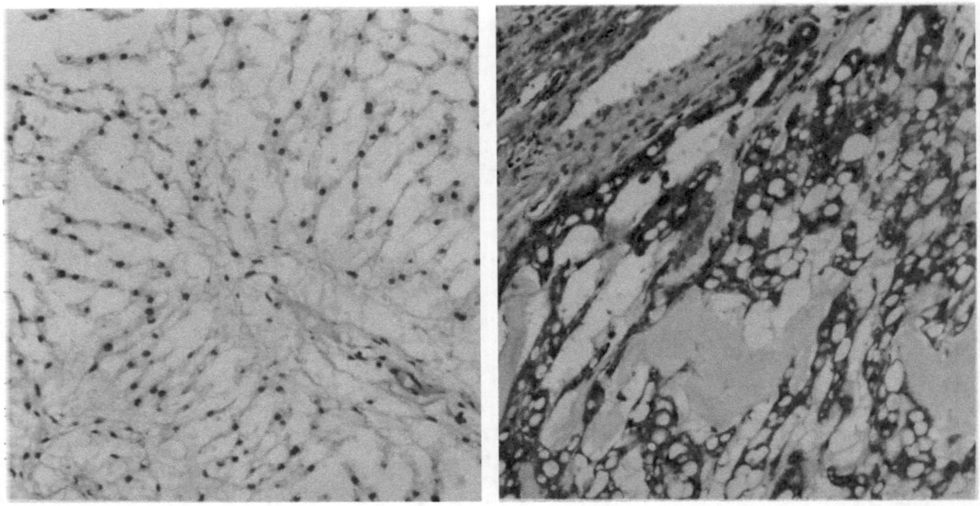

a b

Fig. 10. In contrast to the CK-negative CC (**a**, light), the thick and cohesive cells of chordoma are diffusely CK-positive (**b**, dark). (Brooks et al. 1987)

(Table 2). Both cartilaginous foci and the more myxoid areas with the string pattern failed to stain with epithelial markers (Fig. 10). Antisera to neurofilament and glial fibrillary protein also gave negative reactions.

We have shown that the immunohistochemical profile of CC bears no relationship to that of chordoma and, in fact, is identical to that of chondrosarcoma. Instead, we have shown this tumor to be indistinguishable from chondrosarcoma. These results built upon previous histochemical studies providing the initial evidence that CC may not be related to chordoma (Bottles and Beckstead 1984). Those authors observed the enzyme 5′-nucleotidase within chordomas but not within CC or chondrosarcoma, and also noted the histological similarity between CC and cartilaginous tumors as we did. They thought that CCs were "better considered as cartilaginous tumors rather than as a subtype of chordoma." Our immunohistochemical results were confirmed just recently; Rutherfoord and Davies also failed to detect CK in CC. Although a few CC cases stained "weakly" with epithelial markers according to Abenoza and Sibley, their cases do not appear to be completely acceptable for reasons discussed above. Again, in two recent "CCs" reported as CK-positive by Salisbury (1987), the presence of a chondroid element is not well documented and these cases are also considered to be regular chordomas, albeit somewhat myxoid.

5 Chondroid Chordoma – a Low-Grade Chondrosarcoma

It is clear that the entity called "chondroid chordoma" is morphologically, histochemically, ultrastructurally, and immunohistochemically distinct from chordoma and similar to cartilaginous lesions. Due to all the accumulated evidence, we believe these tumors can now be confidently classified as chondrosarcomas and recommend that the term chondroid chordoma be abandoned and replaced by "low-grade chondrosarcoma." Since their clinical behavior is recognizably different, as originally documented by the Mayo Clinic authors (HEFFELFINGER et al. 1973), these tumors should continue to be separated from typical chordomas as well as high-grade chondrosarcomas. Recognition of them as low-grade chondrosarcomas underscores the frequently indolent course of cartilaginous lesions of the skull base.

Acknowledgments. The authors thank Kathy Snyder for typing the manuscript and Beth Ann Gee for technical assistance.

References

Abenoza P, Sibley RK (1987) Chordoma: an immunohistochemical study. Hum Pathol 17:744–747

Abenoza P, Sibley RK, Rosai J (1985) Immunocytochemistry in the differential diagnosis of chordoma and chondrosarcoma. Lab Invest 52:1 A

Alho A, Connor JF, Mankin HJ, Schiller AL, Campbell CJ (1983) Assessment of malignancy of cartilage tumors using flow cytometry. J Bone Joint Surg 65A:779–785

Angervall L, Enerback L, Knutson H (1973) Chondrosarcoma of soft tissue origin. Cancer 32:507–513

Ariel IM, Verdu C (1955) Chordoma: an analysis of twenty cases treated over a twenty year span. J Surg Oncol 7:27–44

Bonneville J-F, Belloir A, Mawazini H, Manzoni J-M, Runge M, Monnier G, Dietemann J-L (1980) Calcified remnants of the notochord in the roof of the nasopharynx. Radiology 137:373–377

Bottles K, Beckstead JH (1984) Enzyme histochemical characterization of chordomas. Am J Surg Pathol 8:443–447

Brooks JJ, LiVolsi VA, Trojanowski JQ (1987) Does chondroid chordoma exist? Acta Neuropathol 72:229–235

Buckwalter JA (1983) The structure of human chondrosarcoma proteoglycans. J Bone Joint Surg 65A:958–974

Burger PC, Vogel FA (1982) Surgical pathology of the nervous system and its coverings, 2nd edn. Wiley, New York

Chambers PW, Schwinn CP (1979) Chordoma. A clinicopathologic study of metastasis. Am J Clin Pathol 72:765–776

Coltrera MD, Googe PB, Harrist TJ, Hyams VJ, Schiller AL, Goodman ML (1986) Chondrosarcoma of the temporal bone. Cancer 58:2689–2696

Dahlin DC (1967) Bone tumors: general aspects and data on 3, 987 cases. Charles C. Thomas, Springfield

Dahlin DC, MacCarty CS (1952) Chordoma: a study of fifty-nine cases. Cancer 5:1170–1178

Dardick I, Legace R, Carlier MT, Jung RC (1983) Chordoid sarcoma (extra-skeletal myxoid chondrosarcoma). Virchows Arch [A] 399:61–78

Evans HL, Ayala AG, Romstahl MM (1977) Prognostic factors in chondrosarcoma of bone. Cancer 40:818–831

Faraggiana T, Sender B, Glicksman P (1981) Light and electron microscopic study of clear cell chondrosarcoma. Am J Clin Pathol 75:117–121

Faust DB, Gilmore HR, Mudgett CS (1944) Chordomata: a review of literature with a report of a sacro-coccygeal case. Ann Intern Med 21:678–698

Fu YS, Perzin KH (1974) Non-epithelial tumors of the nasal cavity, paranasal sinuses and nasopharynx. A clinico-pathologic study. III. Cartilaginous tumors, chondroma, chondrosarcoma. Cancer 34:453–463

Gardner WJ, Turner O (1941) Cranial chordomas, a clinical and pathologic study. Arch Surg 42:411–425

Harwick RD, Miller AS (1979) Craniocervical chordomas. Am J Surg 138:512–516

Hasegawa M, Nishijima W, Watanabe I, Nasu M, Kamiyama R (1985) Primary chondroid chordoma arising from the base of the temporal bone. A 10-year post-operative follow-up. J Laryngol Otol 99:485–489

Heaton JM, Turner DR (1985) Reflections on notochordal differentiation arising from a study of chordomas. Histopathology 9:543–550

Heffelfinger MJ, Dahlin DC, MacCarty CS, Beabout JW (1973) Chordomas and cartilaginous tumors at the skull base. Cancer 32:410–420

Horwitz T (1941) Chordal ectopia and its possible relation to chordoma. Arch Pathol 31:354–362

Hsu S-M, Raine L, Fanger H (1981) Use of avidin-biotin-peroxidase complex (ABC) in immunoperoxidase techniques: a comparison between ABC and unlabeled antibody (PAP) procedures. J Histochem Cytochem 29:577–580

Huvos AG (1979) Bone tumors: diagnosis, treatment and prognosis, Saunders, Philadelphia, pp 373–391

Jaffe HL (1968) Tumors and tumorous conditions of the bones and joints. Lea and Febiger, Philadelpia, pp 451–462

Kay S, Schatzki PF (1972) Ultrastructural observations of a chordoma arising in the clivus. Hum Pathol 3:403–413

LeCharpentier Y, Forest M, Postel M, Tomeno B, Abelanet R (1979) Clear cell chondrosarcoma: a report of five cases including ultrastructural study. Cancer 44:622–629

Lim GHK (1975) Clivus chordoma with unusual bone sclerosis and brainstem invasion. A case report with review of the radiology of cranial chordomas. Aust Radiol 19:242–250

Marcove RC, Mike V, Hutter RVP, Huvos AG, Shoji H, Miller TR, Kosloff R (1972) Chondrosarcoma of the pelvis and upper end of the femur. J Bone Joint Surg 54A:561–572

Martinez-Tello FJ, Navas-Palacios JJ (1982) Ultrastructural study of conventional chondrosarcomas and myxoid- and mesenchymal-chondrosarcomas. Virchows Arch [A] 396:197–211

Meis J, Raymond A, Evans H, Charles R, Giraldo A (1987) "Dedifferentiated" chordoma: a clinicopathologic and immunohistochemical study of three cases. Am J Surg Pathol 11:516–525

Miettinen M (1984) Chordoma. Antibodies to epithelial membrane antigen and carcino-embryonic antigen in differential diagnosis. Arch Pathol Lab Med 108:891–892

Miettinen M, Lehto E-P, Dahl D, Virtanen I (1983) Differential diagnosis of chordoma, chondroid, and ependymal tumors as aided by anti-intermediate filament antibodies. Am J Pathol 112:160–169

Miettinen M, Lehto V-P, Virtanen I (1984) Malignant fibrous histiocytoma within a recurrent chordoma. A light microscopic, electron microscopic, and immunohistochemical study. Am J Clin Pathol 82:738–743

Miettinen M, Karaharju E, Jarvinen H (1987) Chordoma with massive spindle cell transformation: a light- and electron-microscopic, and immunohistochemical study. Am J Surg Pathol 11:563–570

Muller H (1958) Über das Vorkommen von Resten der Chorda Dorsalis bei Menschen nach der Geburt und über die Verhältnisse zu den Gallertgeschwulsten am Clivus. Z Rationelle Med 2:202–229

Nakamura Y, Becker LE, Marks A (1983) S-100 protein in human chordoma and human rabbit notochord. Arch Pathol Lab Med 107:118–120

Pardo-Mindan FJ, Guillen FJ, Villas C, Vazquez JJ (1981) A comparative ultrastructural study of chondrosarcoma, chordoid sarcoma, and chordoma. Cancer 47:2611–2619

Pena CE, Horvat BL, Risher ER (1970) The ultrastructure of chordoma. Am J Clin Pathol 53:544–551

Perzin KH, Pushparaj N (1986) Nonepithelial tumors of the nasal cavity, paranasal sinuses, and nasopharynx. A clinicopathologic study. XIV. Chordomas. Cancer 57:784–796

Pritchard DJ, Lunke RJ, Taylor WF, Dahlin DC, Medley BE (1980) Chondrosarcoma: a clinical pathologic and statistical analysis. Cancer 45:149–157

Rich TA, Schiller A, Suit H, Mankin HK (1985) Clinical and pathologic review of 48 cases of chordoma. Cancer 56:182–187

Richter HJ, Batsakis JG, Boles R (1975) Chordomas: nasopharyngeal presentation and atypical long survival. Ann Otol Rhinol Laryngol 84:1–6

Robertson DI, Hogg GR (1980) Chordoid sarcoma. Ultrastructural evidence supporting a synovial origin. Cancer 45:520–527

Rutherfoord G, Davies A (1987) Chordomas – ultrastructure and immunohistochemistry: a report based on the examination of six cases. Histopathology 11:775–787

Salisbury JR (1987) Demonstration of cytokeratins and epithelial membrane antigen in chondroid chordoma. J Pathol 153:37–40

Salisbury JR, Isaacson PG (1985) Demonstration of cytokeratins and an epithelial membrane antigen in chordomas and human fetal notochord. Am J Surg Pathol 9:791–797

Sanerkin NG, Gallagher P (1979) A review of the behavior of chondrosarcoma of bone. J Bone Joint Surg 61 B:395–400

Sassin JF, Chutorian Am (1967) Intracranial chordoma in children. Arch Neurol 17:89–93

Sensenig EG (1956) Adhesions of notochord and neural tube in the formation of chordomas. Am J Anat 98:357–370

Sibley R (1985) Metastatic chordoma to lung (case presentation). Surgical Pathology Specialty Conference, International Academy of Pathology, Toronto, March 12

Spjut HJ, Luse SA (1964) Chordoma: an electron microscopic study. Cancer 17:643–656

Spoden JE, Bumsted BM, Warner ED (1980) Chondroid chordoma. Case report and literature review. Ann Otol Rhinol Laryngol 89:279–285

Stewart MJ, Morin JE (1926) Chordoma: A review with a report of a new sacrococcygeal case. J Pathol Bacteriol 29:41–60

Stough DR, Hartzog JT, Fisher RG (1971) Unusual intracranial spinal metastasis of a cranial chordoma. Case report. J Neurosurg 34:560–562

Suit HD, Goitein M, Munzenrider J et al. (1982) Definitive radiation therapy for chordoma and chondrosarcoma of base of skull and cervical spine. J Neurosurg 56:377–385

Sundaresan N, Galicich JH, Chu FCH, Huvos AG (1979) Spinal chordomas. J Neurosurg 50:312–319

Tremblay FG, Lee VM-Y, Trojanowski JQ (1985) Expression of vimentin, glial filament, and neurofilament proteins in primitive childhood brain tumors. A comparative immunoblot and immunoperoxidase study. Acta Neuropathol (Berl) 68:239–244

Valderrama E, Lipper S, Kahn LB, Mare J (1983) Chondroid chordoma. Electron-microscopic study of two cases. Am J Surg Pathol 7:625–632

Virchow R (1857) Untersuchungen über die Entwicklung des Schädelgrundes im gesunden und krankhaften Zustande und über den Einfluss derselben auf Schädelform, Gesichtsbildung und Gehirn. George Reimer, Berlin

Volpe R, Mazabraud A (1983) A clinopathologic review of 25 cases of chordoma (a pleomorphic and metastasizing neoplasm). Am J Surg Pathol 7:161–170

Weiss SW (1976) Ultrastructure of the so-called "chordoid sarcoma". Evidence supporting cartilaginous differentiation. Cancer 37:300–306

Wetzel WJ, Reuhl KR (1980) Microtubular aggregates in the rough endoplasmic reticulum of a myxoid chondrosarcoma. Ultrastruct Pathol 1:519–525

Wold LE, Laws ER (1984) Chordomas in children and young adults. Lab Invest 50:67A

Immunohistochemical Investigation of Chordomas: Histogenetic and Differential Diagnostic Aspects

V. Bouropoulou, A. Bosse, A. Roessner, E. Vollmer, G. Edel, P. Wuisman, and A. Härle

1 Introduction 183
2 Materials and Methods 186
3 Results 188
3.1 Immunohistochemistry 190
4 Discussion 198
4.1 Histogenetic Implications of the Immunohistochemical Findings 199
5 Summary 201
References 201

1 Introduction

Chordomas are tumors of very low incidence. Among 7400 cases collected in the Bone Tumor Registry of Westphalia, only 32 are chordomas, representing 0.4% of the total.

Due to its close topographical relationship to the axial skeleton, chordoma is classified among bone tumors. One year after it had first been described by Luschka, Müller (1858) recognized its origin in persistent remains of the notochord, an opinion now generally accepted. Chordomas mostly develop from ectopic, intraosseous, rarely perisacral notochordal residues, and very rarely from the central parts of the intervertebral disks (Ashley 1978). Accordingly, 50% of all chordomas are found in the sacrococcygeal region, 35% in the spheno-occipital area, and 15% in the vertebral column. The chordomas collected in the Bone Tumor Registry of Westphalia show a corresponding distribution pattern (Fig. 1).

Chordomas are slowly invasive and destructive. They may extend from their primary localization to the mediastinum, retroperitoneum, spinal canal, and the antero- and retrosacral areas. Involvement of the paranasal sinuses has also been reported in cases of spheno-occipital chordoma. About 30% of all chordomas metastasize, mostly those of the anaplastic type and of sacrococcygeal or vertebral origin. Metastasis occurs during the phase of recurrent disease, and an exceptionally high rate of skin metastases has been reported, apart from bone, lung, and lymph node involvement, sometimes even as the primary manifestation of the disease (Chambers and Schwinn 1979).

Chordomas may arise at any age, with the peak incidence of sacrococcygeal chordomas in the fifth decade, and that of spheno-occipital chordomas in the

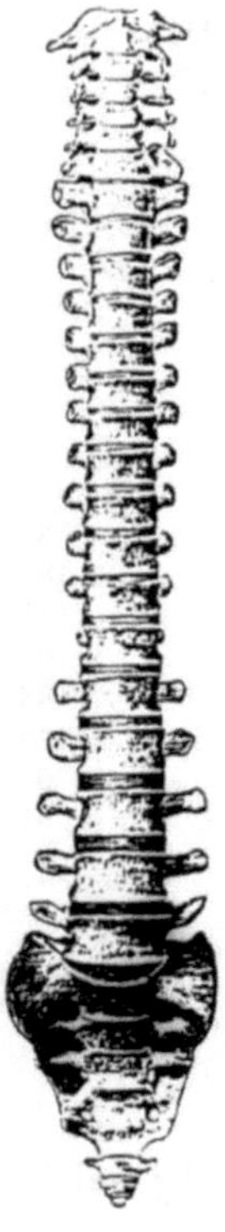

Fig. 1. Topography of chordomas collected in the Bone Tumor Registry of Westphalia, 1974–1986

fourth (HEFFELFINGER et al. 1973). The disease is twice as common in males. Pain caused by nerve compression and destruction, accompanied by motor and sensory deficiency symptoms, is a constant sign of sacrococcygeal and vertebral chordomas. The cranial subtype usually becomes manifested through cranial nerve dysfunction. With an average survival period of 4 years, chordoma of the skull shows the poorest prognosis, the localization close to vital structures generally preventing the therapy of choice, complete surgical removal (HEFFELFINGER et al. 1973). The radiological picture of chordoma is uncharacteristic. We often find indistinctly outlined osteolytic areas with cortical destruction and a large soft tissue shadow.

Macroscopically, the ordinary chordoma is a lobulated, fairly well-encapsulated, partially translucent mucoid tumor. The lobules, often grossly visible, are similar to those of cartilaginous tumors and measure up to 2 or 3 cm in diameter. The smallest lobules are grossly invisible and are not infrequently found in microscopic sections of tissue beyond the gross "capsule." Small calcified masses may be present throughout the tumor. Hemorrhagic areas may be prominent and often convert the translucent lobules into currant-jelly-like masses. The tumor may be almost liquid in consistency and is rarely very firm. Best seen in the sacrum, the neoplasm expands and destroys bone and the gross extent of involvement of bone may be difficult to determine. Soft tissue structures are usually pushed ahead of, and suffer by pressure from, the growing tumor. Mucus-producing adenocarcinomas and soft chondromas or chondrosarcomas may grossly simulate chordoma.

Although the histogenesis of the tumor from the notochord is generally accepted, the exact plastodermic layer to which this primitive structure (and hence its neoplastic counterpart) should be ascribed is still a matter of controversy (ASHLEY 1978). This is mainly due to the early and close relationship of the notochord to all three germinal layers (JAFFE 1958; LICHTENSTEIN 1977). Thus, the various histological patterns observed in chordomas might reflect steps in the notochord's evolution, thereby indicating the origin of the tumor from this specific embryonic structure (ASHLEY 1978). Epithelial and mesenchymal differentiation of the cells of chordoma results in a variable histological appearance of the tumor tissue, which may cause differential diagnostic problems. Areas of homogeneous ground substance, stained light blue in the H & E staining technique, with scattered tumor cells or small cell clusters may suggest a cartilage tumor such as chondroma, chondrosarcoma, or chondromyxoid fibroma. But cartilage tumors have no epithelial-like cell picture or the marked vacuolization of the cytoplasm as in chordomas, with the exception, however, of chordoid sarcoma and myxoid chondrosarcoma. These, too, have a lobular structure and may contain epithelial-like and multivacuolated cells as well as a large amount of myxoid ground substance. Large calcified areas can often be demonstrated in chondroma or chondrosarcoma. Chondromyxoid fibroma, which also has a lobular structure, often shows a large number of multinucleated giant cells. The difficult differentiation, especially from extraskeletal myxoid chondrosarcoma, is reflected in the rather confusing nomenclature: chordoid sarcoma, parachordoma, chordoma periphericum (BYERS 1981; HEFFELFINGER et al. 1973; MIETTINEN et al. 1983; MIETTINEN 1984; PARDO-MINDAN et al. 1981; MEHIO and FERENCZY 1978).

A special variant seen mostly in spheno-occipital chordomas contains a varying chondromatous or chondrosarcomatous component tending to focal calcification. This subtype, labeled chondroid chordoma, differs from the conventional chordoma by its better prognosis despite the often malignant appearance of the cartilage portions and by a nearly equal sex ratio (HEFFELFINGER et al. 1973). Atypical intracranial primary localizations, such as os temporale and foramen jugulare, have been reported (HASEGAWA et al. 1985; IRACI et al. 1973).

Ultrastructural characteristics of chordoma such as the occurrence of star-shaped and physaliphorous cells, complexes of mitochondria-associated endoplasmatic reticulum, and amorphous or fine granulated ground substance help in the differential diagnosis, especially of chondrosarcoma and chordoid sarcoma (PARDO-MINDAN et al. 1981). The electron microscopic technique, however, is too demanding for daily routine. Immunohistochemistry presents a helpful and sophisticated method in the differential diagnosis of histologically uncertain tumors, especially if only a little biopsy material is available.

Immunohistochemistry also offers a convenient and helpful method for verifying the diagnosis of tumors with inconclusive histological features (DU BOULAY 1985). Special attention should be paid to the immunohistochemical identification of intermediate filaments, of which cytokeratin characterizes epithelial

Table 1. Distribution of the 32 cases of chordoma according to age and sex

Nr.	Localization	Age	Sex	Nr.	Localization	Age	Sex
1	Skull	51	F	17	Lumbar	15	F
2	Skull	12[a]	F	18	Lumbar	47	F
3	Cervical	40	F	19	Sacrococcygeal	16	F
4	Cervical	64	F	20	Sacrococcygeal	36	F
5	Cervical	53	M	21	Sacrococcygeal	55[a]	M
6	Cervical	73	F	22	Sacrococcygeal	56	M
7	Thoracic	60	M	23	Sacrococcygeal	58	F
8	Thoracic	54	M	24	Sacrococcygeal	63[a]	M[c]
9	Thoracic	53	M[b]	25	Sacrococcygeal	69	F
10	Thoracic	22	F[c]	26	Sacrococcygeal	71	M
11	Thoracic	53	M	27	Sacrococcygeal	72	M[b,c]
12	Lumbar	57	M	28	Sacrococcygeal	52	M
13	Lumbar	53	F[b]	29	Sacrococcygeal	60	F
14	Lumbar	52	F[b]	30	Sacrococcygeal	64	M
15	Lumbar	55	F	31	Sacrococcygeal	72	M
16	Lumbar	61	F	32	Sacrococcygeal	19	F

[a] Death
[b] Recurrence
[c] Metastasis

tumors and vimentin those of mesenchymal origin (GABBIANI et al. 1981). In a number of tumors, such as pleomorphic adenoma, spindle cell mesothelioma, renal cell carcinoma, and cystadenocarcinoma, there is simultaneous immunohistochemical evidence for both vimentin and cytokeratin (CASELITZ et al. 1982; CONNEL and RHEINWALD 1983). Recent studies have also shown this bimodal pattern of immunoexpression in chordomas (ABENOZA et al. 1985; VOLLMER et al. 1985). If differential diagnosis of such tumors is difficult, the application of additional antibodies is needed for unequivocal classification.

In this report we shall present the results of the immunohistochemical study which is a part of an extensive investigation of chordomas carried out during the last 2 years. The main purpose of this report was the evaluation of the contribution of immunohistochemistry in the elucidation of the tumor histogenesis and also in the differential diagnosis of chordoma from other epithelial and mesenchymal tumors.

2 Materials and Methods

The study is based on 32 cases of chordoma diagnosed and collected in the Bone Tumor Registry of Westphalia at the Institute of Pathology of Münster University between 1974 and 1986. The age and sex distributions of these cases as well as the tumor localization are presented in Table 1.

Multiple sections from each tumor were stained with H & E and sample sections were stained by histochemical procedures detecting lipid and carbohy-

Table 2.

Reaction	Color	Substance
Alcian blue (pH 2.5) – PAS	Red	Neutral mucins, glycogen, compound lipids
	Blue	Acidic mucosubstances
Diastase[a] pretreatment		
AB (pH 2.5) – PAS	Red	Neutral mucins, compound lipids
	Blue	Acidic mucosubstances
Sudan black B (McManus)	Black	Compound lipids
Alcian blue (pH 1.0)		
Alcian yellow (pH 2.5)	Blue	Sulfated acid mucopolysaccharides
	Green	Mixed acid mucopolysaccharides, sulfated sialomucins
	Yellow	Nonsulfated acid mucopolysaccharides Nonsulfated sialomucins
Sialidase[b] pretreatment		
AB (pH 1.0) – AY (pH 2.5)	Blue	Sulfated acid mucopolysaccharides
	Green	Mixed acid mucopolysaccharides
	Yellow	Nonsulfated acid mucopolysaccharides
Testicular hyaluronidase[c] pretreatment		
AB (pH 1.0) – AY (pH 2.5)	Loss of the color reaction due to hyaluronic acid and chondroitin sulfate A and C	
Chondroitinase AC[d] pretreatment		
AB (pH 1.0) – AY (pH 2.5)	Loss of the color reaction due to chondroitin sulfate AC	
Chondroitinase ABC[e] pretreatment		
AB (pH 1.0) – AY (pH 2.5)	Loss of the color reaction due to chondroitin sulfate AC and B	

[a] Malt diastase (1:100) 1 h at 37 °C
[b] Sialidase (neuraminidase) 100 units/ml 24 h at 37 °C
[c] Testicular hyaluronidase +mg/ml 3 h at 37 °C
[d,e] Chondroitinases AC and ABC 1.25 units/ml 2 h at 37 °C

drate elements in the cytoplasm as well as in the extracellular matrixes according to Cook (1974), Culling (1974), and Filipe and Brian (1983), as these have been presented in previous papers (Bouropoulou et al. 1987, 1988). The methods are listed in Table 2.

Immunohistochemistry was performed on (a) paraffin sections from formalin-fixed material, and (b) frozen sections from fresh material snap-frozen in liquid nitrogen, immediately sealed in small platic bags, and stored at −80 °C

Table 3.

Antigen	Source	Dilution
Intermediate filaments		
Cytokeratin CK5 (monoclonal)	BIOMAKOR	1:50
Keratin wide spectrum	DAKO	1:100
Vimentin V9 (monoclonal)	BIOMAKOR	1:50
GFAP	DAKO	1:100
Desmin (monoclonal)	DAKO	1:50
Oncofetal antigens		
CEA	DAKO	1:200
AFP	DAKO	1:100
Epithelial antigens		
EMA (monoclonal)	DAKO	1:100
SC	DAKO	1:100
Other proteins		
S-100	DAKO	1:300
NSE	DAKO	1:300

in a deep freezer. Frozen sections were cut on a freezing microtome (Frigocut 2700, R. Jung, Heidelberg) and mounted on poly-L-lysine-coated (Sigma, Munich) slides. A panel of monoclonal and polyclonal antibodies was used which are listed in Table 3 together with the source and the working dilutions. The indirect peroxidase labeled (frozen sections) and the unlabeled antibody peroxidase-antiperoxidase (paraffin sections) methods were used. Endogenous peroxidase activity was blocked by the application of either 3% aqueous hydrogen peroxide for 10 min or $NaNO_3$, except for carcinoembryonic antigen (CEA), for which a 1% periodic acid solution was used according to ISAACSON and JUDD (1977). The reactions were performed at 37 °C in a moist chamber and the color precipitate was developed using the substrates 3,3-diaminobenzidine tetrahydrochloride or 3-amino-9-ethylcarbazole. Secondary and tertiary antibodies were products by Sigma, Dakopatts, Biomakor, and Dianova. Phosphate buffer saline (PBS) was used for the dilutions and the washings and the same PBS buffer was applied in control sections instead of the specific primary antisera. For electron microscopy the tissue was prepared according to ROESSNER et al. (1988).

3 Results

For a better interpretation of our immunohistochemical results, a brief reference to our histological and histochemical findings seems necessary.

The tumor tissue consisted mainly of lobulated masses of varying size, surrounded by fibrovascular connective tissue septa branching off into the neoplastic lobules. The latter were composed of a mixture of different cell types, and

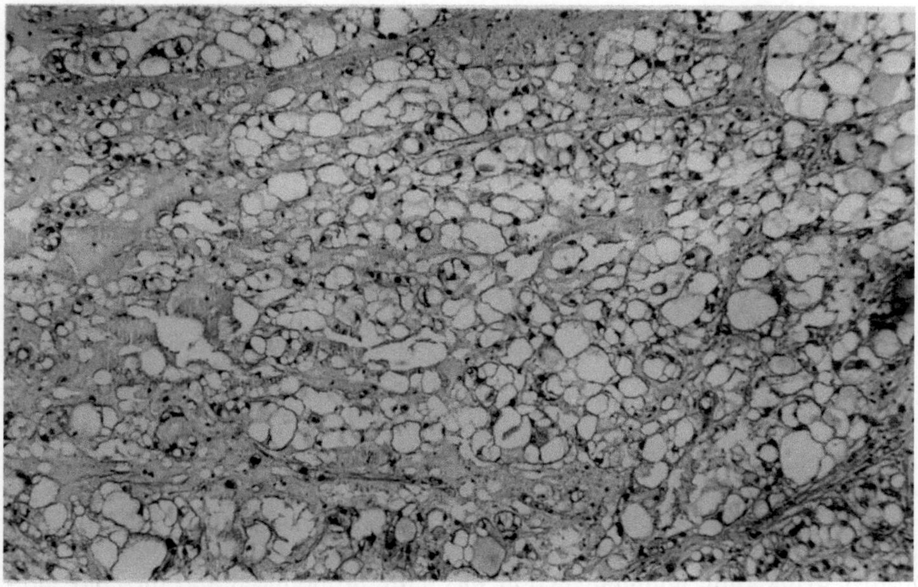

Fig. 2. Chordoma with physaliphorous cells and mucoid ground substance (H & E, ×120)

so the appearance of the neoplastic tissue varied from one tumor to another, in different areas of the same tumor, and even within the same neoplastic lobule. Three types of cells were observed. The cell considered to be the most characteristic was the so-called physaliphorous cell. It was found mainly in the center of the neoplastic lobules which were composed of large vacuolar cells containing a small, hyperchromatic, eccentrically located nucleus, surrounded by a myxoid ground substance, lobulated by a fibrovascular stroma (Figs. 2, 3). Electron microscopically, the walls of the large physaliphorous cells were formed by long cytoplasmic branches, joined by desmosomes, thus separating large extracytoplasmic areas which then appeared as cell vacuoles (Fig. 4). This physaliphorous cell type is to be interpreted as a degenerate terminal stage with decondensation and membrane destruction of the cell organelles and the formation of characteristic mucous areas. Another cell type frequently encountered in most chordomas was smaller, arranged in trabeculae, but also in cords and pseudoacinar or spherical structures. The cytoplasm of the cell was eosinophilic, homogeneous, or granular and in some of the cells slightly or moderately vacuolated. This cell type was found mainly in the periphery of the physaliphorous cells, and it was separated by mucoid extracellular matrix (Fig. 5).

A third cell type was observed in the outmost part of some neoplastic lobules. This cell was small, undifferentiated, with a high nuclear/cytoplasmic index. Its cytoplasm was radially condensed around a centrally located nucleus in a somewhat stellate appearance. This cell type is called "star-like" and is considered to be the proper tumor stem cell, which is also suggested by immunohistochemical investigations using the proliferation antibody (Vollmer et al. 1985) Ki-67 (Figs. 6, 7).

Most tumor cells of the chordomas in our study were found to contain glycogen granules. These were found to be more abundant and diffusely dispersed throughout the cytoplasm of the second cell type while the stellate and the physaliphorous cells contained fewer granules, occupying the cytoplasmic rim surrounding the nucleus. The type of glycosaminoglycans (GAG) of the extracellular matrix varied also according to the cell type. The stellate cells were associated with a stroma containing almost exclusively hyaluronic acid, while cells arranged in trabeculae and physaliphorous cells were found to lie in a stroma rich in sulfated acidic GAG belonging to the group of chondroitin sulfate A and C, with the participation of dermatan sulfate.

3.1 Immunohistochemistry

Immunoreactivity with antisera to cytokeratin was evident in almost all tumor cells, although the intensity of the reaction was not evenly distributed in all cells and in all tumors. Differences were found in relation to the type of antisera used (monoclonal/polyclonal) as well as between fixed and frozen sections. The positive cytokeratin immunoreaction was more pronounced and the color precipitate more widely distributed throughout the cytoplasm of the second cell type. The physaliphorous cells as well as the stellate cells showed a positive reaction in the cytoplasmic rim surrounding the nucleus or the vacuoles (Fig. 8). The mesenchymal structures of the fibrovascular septa were negative.

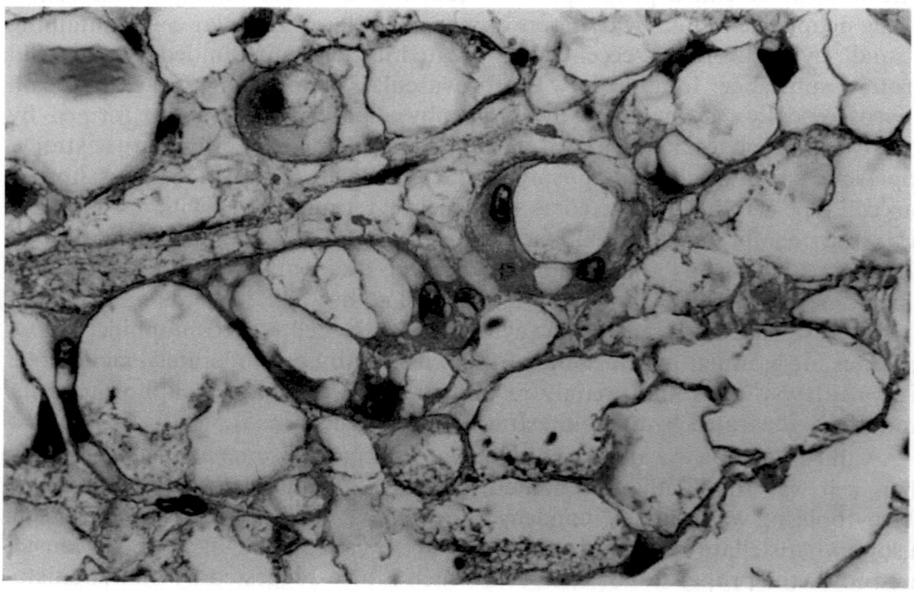

Fig. 3. Typical physaliphorous chordoma cells with long cytoplasmic processes and formation of vacuoles (H & E, × 1000)

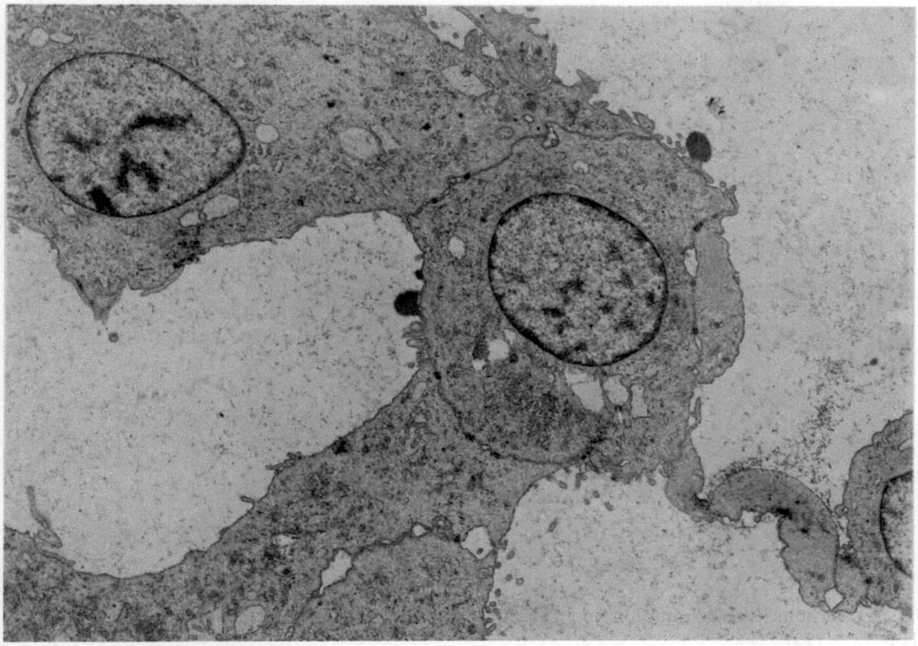

Fig. 4. Low power electron microscopy of chordoma. The cells are connected by cytoplasmic bridges and desmosomes. The cytoplasmic processes of the tumor cell separate large vacuoles with electron-lucent contents, which give the appearance of "physaliphorous" cells in light microscopy. (×4900)

Most tumor cells also displayed a strong immunoreactivity with vimentin antiserum. When comparing parallel sections incubated with antibodies for both cytokeratin and vimentin, we were unable to identify different cell populations reacting with each one of these antibodies (Fig. 9). Vimentin was also found to be strongly positive in nearly all mesenchymal cells of the septa. Desmin and GFAP were always negative.

Both CEA and α-fetoprotein (AFP) were found positive in the tumor cells of all chordomas examined. The reaction precipitate decorated the cytoplasm, while the extracellular matrix was negative (Figs. 10, 11).

Epithelial membrane antigen (EMA) and secretory component (SC) were found to be expressed by most chordoma cells of all tumors of our series (Figs. 12, 13). The distribution of the color precipitate was intracytoplasmic for both markers, while SC also presented some extracellular staining of the stromal mucosubstances.

S-100 protein was positive in all cells of chordoma, with the exception of the small undifferentiated cells of the stellate type. The reaction was intense in the cytoplasm of the neoplastic cells arranged in cords and separated by abundant stroma rich in acidic sulfated GAG, as well as in the physaliphorous cells (Fig. 14). However, neuron-specific enolase (NSE) positivity was displayed by all types of tumor cells, though the reaction was particularly strong in the cells forming trabeculae (Fig. 15). Finally the neoplastic cells in all tumors dis-

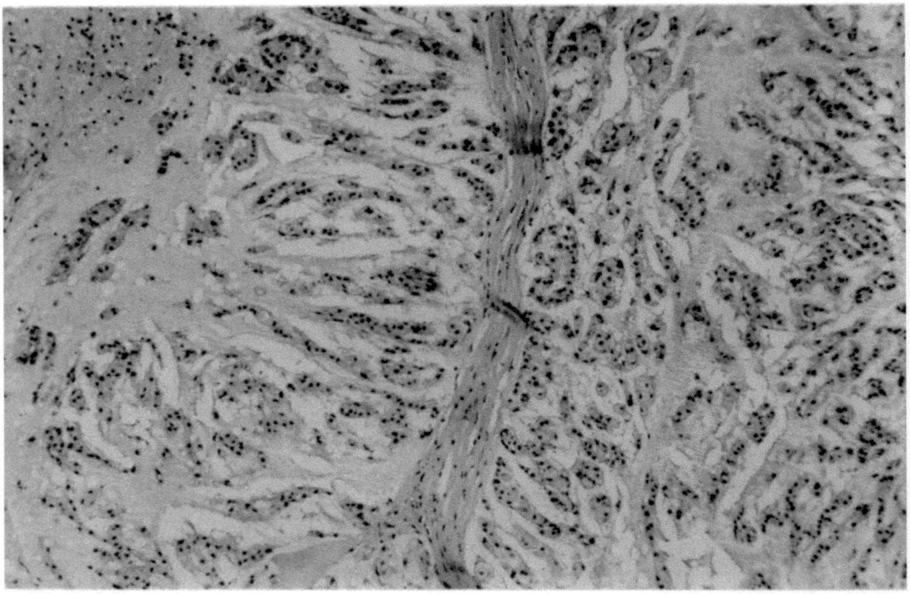

Fig. 5. Chordoma with column-like and trabecular structure with large intracellular mucous formation (H & E, $\times 120$)

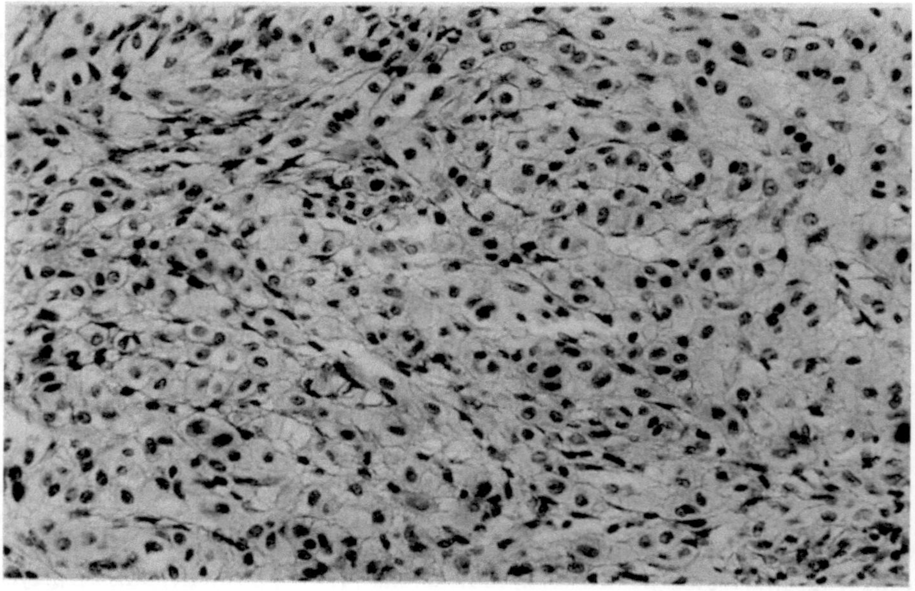

Fig. 6. Chordoma with star-like densely packed eosinophilic cells, no interstitial mucous formation (H & E, $\times 350$)

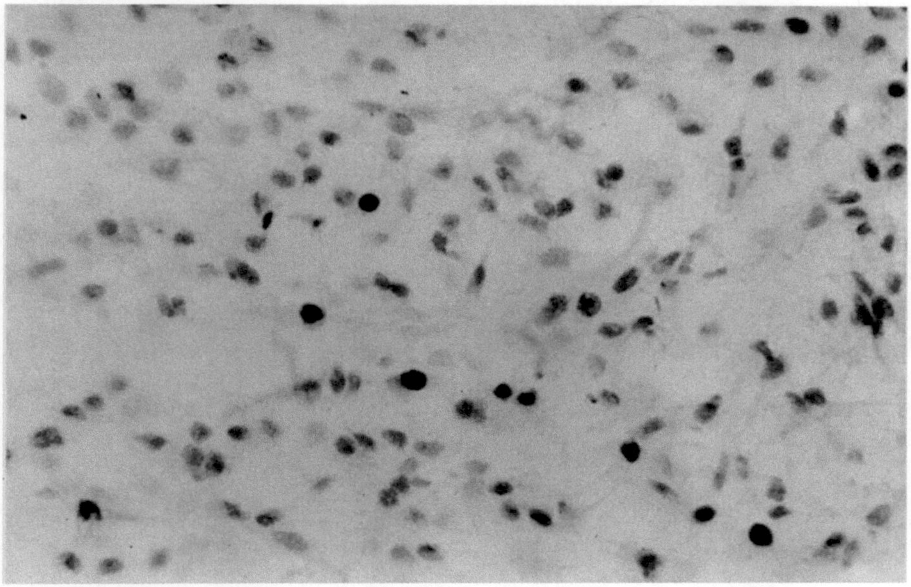

Fig. 7. Marked positive reactions in a star-shaped chordoma area with the proliferation antigen Ki-67 (×480)

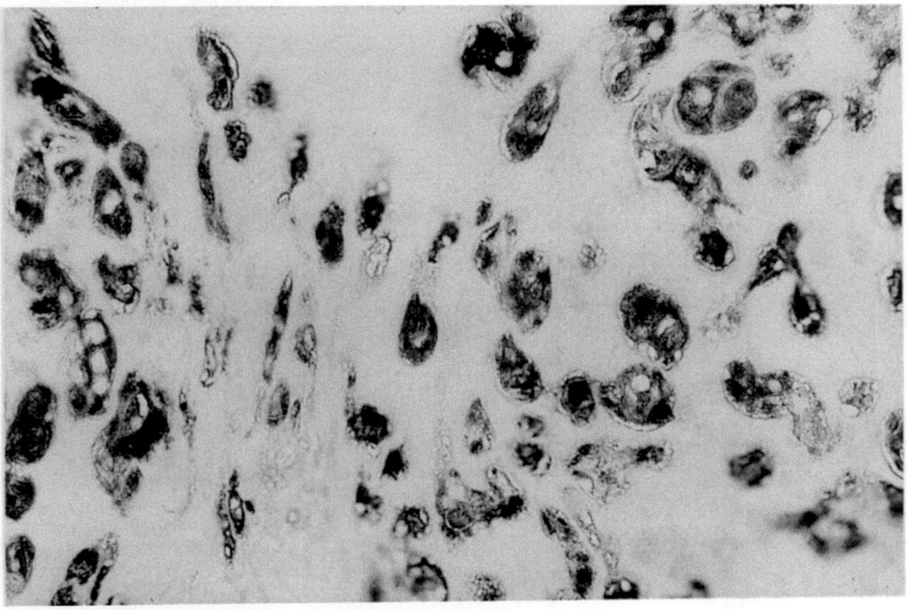

Fig. 8. Positive cytokeratin reaction in chordoma cells (×250)

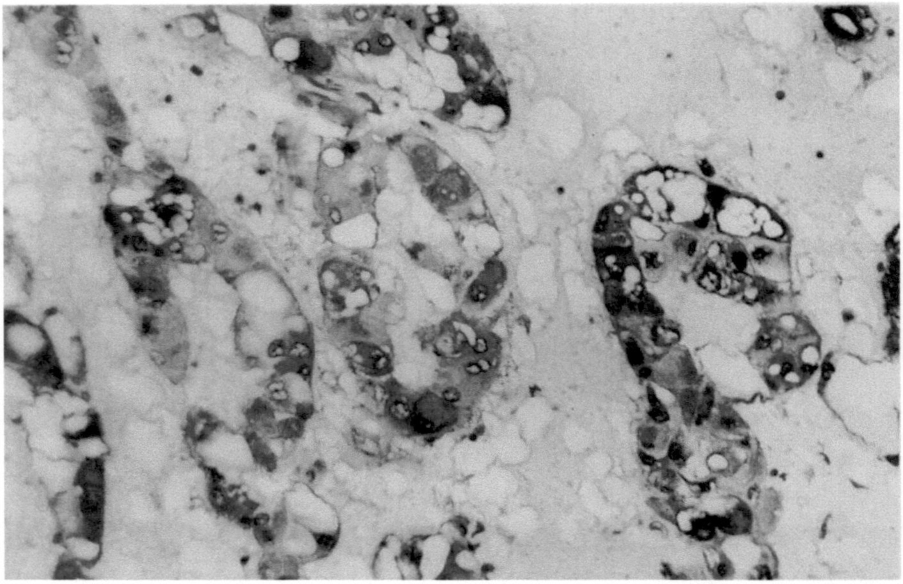

Fig. 9. Positive vimentin reaction in chordoma cells and in basilar mesenchymal connective tissue cells (× 250)

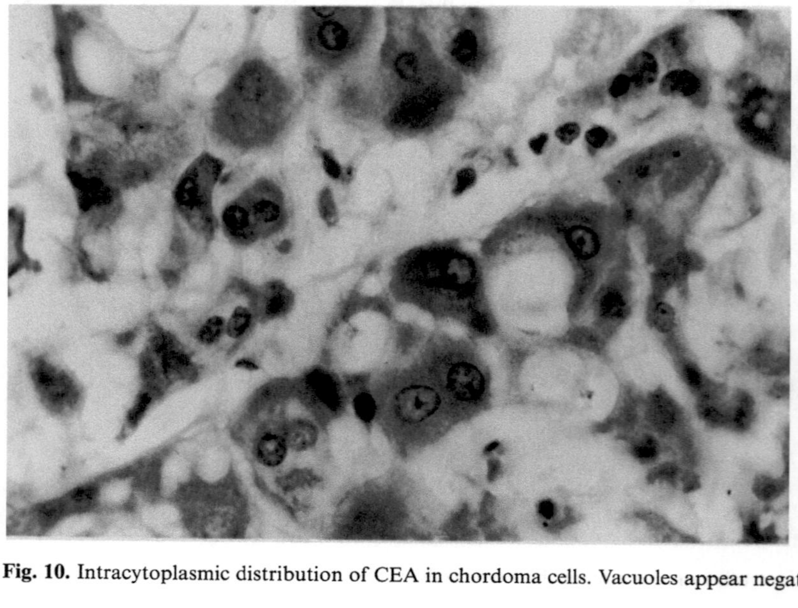

Fig. 10. Intracytoplasmic distribution of CEA in chordoma cells. Vacuoles appear negative (× 480)

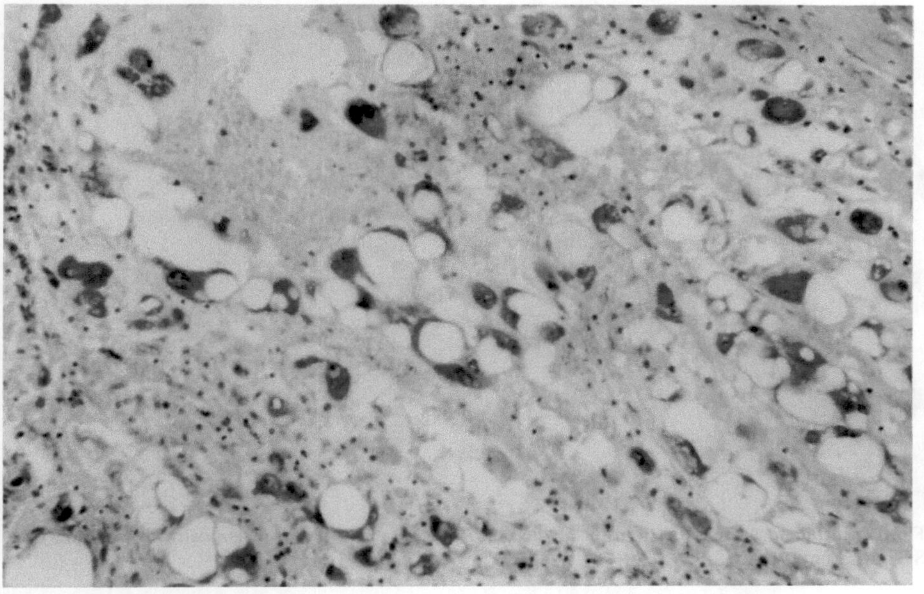

Fig. 11. Strongly positive immunoreaction of the tumor cells with AFP antiserum (× 250)

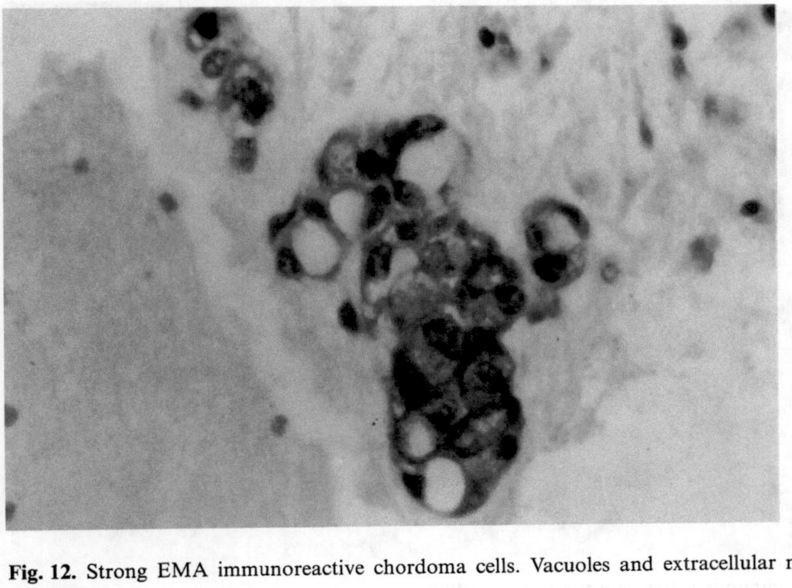

Fig. 12. Strong EMA immunoreactive chordoma cells. Vacuoles and extracellular matrix negative (× 480)

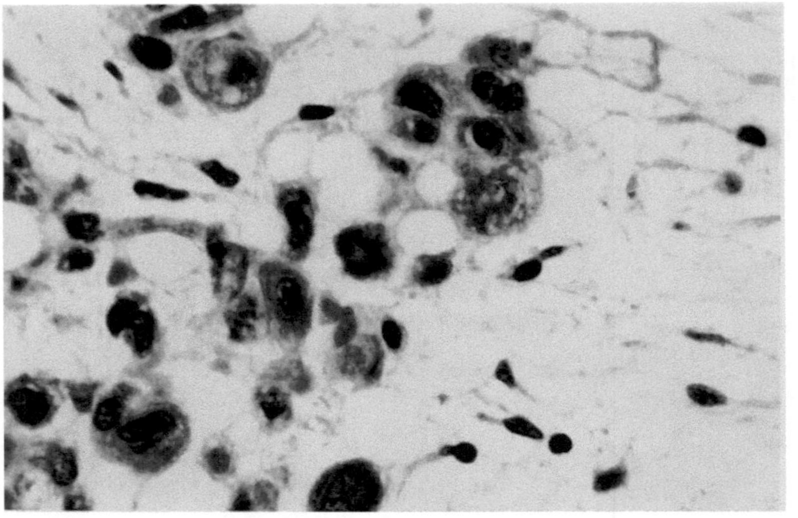

Fig. 13. Intracytoplasmic distribution of the color precipitate in tumor cells positively reacting with SC antiserum (× 480)

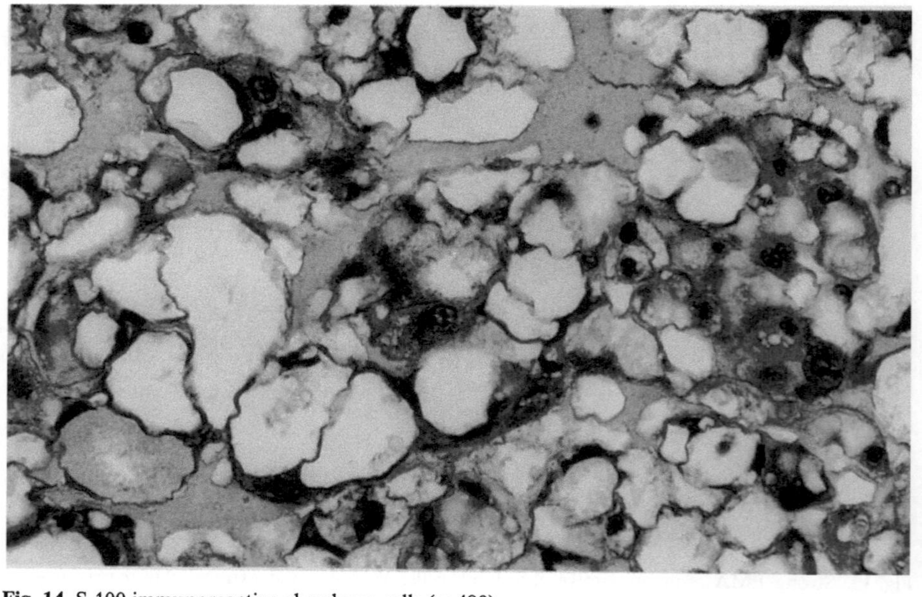

Fig. 14. S-100 immunoreactive chordoma cells (× 480)

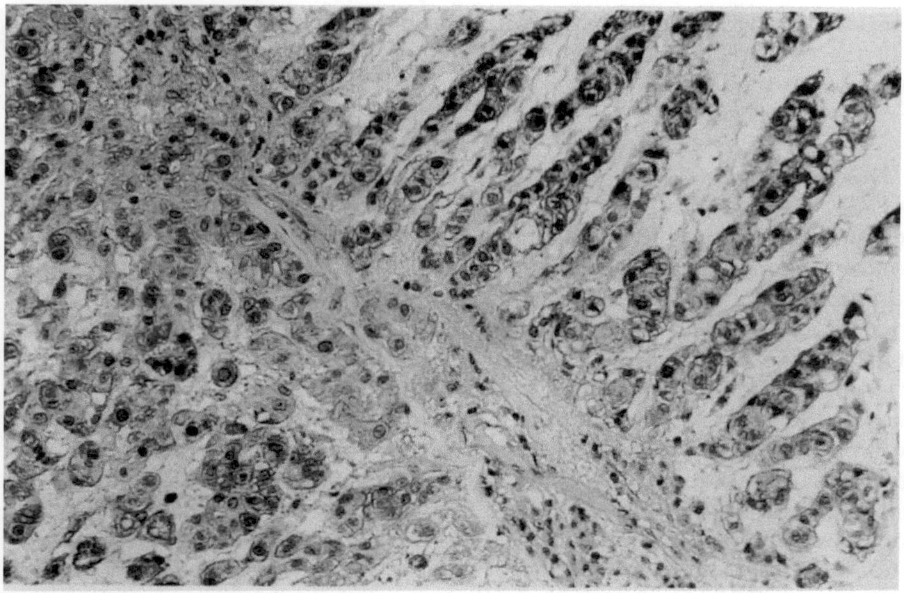

Fig. 15. Positive immunoreaction with NSE in chordoma cells arranged in trabeculae (× 250)

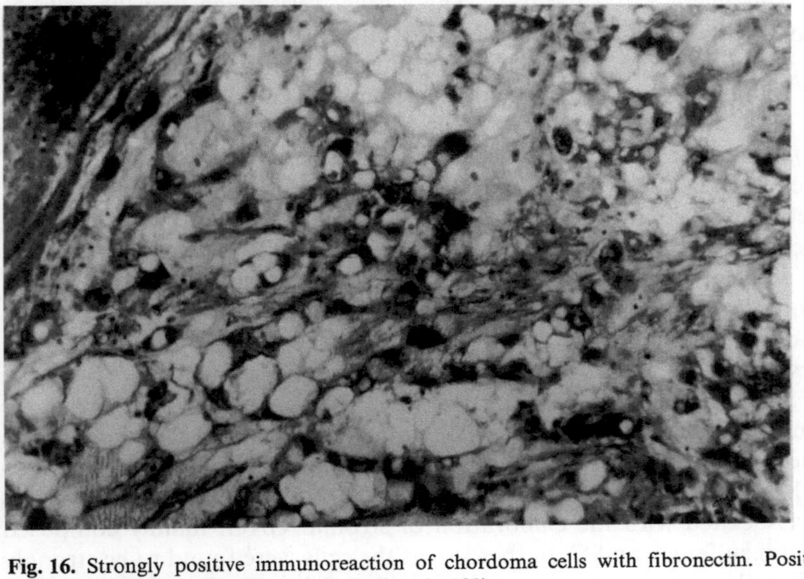

Fig. 16. Strongly positive immunoreaction of chordoma cells with fibronectin. Positively stained mesenchymal cells in the fibrovascular septa. (× 120)

played a strong immunoreactivity with fibronectin. The color precipitate decorated the cytoplasm of the tumor cells, but also the mesenchymal cells of the fibrovascular septa (Fig. 16).

4 Discussion

Previous studies have revealed that S-100 protein is positive in chordomas, chondrosarcomas, and pleomorphic adenomas of the salivary glands (Abenoza and Sibley 1986; Bouropoulou et al. 1987, 1988; Vollmer et al. 1985; Nakazato et al. 1982). This finding cannot be ascribed to the common histogenetic origin of these tumors. Since all the above-mentioned tumors are characterized by the production of intercellular matrix of the myxoid and/or chondroid type, the possibility of a relationship between S-100 protein immunoreactivity and the type of stromal GAG seems evident. Our findings strongly support this view (Bouropoulou et al. 1988). We found that S-100 was negative in the closely packed cells of the notochord of the 1.5 cm long embryo where no intercellular stroma was observed. However, the elaboration of stromal GAG and the participation of sulfated mucopolysaccharides were associated with a strongly positive reaction with S-100 protein in the cytoplasm of the cells composing the notochordal remnants. Nakamura et al. (1983) noticed that the cells of human notochord gave a weaker and sometimes negative reaction with S-100 antiserum when compared to cells from rabbit notochords, but they made no correlation of this finding with the age of the embryos or the evolutional stage of the notochords of either species.

The immunoreactivity of chordoma cells with S-100 seems to correlate with their morphology, which also reflects their functional status. We observed that the stellate cells were S-100 negative. These cells, very much like the cells of the primitive notochord, are closely packed in a stroma devoid of mucosubstances or containing small amounts of hyaluronic acid. Evidence exists that hyaluronic acid enhances tissue growth by promoting cell proliferation, as well as cellular infiltration, by increasing tissue hydration (Iozzo 1984; Nakazato et al. 1982). The presence of hyaluronic acid only in areas composed of stellate cells further supports the view also expressed by others (Mikuz et al. 1987; Vollmer et al. 1985) that these cells are stem cells with proliferative properties.

The second type of cell was characterized by abundant glycogen granules and by its association with variable amounts of extracellular mucosubstances, mainly composed of sulfated GAG of the chondroitin sulfate A and C type. This type of cell was strongly S-100 positive. A strong positive reaction was also observed in the physaliphorous cells. Our findings further support the view that S-100 protein cannot be considered as a marker with cytogenetic implications, at least for chordomas. We found that primitive notochord, as well as the stellate stem cells of chordomas, were S-100 negative. We also observed that evolutional changes taking place in both normal and neoplastic tissue are associated with the elaboration of stromal GAG, mainly composed of chondroitin sulfate A and C. In these areas the cells were found to be strongly positive. The absence of immunoreactivity of chordoma cells with GFAP as well as with neurofilaments (COINDRE et al. 1986) could be considered as an argument against the neural origin or neuroectodermal differentiation of the tumor cells.

The differential diagnosis of chordomas arising in the spheno-occipital region should also include pleomorphic adenomas of the salivary glands (BYERS 1981; HEFFELFINGER et al. 1973; MIKUZ et al. 1977). The double expression of cytokeratin and vimentin was of no use for the differentiation between these tumors, since the cells of pleomorphic adenomas also show positive results in both reactions (CASELITZ et al. 1981, 1982; ERLANDSON et al. 1983). The same is also true for other markers, such as S-100 and NSE (BOUROPOULOU et al. 1987; NAKAZATO et al. 1982). Therefore, the differential diagnosis between these two neoplasms should be based upon the reactivity of chordoma cells with CEA and AFP (BOUROPOULOU et al. 1987).

Vertebral metastatic deposits from mucinous adenocarcinomas may present differential diagnostic problems from chordomas (CHAMBERS and SCHWINN 1979; MIETTINEN 1984). The distinction should be based upon the positive immunoreaction of the tumor cells with vimentin and fibronectin. In addition, positive immunoreaction of chordoma cells with AFP, S-100, and NSE may facilitate the differential diagnosis from mucinous adenocarcinomas (BOUROPOULOU et al. 1987).

Sacrococcygeal chordomas may sometimes be confused with myxopapillary ependymomas of the filum terminale (BOTTLES and BECKSTEAD 1984; MIETTINEN et al. 1983). The positive reaction with all epithelial markers (EMA, CEA, AFP, SC), the cytokeratin intermediate filament (IF) expression, and the lack of reactivity with GFAP, permit a clear distinction between the two tumors (BOUROPOULOU et al. 1987; MIETTINEN 1984; MIETTINEN et al. 1983).

The mesenchymal differentiation of the tumor cells frequently observed in chordomas and the production of abundant myxoid and/or chondroid extracellular matrix may lead to the erroneous diagnosis of conventional chordoma or chondrosarcoma, especially of the myxoid variety (FLETCHER et al. 1986; MEHIO and FERENCZY 1978; PARDO-MINDAN et al. 1981). There is no doubt that the myxoid variant of chondrosarcoma poses the most demanding and difficult differential diagnosis. Here, differentiation from chordoma – especially with regard to fine needle biopsy – is extremely difficult, due to the large number of pyknotic cell nuclei, embedded in a largely vacuolated ground substance. However, the positive reaction of chordoma with all epithelial tumor markers allows a clear differentiation from chondrosarcoma, which, unlike chordoma, does not express cytokeratin.

All tumor cells are characterized by a bimodal expression of IF (cytokeratin and vimentin) as well as by a strong immunoreactivity with both oncofetal markers (CEA and AFP). We suggest that these properties should be ascribed to the origin of the tumor from remnants of the notochord.

4.1 Histogenetic Implications of the Immunohistochemical Findings

Chordoma is composed of an admixture of cell types forming structures which seem to imitate the evolutional stages of the development and fate of human notochord (Huvos 1979; Jaffe 1958; Wellinger 1975). All three phenotypically different cell types observed in chordomas presented identical intermediate filament composition, reacting positively with both cytokeratin and vimentin antisera (Abenoza et al. 1985; Abenoza and Sibley 1986; Coindre et al. 1986; Vollmer et al. 1985). The phenomenon of the coexpression of more than one IF protein system is well known and the list of normal and neoplastic cells presenting a bimodal IF expression is growing (Caselitz et al. 1981, 1982; Connel and Rheinwald 1983; Holthöfer et al. 1983; Miettinen et al. 1983; Vialle 1987; Vollmer et al. 1985). A possible explanation for this coexpression in chordoma might be ascribed to the origin of the tumor from remnants of the notochord. Since notochordal tissue emerges from ectodermal primitive streak, its cells are epithelial in nature and thus synthesize cytokeratin filaments (Kempler et al. 1981). Later on, during the evolution of the organ, the cells of the notochord participate in the development of the mesoderm and the mesenchyme. It is suggested that the cells of the notochord, once formed, lose their epithelial organization and start to behave like mesodermal–mesenchymal elements (Ashley 1978). This mesodermal–mesenchymal differentiation is probably accompanied by the acquisition of vimentin IF, which is the first IF protein type expressed by nearly all nonepithelial cells, from the very early stages of the embryonal development (Bannasch et al. 1982; Denk et al. 1983; Lane et al. 1983).

The epithelial nature of the neoplastic cells of chordoma is well documented by the expression of cytokeratin IF, detected by immunohistochemical methods. Besides cytokeratin positivity, the ectodermal origin of chordoma is further supported by the immunoreactivity of the tumor cells with other epithelial markers, such as EMA and SC (Bouropoulou et al. 1987; Coindre et al. 1986; Miettinen 1984; Vollmer et al. 1985). However, the coexpression of vimentin and the intracytoplasmic distribution of fibronectin imply a certain degree of mesenchymal differentiation (du Boulay 1985).

The immunohistochemical profile of chordoma cells indicates that, in spite of their phenotypic differences, these cells belong to the same line of primitive embryonal cells and this suggestion seems to be further supported by the detection of both oncofetal antigens (CEA and AFP) in the tumor cells.

The immunoreactivity of chordoma cells with S-100, also maintained by others (Abenoza et al. 1985; Coindre et al. 1986; Nakamura et al. 1983), may have two possible explanations. It might be interpreted as pointing toward a close relationship of notochord to neuroectodermal tissues, and even more toward a common origin (Nakamura et al. 1983). However, in a combined histochemical and immunohistochemical study of notochord and chordomas, we observed that the immunoreactivity of the cells in both structures is related to the type of extracellular matrix and to the metabolic activity of the cells rather than to the origin of the cells from the neuroectoderm (Bouropoulou et al. 1987).

These immunohistochemical investigations have shown that in tumors with bimodal expression of vimentin and cytokeratin, the use of several other antibodies offers a reliable differential diagnostic tool. In diagnostic routine, immunohistochemistry will support histology by substantiating and enlarging morphological evaluation. The identification of a "marker profile" by the use of commercial antisera is of value in distinguishing chordoma from other epithelial or mesenchymal tumors.

5 Summary

Chordomas are rare tumors of neuroectodermal origin and often show a very heterogeneous histological picture. In a combined histochemical and immunohistochemical study of 32 chordomas collected in the Bone Tumor Registry of Westphalia we were able to show that the immunoreactivity of the cells in both chordoma and notochordal structures are in close relationship with the extracellular matrix and depends more on the metabolic activity of these cells than on the origin of the cells of the neuroectoderm. All tumor cells show a bimodal immunoreaction with cytokeratin and vimentin, as well as a strong immunoreaction with the oncofetal markers CEA and AFP. The differentiation of chordomas from other malignant tumors, mainly the myxoid variant of chondrosarcoma, may cause major difficulties, especially if only a little biopsy material is available. Here we can see that in tumors with bimodal immunoexpression of vimentin and cytokeratin, as can be found in chordomas, the further use of antibodies offers a reliable differential diagnostic tool. The positive reaction of chordomas with all epithelial tumor markers offers a clear differentiation from chondrosarcomas, which, unlike chordomas, do not express cytokeratin. The identification of a marker profile by employing common antisera is of major value in the differentiation of chordoma from other epithelial or mesenchymal tumors.

References

Abenoza P, Sibley RK (1986) Chordoma: an immunohistochemical study. Hum Pathol 17:744–747

Abenoza P, Sibley KA, Rosai J (1985) Immunohistochemistry in differential diagnosis of chordoma and chondrosarcoma (abstract). Lab Invest: 52 1 A

Ashley D (1978) In: Evan's histological appearances of tumors, 3rd edn. Churchill Livingstone, Edinburgh

Bannasch P, Zerban H, Mayer D (1982) The cytoskeleton in tumor cells. Pathol Res Pract 175:196–211

Bottles K, Beckstead HJ (1984) Enzyme histochemical characterization of chordomas. Am J Surg Pathol B:443–447

Bouropoulou V, Kontogeorgos G, Papamichales G, Bosse A, Roessner A, Vollmer E (1987) Differential diagnosis of chordoma. Immunohistochemical aspects. Arch Anat Cytol Pathol 35:35–40

Bouropoulou V, Kontogeorgos G, Papamichales G, Milas P, Roessner A, Vollmer E, Grundmann E (1988) S-100 protein and neuron specific enolase expression by chordomas in relation to the composition of their stromal mucosubstances. Pathol Res Pract 183:256–261

Byers PD (1981) A study of histological features distinguishing chordoma from chondrosarcoma. Br J Cancer 43:229–232

Caselitz J, Osborn M, Seifert G, Weber K (1981) Intermediate-sized filament protein (prekeratin, vimentin, desmin) in normal parotid gland tumors. Immunofluorescence study. Virchows Arch [A] 393:273–286

Caselitz J, Osborn M, Wustrow J, Seifert G, Weber K (1982) The expression of different intermediate-sized filaments in human salivary glands and their tumors. Pathol Res Pract 175:266–278

Chambers P, Schwinn C (1979) Chordoma. A clinico-pathologic study of metastases. Am J Clin Pathol 72:765–776

Coindre JM, Rivell J, Trojani M et al. (1986) Immunohistological study of chordomas. J Pathol 150:61–63

Connel ND, Rheinwald JG (1983) Regulation of the cytoskeleton in mesothelial cells: reversible loss of keratin and increase in vimentin during rapid growth in culture. Cell 34:245–253

Cook HC (1974) Manual of histological demonstration techniques. Butterworths, London

Culling CFA (1974) Handbook of histopathological and histochemical techniques, 3rd edn. Butterworths, London

Denk H, Krepler R, Artlieb V et al. (1983) Protein of intermediate filaments. An immunohistochemical and biochemical approach to the classification of soft tissue tumors. Am J Pathol 110:193–208

Du Boulay CEH (1985) Immunohistochemistry of soft tissue tumors: a review. J Pathol 146:77–94

Erlandson RA, Cordon-Cardo C, Higgins P (1983) Coexpression of cytokeratin (CK), vimentin and actin in cells composing pleomorphic adenomas of salivary glands. An immunohistochemical and ultrastructural study. J Cell Biol 97:219a

Filipe MI, Brian L (1983) Histochemistry in pathology. Churchill Livingstone, Edinburgh

Fletcher CDM, Powell G, McKee PH (1986) Extraskeletal myxoid chondrosarcoma: a histochemical and immunohistochemical study. Histopathology 10:489–499

Gabbiani G, Kapanchi Y, Barazzone P, Franke WW (1981) Immunochemical identification of intermediate-sized filament in human neoplastic cells: a diagnostic aid for the surgical pathologist. Am J Pathol 104:206–216

Hasegawa M, Nishiyima W, Watanabe I, Nasu M, Kamiyama R (1985) Primary chondroid chordoma arising from the base of the temporal bone. J Laryngol Otol 99:485–489

Heffelfinger MJ, Dahlin DC, MacCarthy CS, Beabout JW (1973) Chordomas and cartilaginous tumors at the skull base. Cancer 32:410–420

Holthöfer H, Miettienen A, Paasivuo R et al. (1983) Cellular origin and differentiation of renal carcinomas. A fluorescence microscopic study with kidney-specific antibodies, anti-intermediate filament antibodies and lectins. Lab Invest 49:317–326

Huvos GA (1979) Bone tumors. Diagnosis, treatment and prognosis. Saunders, Philadelphia

Iozzo VR (1984) Proteoglycans and neoplastic-mesenchymal cell interactions. Hum Pathol 15:2–10

Iraci G, Gerosa M, Pardatscher K (1973) Isolated Vernet's syndrome: an unusual manifestation of intracranial chordoma. Surg Neurol 1:259–298

Isaacson P, Judd AM (1988) Immunohistochemistry of carcinoembryonic antigen: characterization of cross-reactions with other glycoproteins. Gut 18:779–785

Jaffe AG (1958) Tumors and tumorous conditions of bones and joints. Lea & Febinger, Philadelphia

Kempler R, Brulet P, Schnebelen MT, Gaillard J, Jacob (1981) Reactivity of monoclonal antibodies against intermediate filament proteins during embryonic development. J Embryol Exp Morphol 64:45–60

Lane EB, Hogan BLM, Kurkinen M, Garrels JI (1983) Coexpression of vimentin and cytokeratins in parietal endoderm cells of early mouse embryo. Nature 303:701–704

Lichtenstein L (1977) Bone tumors, 5th edn. CV Mosby, St. Louis

Luschka H (1857) Über gallertartige Auswüchse am Clivus Blumenbachii. Virchows Arch [Path Anat Physiol] 11:8–12

Mehio AR, Ferenczy A (1978) Extraskeletal myxoid chondrosarcoma with chordoid features (chordoid sarcoma). Am J Clin Pathol 70:700–705

Miettinen M (1984) Chordoma: antibodies to epithelial membrane antigen and carcinoembryonic antigen in differential diagnosis. Arch Pathol Lab Med 108:891–892

Miettinen M, Lehto VP, Virtanen I (1983) Differential diagnosis of chordoma, chondroid, and ependymal tumors as aided by anti-intermediate filament antibody. Am J Pathol 112:160–160

Mikuz G, Mydla F, Gutter K (1977) Ultrastrukturelle biochemische und cytomorphometrische Befunde beim Chordom. Beitr Pathol 161:150–165

Müller H (1858) Über das Vorkommen von Resten der Chorda dorsalis bei Menschen nach der Geburt und über ihr Verhältnis zu den Gallertgeschwülsten am Clivus. Z Rat Med 2:202–229

Nakamura Y, Becker L, Marks A (1983) S-100 protein in human chordomas and in human and rabbit notochord. Arch Pathol Lab Med 107:118–120

Nakazato Y, Ishizeki J, Takahashi K et al. (1982) Localization of S-100 protein and glial fibrillary acidic protein-related antigen in pleomorphic adenoma of the salivary glands. Lab Invest 46:621–626

Pardo-Mindan FJ, Guillen FJ, Villas C, Vasques JJ (1981) A comparative ultrastructural study of chondrosarcoma, chondroid sarcoma and chordoma. Cancer 47:2611–2619

Roessner A, Vollmer E, Zwadlo G et al. (1988) The cytogenesis of macrophages and osteoclast-like giant cells in bone tumors with special emphasis on the so-called fibrohistiocytic tumors

Vialle G (1987) Co-expression of different intermediate filament proteins by human tumors (Abstr IX Europ Congr Path, Prague). Pathol Res Pract 182:573

Vollmer E, Bouropoulou V, Roessner A et al. (1985) Immunhistologische und elektronenmikroskopische Untersuchungen an Chordomen. Verh Dtsch Ges Pathol 69:633

Wellinger C (1975) Le chordome rachidien. Revue de la litterature depuis 1960. Rev Rhum Mal Osteoart 42:106–116, 196–204, 287–295

The Cytogenesis of Macrophages and Osteoclast-like Giant Cells in Bone Tumors with Special Emphasis on the So-Called Fibrohistiocytic Tumors

A. Roessner, E. Vollmer, G. Zwadlo, C. Sorg, M. Kolve, D.B. v. Bassewitz, P. Wuisman, A. Härle, and E. Grundmann

1 Introduction 205
2 Special Methods 206
3 Distribution of Macrophages in Bone Tumors 208
3.1 Macrophage Reaction in Different Bone Tumors 208
4 Phenotypic Characterization of Osteoclast-like Giant Cells 214
5 The Proliferation Behavior of Macrophages as Compared with Fibroblastic Cells in Malignant Fibrous Histiocytoma and Giant Cell Tumor of Bone 217
6 Summary 223
References 225

1 Introduction

The osteoclast was first described in 1873 by Kölliker as a "bone resorbing cell." Its origin, however, remained obscure. Osteoblasts and osteoclasts were first believed to have a common origin, a precursor descending from the connective tissue of bone (Tonna and Cronkite 1961). Later observations and experimental results prompted a search for osteoclast precursors in the mononuclear phagocyte system (Fishman and Hay 1962; Jee and Nolan 1963; Hanaoka et al. 1970; Chambers 1978; Byers et al. 1975; Kasahara et al. 1979). Morphological and enzyme histochemical investigations revealed several similarities between macrophages and multinucleated giant cells in bone tumors, as far as their histological appearance and their intracellular enzymatic pattern were concerned (Chambers 1978; Aparisi et al. 1977; Steiner et al. 1972; Schajowicz 1961; Yoshida et al. 1982). Osteoclasts and tumor-associated giant cells were found to share the presence of the enzymes nonspecific esterase and acid phosphatase, which are both equally characteristic of macrophages (Chambers 1978; Schajowicz 1961). Experimental cell analysis in studies of thorotrast-stained peritoneal macrophages from healthy rats, transfused into histocompatible rats with experimental fractures (Göthlin and Ericsson 1976), as well as studies of osteopetrotic mice (Loutit and Sansom 1976), further advanced the research. Quail-chick chimera experiments suggested that osteoclasts are differentiated descendants of the multipotential hematopoietic stem cell of the bone marrow (Ash et al. 1980).

The immunohistochemical finding of an absence of F_c and C_3 receptors (Hogg et al. 1980) and a lack of macrophage specific antigens on giant cells (Horton et al. 1984) as well as further cell transplantation experiments (Loutit and NISBET 1982) initiated the discussion of a nonhematopoietic origin for the polykaryons, in contrast to the suggestion of a hematopoietic descent (HANAOKA and YABE 1985).

Recent immunohistochemical data from experimental results again confirm a close relationship between the hematopoietic system, especially cells of the mononuclear phagocyte system, osteoclasts, and the multinucleated giant cells found in giant cell tumors of bone (BURGER et al. 1984; ATHANASOU et al. 1985; OURSLER et al. 1985). Thus osteoclasts derived from hematopoietic cells of mononuclear phagocytic origin and osteoblasts derived from local mesenchymal cells are of different cytogenetic origin. However, they have a close functional relationship. As most bone tumors are derived from local mesenchymal cells (ROESSNER 1984; ROHOLL et al. 1985), the relationship between hematopoietically derived giant cells and local mesenchymal cells finds its neoplastic counterpart in bone tumors in the so-called osteoclast-like giant cells that are found in most bone tumors. While the occurrence of these giant cells is well documented, little is known about the distribution of mononuclear macrophages. They can hardly be visualized with routine histological methods, but may be reliably demonstrated by enzyme histochemical or electron microscopic methods. In recent years immunohistology was found to be a more appropriate tool for demonstrating macrophages (KINDBLOM et al. 1982; NASH 1982; PERMANETTER and MEISTER 1984; ROESSNER et al. 1987).

The cells of the mononuclear phagocyte system in bone tumors are of special interest with regard to their role in the so-called fibrohistiocytic tumors of bone (HUVOS 1979). As many important bone tumor entities are considered to be of fibrohistiocytic type (malignant fibrous histiocytoma, benign fibrous histiocytoma, giant cell tumor of bone, nonossifying fibroma), the key to understanding the histogenesis and relationship between these different tumor entities lies in the impact of cells of the mononuclear phagocyte system.

The present study therefore, focuses on the distribution of macrophages in the different bone tumor entities. In another section, the role and cytogenesis of osteoclast-like giant cells in bone tumors will be investigated with advanced immunohistological methods. Finally, the investigation focuses on the proliferation behavior of macrophages and giant cells in bone tumors when compared with the local mesenchymal cells. The conclusions which can be drawn on the basis of these different approaches will facilitate the understanding of the different so-called fibrohistiocytic tumor entities in bone, and of the roots of their close relationship.

2 Special Methods

For *electron microscopy*, tissue samples were taken from various areas of each tumor, fixed immediately after excision for 2 h at 4° C in 2.5% glutaraldehyde (0.05 M phosphate buffer), and then rinsed for 24 h in the same buffer. Fixation was carried out in 1.35 osmic acid solution, in 0.05 mol phosphate buffer (pH 7.4) for 2 h. The samples were dehydrated in graded ethanols and embedded in Epon 812. Semithin sections were cut with glass knives on a Porter-Blum microtome and stained with toluidine blue. Ultrathin section were cut on a Porter-Blum microtome using diamond knives, then mounted on unfilmed copper grids and stained for 15 min with uranyl acetate and for 3 min with lead citrate. The sections were examined with a Philips EM 400.

For *autoradiography* small cubes of 1 m^3 were excised from the tumor tissue during surgery and immediately immersed in 8 ml medium cooled at 4° C (TC medium 199 W/O phenol red, Difco, Detroit). The cubes were then incubated in 8 ml ^{3}H-thymidine (Amersham/Buchler, Braunschweig), dissolved with Tc 199 (activity 4 µc/ml medium). Incubation lasted 20 min at 37° C 2 bar O_2. Between tissue sampling and incubation the maximum delay was only 8 min. To stop incubation the specimens were rinsed twice in Tc 199 medium at 4° C for 2 min, then three times in the same medium at 4° C for 4 min. After fixation in glutaraldehyde the processing followed the usual routine methods. Preselected 1-mm sections were prepared. Ilford K2 emulsion was applied using the dipping method. The dipped slides were transferred to lightproof plastic boxes containing dried silica gel. The emulsion-coated sections were exposed for 7 weeks at 4° C. After fine-grain development with Kodak D 19, the sections were stained with toluidine blue. Ultrathin sections were prepared from selected blocks and mounted on uncoated silver grids. Ilford emulsion was applied using glass loops. After 6 weeks' exposure at 4° C, the coated sections were developed according to the Gevaert 210 formula with subsequent multiple washing in aqua bidest. The sections were stained without gelatin removal for 2 min with lead citrate.

For immunohistochemical analysis, the tissue was snap-frozen in liquid nitrogen immediately after excision. Peroxidase-antiperoxidase or indirect immunoperoxidase techniques were applied to frozen sections. In addition a modified APAAP method (CORDELL et al. 1984) was used for immunohistochemical double labeling. Antibodies to mononuclear phagocyte system (MPS) were used as listed in Table 1. A monoclonal antibody to a proliferation-associated nuclear antigen (Ki-67) was also used (GERDES et al. 1984). Our results in determining the proliferation rates in bone tumors with this antibody have been published (VOLLMER et al. 1986).

Table 1. Specificity of the monoclonal antibodies used in the series of experiments

Antibody	Specificity	Reference
27-E-10	Blood monocytes	ZWADLO et al. 1987
25-F-9	Mature macrophages	ZWADLO et al. 1985
RM 3/1	Macrophages	ZWADLO et al. 1986
Ki M1	Monocytes/macrophages	RADZUN and PARWARESCH 1983
Ki M2	Monocytes/macrophages	RADZUN and PARWARESCH 1983
Leu M3	Monocytes/macrophages	DIMITRIOU-BONA et al. 1983
OKM 5	Monocytes/macrophages	KNOWLES et al. 1984

3 Distribution of Macrophages in Bone Tumors

The occurrence of histiocytic giant cells in bone tumors is well documented since these cells are readily recognized by conventional histology. Little is known, however, about mononuclear macrophages in bone tumors. They can be demonstrated reliably only by enzyme histochemical or electron microscopic methods. In the past few years, immunohistology has become a more appropriate tool for demonstrating macrophages (NASH 1982; KINDBLOM et al. 1986; PERMANETTER and MEISTER 1984; ZWADLO et al. 1985, 1986).

First we used the monoclonal antibodies specific against lysozyme, α_1-antitrypsin (α_1-AT) and α,-antichymotrypsin (α_1-ACT), for an orientating analysis since they have been recommended as markers for histiocytes in various tumors and organs (MEISTER and NATHRATH 1981; KINDBLOM et al. 1982; NASH 1982; PERMANETTER and MEISTER 1984). These antibodies, however, are not specific for cells of the mononuclear phagocyte system, and so their value for our special purpose was rather limited. Lysozyme, often used for demonstrating macrophages (MASON and TAYLOR 1975), also shows strong positivity in cells of the granulocytic series. α_1-AT, also introduced as a marker for macrophages (ISAACSON et al. 1979), is positive in some macrophages and in some granulocytes, but not in the majority of macrophages analyzed in our study. Our results have further shown that α_1-ACT does stain the majority of macrophages, but not the cells of the granulocytic series.

Generally, these results agree with those of MOTO et al. (1980), who analyzed histiocytes and other cellular elements in the lymph node with the polyclonal marker used here. However, we are reluctant to confirm the results of MEISTER and NATHRATH (1981), MEISTER (1984), and KINDBLOM et al. (1982), who were generally inclined to consider as histiocytic differentiations all those cells positively staining with these polyclonal antibodies. It still appears unsafe to draw diagnostic conclusions from this assumption (ERLANDSON 1984).

As monoclonal antibodies against cells of the mononuclear phagocyte system (BREARD et al. 1980; UGOLINI et al. 1980; DIMITRIOU-BONA et al. 1983; RADZUN and PARWARESCH 1983; RADZUN 1985; SHEN et al. 1983; TALLE et al. 1983; ZWADLO et al. 1985, 1986) are much more specific for characterizing and differentiating mononuclear phagocytes, we applied antibodies against blood monocytes and inflammatory monocytes (27-E-10), ZWADLO et al. 1986, and 25-F-9 against mature tissue macrophages (ZWADLO et al. 1985), on a larger panel of different bone tumor entities. Our results showed that in all bone tumor entities investigated, the antibody 27-E-10 against blood monocytes generally evoked a negative reaction. The best staining of macrophages was obtained with the antibody 25-F-9 against mature tissue macrophages. The number of cells staining positively with 25-F-9 varied from tumor to tumor.

3.1 Macrophage Reaction in Different Bone Tumors

Sixteen osteosarcomas were analyzed. They belong to different subtypes: four were anaplastic, five mostly osteoblastic, four fibroblastic and two chondroblas-

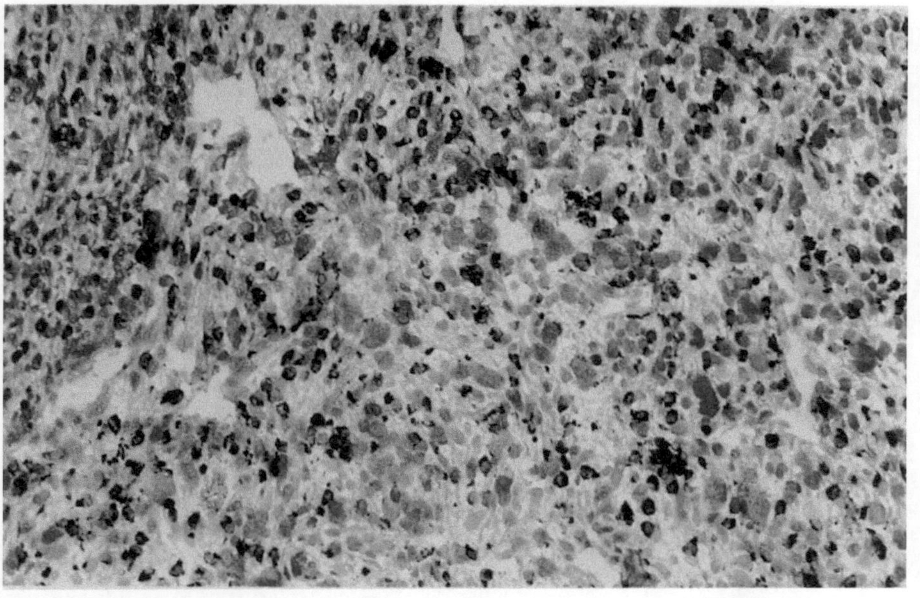

Fig. 1. Anaplastic osteosarcoma of bone after staining with the antibody 25-F-9 directed against mature tissue macrophages. Clusters of macrophages can be observed between negatively staining anaplastic tumor cells. (× 136)

tic. One osteosarcoma was of the telangiectatic type. In anaplastic osteosarcomas the mature macrophages positively staining with 25-F-9 were scattered over the whole tissue in some areas; in others they appeared localized in clusters (Fig. 1). In osteoblastic osteosarcomas, the macrophage content was similar to that of anaplastic areas, decreasing with the advancing differentiation of osteoid. In the fibroblastic region the pattern of macrophage infiltration was similar to that of anaplastic areas. The spindle-shaped fibroblastic cells reacted negatively. The lowest macrophage content was found in the chondroblastic osteosarcomas. Areas with entirely chondroblastic differentiation were completely devoid of macrophages, but some were found in adjacent anaplastic areas. In the telangiectatic type of osteosarcoma the macrophage content was also comparatively low.

Three osteosarcomas contained considerable amounts of histiocytic giant cells. In these cases, the content of mononuclear macrophages appeared comparatively higher than in the other osteosarcomas.

In chondroblastic tumors (chondromas and chondrosarcomas) macrophages were rare, corresponding to the chondroblastic areas of osteosarcomas (Fig. 2). In those chondroblastomas, however, which contained typical histiocytic giant cells, a moderate number of macrophages were found.

Of greatest interest were the so-called fibrohistiocytic tumors [malignant fibrous histiocytoma (MFH), giant cell tumor of bone (GCT), nonossifying fibroma (NOF)], because the histogenesis of this entity is not clearly understood. The content of macrophages in these tumors was most pronounced in MFH,

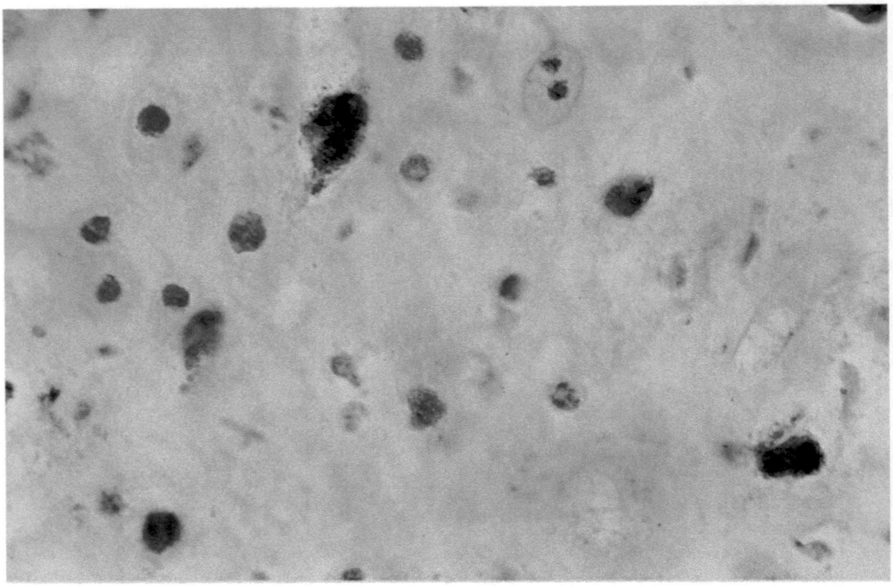

Fig. 2. Chondrosarcoma grade I of bone after staining with the antibody 25-F-9 against mature tissue macrophages. Only a few scattered macrophages can be observed between chondroblastic tumor cells. (×330)

but here, too, the cells appeared as an infiltrate when stained with 25-F-9, between completely negative spindle-shaped tumor cells (Fig. 3). Generally, not more than 10%–20% of all cells were positive macrophages. Sometimes, dense clusters of positive macrophages could be observed (Fig. 4). The NOFs showed a similar behavior: positive macrophages infiltrated between negative fibroblastic cells. In GCT there was also a large number of macrophages, which could be demonstrated with antibodies against α_1-ACT (Fig. 5). In some cases, they were localized around the giant cells when stained with 25-F-9, which points to a close relationship between giant cells and mononuclear macrophages. Here, too, mononuclear tumor cells were negative.

Aneurysmal bone cysts contained a considerable number of histiocytic giant cells. Their content of mononuclear macrophages was also rather high (Fig. 6). Spindle-shaped cells were negative, and so were the endothelial-like cells lining the cyst walls. In *Ewing's sarcoma*, macrophage content was comparatively low, but clusters were observed between the negative round cells after primary chemotherapy (Fig. 7). In contrast to MFH, *fibrosarcomas* contained only a few macrophages, and the neoplastic fibroblasts were negative, corresponding to the negative spindle cells in MFH. In *desmoplastic fibroma* and in *fibrous dysplasia* the macrophage content was quite low, like that in malignant *hemangioendothelioma*.

Summarizing these results we found the antibody 25-F-9 to be most appropriate for evaluating the extent of macrophage infiltration in different bone

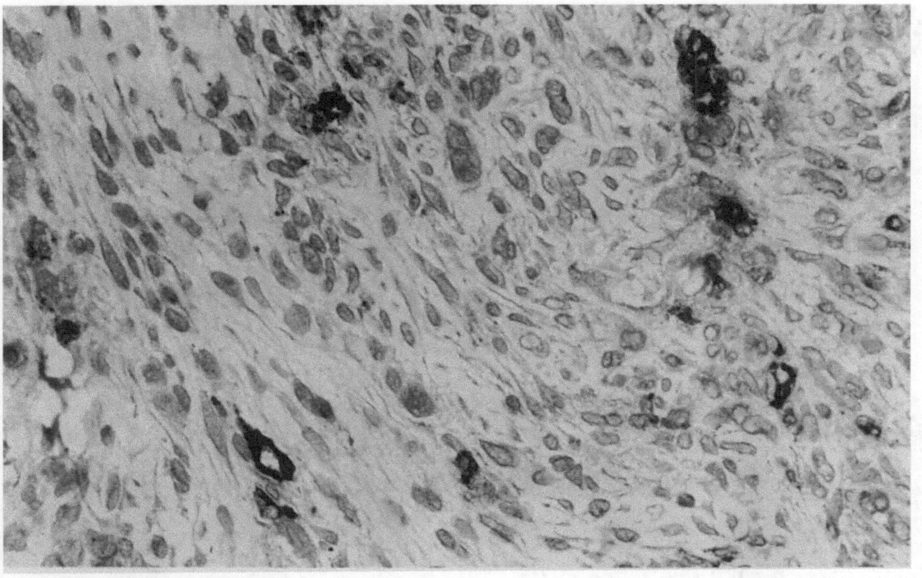

Fig. 3. MFH after staining with the antibody 25-F-9 against mature tissue macrophages. Regularly macrophages can be observed between negatively staining spindle-shaped tumor cells. (× 330)

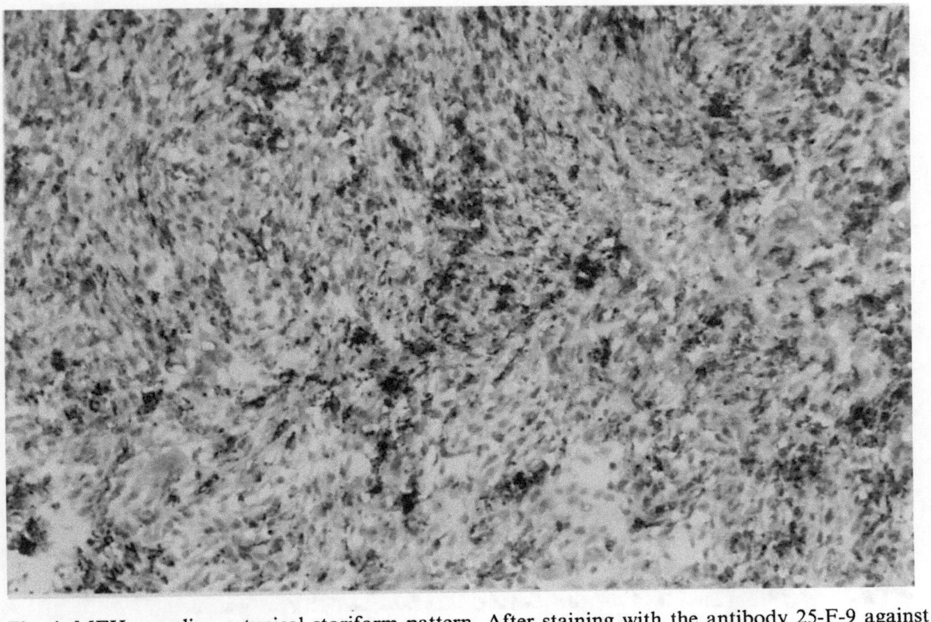

Fig. 4. MFH revealing a typical storiform pattern. After staining with the antibody 25-F-9 against mature tissue macrophages, clusters of macrophages can be observed between spindle-shaped tumor cells. (× 136)

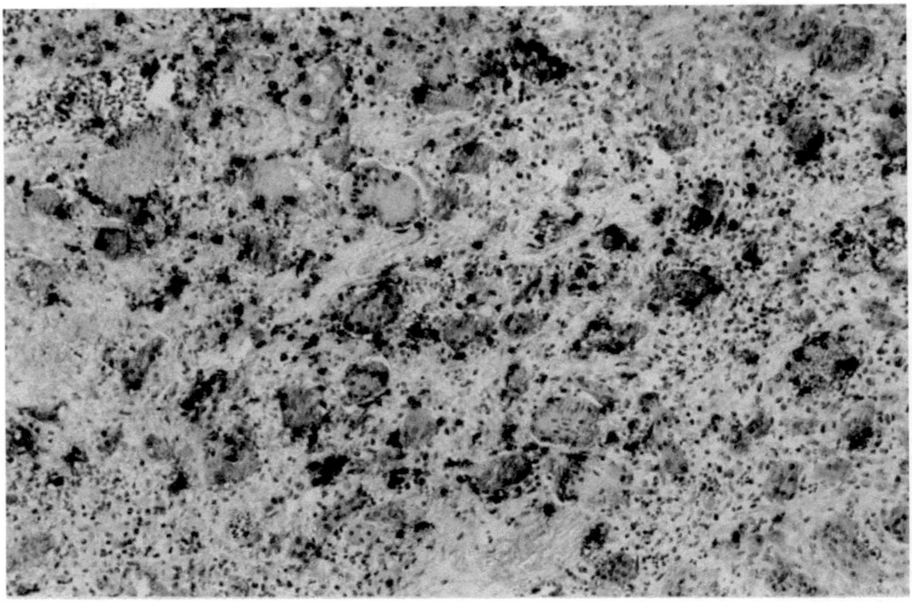

Fig. 5. GCT after staining with an antibody against α_1-ACT. Abundant macrophages can be observed between negative tumor cells. Some osteoclast-like giant cells show a faint reaction. (× 330)

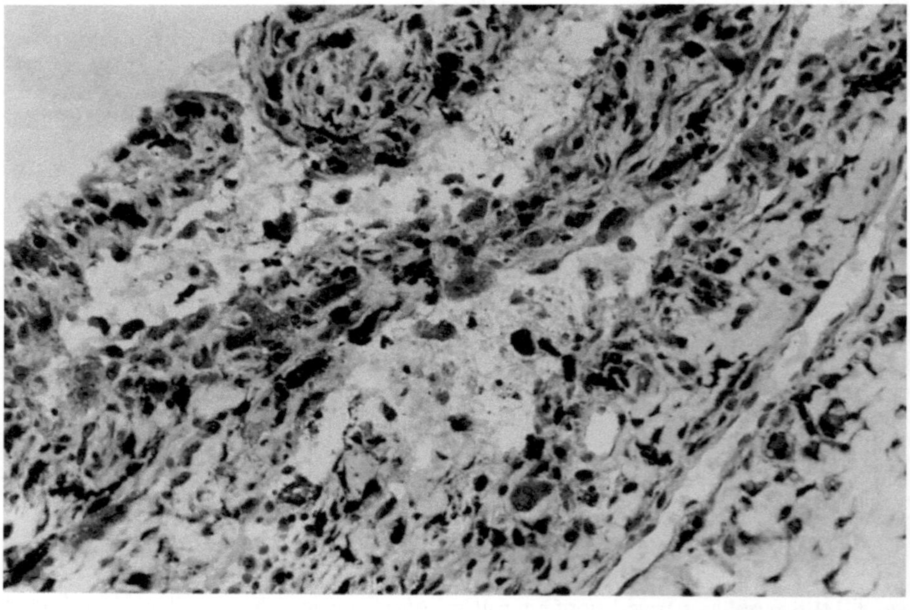

Fig. 6. Aneurysmal bone cyst. After staining with 25-F-9 against mature tissue macrophages, clusters of macrophages can be observed in the cyst walls of the aneurysmal bone cyst. (× 330)

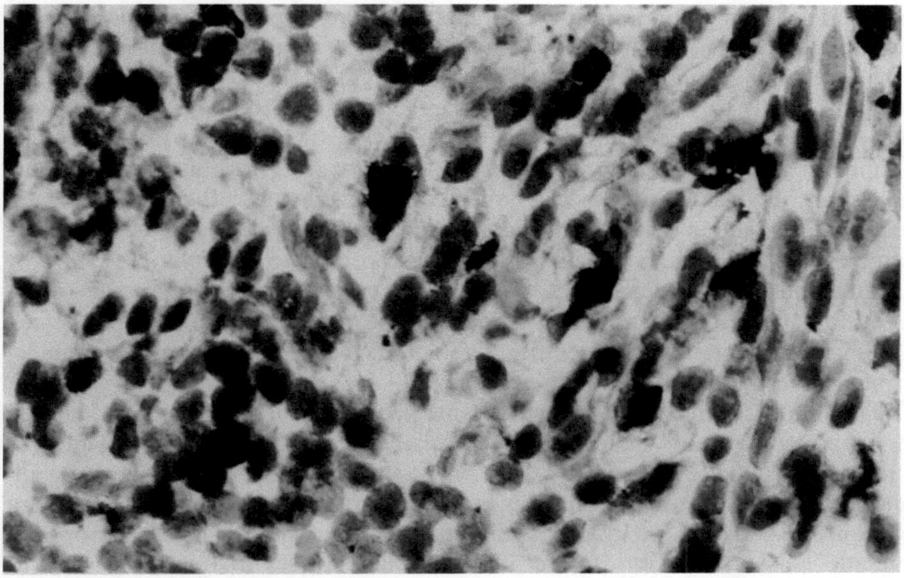

Fig. 7. Ewing's sarcoma after chemotherapy reveals viable areas of anaplastic tumor round cells and a moderate infiltration of macrophages after staining with the antibody 25-F-9 against mature tissue macrophages. (×330)

tumor entities. The value of polyclonal markers appears restricted as they are not specific for cells of the mononuclear phagocyte system.

We have demonstrated mature macrophages in all 16 osteosarcomas. In tumors that revealed a higher number of nonneoplastic osteoclast-like giant cells, the number of mononuclear phagocytes was comparatively high. This may point to a closer relationship between these giant cells and the mononuclear macrophages.

The group of so-called fibrohistiocytic tumors is of special interest with regard to its relationship to the mononuclear phagocyte system. According to the current histogenetic concept of these tumors, a tumor of bimodal differentiation into either a fibroblastic or a histiocytic cell is considered their stem cell (Alguacil-Garcia et al. 1978; Brooks and Pascal 1984; Iwasaki et al. 1982; Katenkamp and Stiller 1981; Kindblom et al. 1982). In the bone, MFH, GCT, and NOF are thought to be of this origin.

We recorded positive staining of macrophages with different markers, especially the monoclonal antibody 25-F-9, whereas the majority of tumor cells were found to be strictly negative in the fibrohistiocytic tumors. As 25-F-9 has been observed so far practically exclusively in mature macrophages, it appears probable that macrophages in fibrohistiocytic tumors are truly mature macrophages. Roholl et al. (1985) have found similar results in MFH.

For a general conclusion from these observations we want to emphasize first that macrophages in these tumors are generally mature tissue macrophages, but not developing blood monocytes. This inference is in good accordance with preliminary studies of macrophage infiltration in various carcinomas (Zwadlo et al. 1985). The second important point is the negative reaction of the mesenchymal tumor cells to the different antibodies against macrophages tested in our study. All bone tumor entities showed this behavior, including the fibrohistiocytic tumors. Thus, it appears plausible that the so-called fibrohistiocytic lesions should not be considered as special bone tumor entities, but rather as fibroblastic or spindle cell tumor with a considerable reactive infiltration of osteoclast-like giant cells and mature tissue macrophages. According to this hypothesis, fibrosarcoma and MFH, for instance, would not be considered as separate nosological entities, but rather as manifestations of histogenetically similar spindle cell sarcomas differing only in the degree to which they are infiltrated by mononuclear phagocytes and osteoclast-like giant cells.

The role of the macrophage and its possible function in bone tumors certainly deserves further study. Positive correlations between the occurrence of macrophages and osteoclast-like giant cells point to their role as mononuclear progenitors of the giant cells. It has not been possible, however, to confirm a significant relationship between the grade of malignancy in a tumor and its macrophage content. This may be due to the low number of cases in our study. As the majority of macrophage markers can be readily applied to paraffin sections, the question should be studied in a significant number of cases.

4 Phenotypic Characterization of Osteoclast-like Giant Cells

As mentioned earlier, recent immunohistochemical and experimental results confirm the close relationship between the hematopoietic system, especially the phagocytic macrophages, osteoclasts, and the multinucleated giant cells of GCTs (Burger et al. 1984; Athanasou et al. 1985; Oursler et al. 1985). We have therefore characterized the phenotypic features of tumor-associated giant cells in GCT osteosarcoma, and aneurysmal bone cysts using monoclonal antibodies with monocyte/macrophage specificity. We analyzed the reactivity of the polykaryons compared with the immunological staining of the tumor-associated macrophages in order to obtain further information about the relationship between these cells. The different antibodies are plotted in Table 1.

Giant Cell Tumor of Bone. Cryostat sections taken from five GCTs were treated with different macrophage/monocyte specific antibodies in order to establish the existence of cell surface antigens on tumor-associated giant cells, demonstrating a relation between macrophages and giant cells. The results are summarized in Table 2. Using the antibody 25-F-9 specific for mature macrophages, giant cells stained positive in two of the five cases (Fig. 8). In one of five tumor specimens the reaction was positive for RM 3/1 and Ki M1 respectively, whereas in the same sections other multinucleated cells remained unstained. Immunohistochemical demonstration of macrophage/monocyte specific cell surface antigens with other antibodies was not possible.

Osteosarcomas. Among eight osteosarcomas, reactivity of giant cells with the antibody 25-F-9 could be established in five cases (Fig. 9). The reaction between

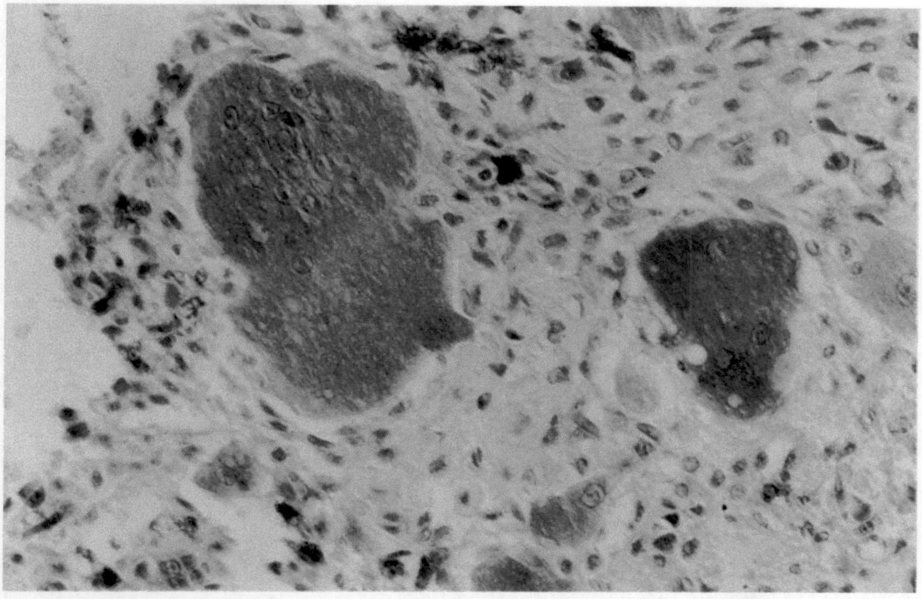

Fig. 8. GCT after staining with the antibody 25-F-9 against mature tissue macrophages. The giant cells show a comparatively strong reaction, pointing to the relationship with the mononuclear phagocyte system. Some mononuclear cells, obviously macrophages, show a strong reaction. (×330)

Table 2. Reactivity of tumor-associated giant cells in eight osteosarcomas, five giant cell tumors of bone, and one aneurysmal bone cyst with seven specific monoclonal antibodies

Antibody	Specificity	Osteosarcoma	Giant cell tumor	Aneurysmal bone cyst
25-F-9	Mature macrophages	5/8	2/5	1/1
RM 3/1	Macrophages	1/8	1/5	0/1
Ki M1	Monocytes/macrophages	1/8	1/5	0/1
Ki M2	Monocytes/macrophages	0/8	0/5	0/1
Leu M3	Monocytes/macrophages	0/8	0/5	0/1
27-E-10	Blood monocytes	0/8	0/5	0/1
OKM 5	Monocytes/macrophages	0/8	0/5	0/1

giant cells and the antibodies RM 3/1 and Ki M1 showed positive results in one case each. There was no positive staining in osteosarcomas and GCTs with other antibodies employed in this series.

Aneurysmal Bone Cyst. In this tumor-like lesion the giant cells showed strong staining with the antibody 25-F-9. All other antibodies revealed no detectable reactivity.

Analysis of the results concerning the osteoclast-like giant cells reveals varying patterns of cell reactivity. Among the panel of monocyte/macrophage specific antibodies only the antibody 25-F-9 specific for mature phagocytic macro-

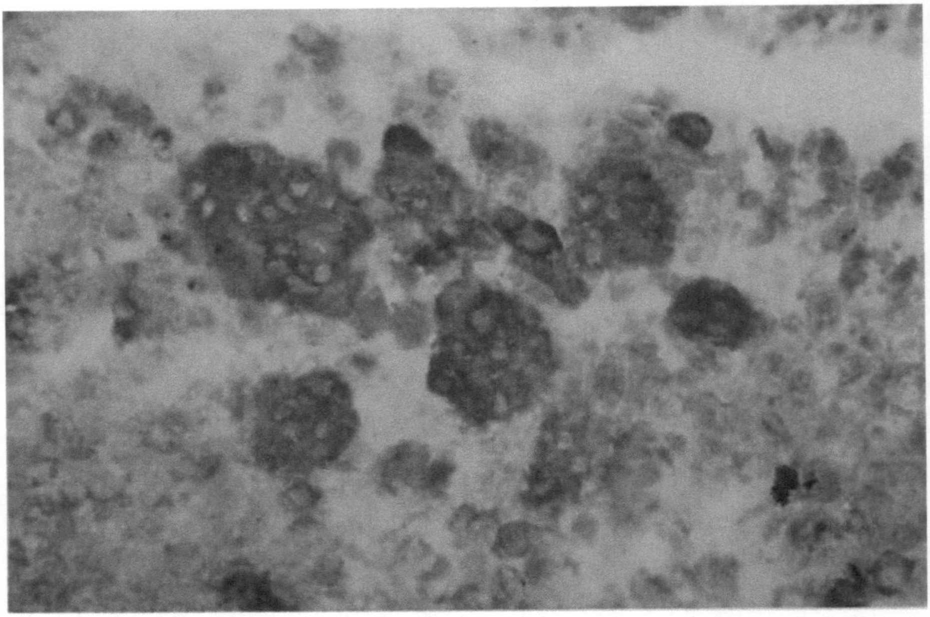

Fig. 9. Anaplastic area of giant cell containing osteosarcoma after staining with the antibody 25-F-9 against mature tissue macrophages. The giant cells show a strong reaction. (Frozen section, ×330)

phages displayed convincing reactivity with the giant cell-associated determinants. The other macrophage-specific antibodies RM 3/1 and Ki M1 showed but slight reactivity in one case each. The staining of giant cells in mononuclear phagocytes with 25-F-9 enables the distinct differentiation of these reactive cells from the neoplastic spindle-shaped tumor cells. Therefore the polykaryons are not of neoplastic origin, but seem to have an antigenic relationship with mononuclear phagocytes. Although this positive labeling could not be found in all tumor specimens – there were some cases without stained giant cells and others with both positive and unstained giant cell – the common antigen labeled by the antibody 25-F-9 indicates a close cell relation.

In order to explain the absence of giant cell labeling in some tumor specimens it has to be considered that in cellular fusion leading to the formation of multinucleated cells a part of the outer cell membrane is incorporated. This mechanism of cell fusion reduces the number of cell surface antigens as observed on histiocytic giant cells in granuloma (HORTON et al. 1984). A second explanation for the lack of 25-F-9 staining may be the loss of the immunological receptors in physiological aging of the cells, including degeneration of cell components (LOUTIT and NISBET 1982; OURSLER et al. 1985).

As regards the antigenic shift on macrophages during their maturation to differentiated cells with cell-specific functions, a change of antigenic determinants combined with giant cell differentiation is possible. The giant cells and the osteoclasts are considered to be the final differentiated functional cells at the end of the monocyte/macrophage lineage (Loutit and Nisbet 1982; Todd et al. 1985). Cell differentiation, together with a change in the antigenic pattern of the cell surfaces, would explain the absence of immunohistochemical labeling with most of the monoclonal antibodies and also the lack of 25-F-9 staining on some multinucleated giant cells.

In accordance with other authors our experimental results corroborate the theory of a hematopoietic origin of the tumor-associated giant cells, based on the close relationship between phagocytic macrophages and the polykaryons. By means of immunohistochemical analysis, Athanasou et al. (1985) found a cell surface antigen common to the multinucleated cells and the macrophages stained by the monoclonal antibody EBM 11 in giant cell tumors of bone and in osteoclasts of fetal bone tissue. From this they concluded that the osteoclasts and the tumor-associated giant cells had phenotypic and functional similarities and seem to have a common origin in the phagocytic macrophages. Oursler et al. (1985) analyzed osteoclasts, tumor-associated giant cells, and macrophages using osteoclast-specific antibodies. They were able to demonstrate the close relationship between these three cell types but pointed out that each cell type has to be clearly distinguished from the others as to its functional and antigenic behavior. These authors believe there is a progenitor of osteoclasts, giant cells, and mononuclear macrophages. The giant cells are regarded as multinucleated phagocytes having lost macrophage-typical features and having gained new giant cell specific characteristics.

These phenotypic characterizations indicate, in accordance with the results of Athanasou et al. (1988), the hematopoietic origin of the tumor-associated phagocytes and the osteoclasts, whereas Horton et al. (1985) suggest a nonhematopoietic descent, after immunohistochemical investigations on giant cell tumors with several monoclonal antibodies of leukocyte specificity.

Burger et al. (1984) classified the giant cells as hematopoietic cells, but considered a population of immature macrophages of the bone marrow to be precursors of the giant cells.

Summarizing our results, immunohistochemistry reveals a relationship between the tumor-associated mature macrophages and the multinucleated giant cells. The cells share common antigenic features. However, phenotypic analysis also reveals differences in the cell surface structure of macrophages and giant cells. The different behavior toward certain antibodies may suggest a final differentiation of the polykaryons to specific functional cell forms including a loss of precursor features. Further investigations would be helpful, such as the cultivation of osteoclast specific antibodies in order to characterize the phenotype of the multinucleated giant cells in detail.

5 The Proliferation Behavior of Macrophages as Compared with Fibroblastic Cells in Malignant Fibrous Histiocytoma and Giant Cell Tumor of Bone

The results of the present study have made it seem probable that macrophages and osteoclast-like giant cells in bone tumors are a reactive phenomenon and not proliferating tumor cells. This is in good accordance with the results of other authors (ROHOLL et al. 1985; LAWSON et al. 1987; DEHNER 1988). In order to substantiate this assumption further, we have analyzed GCTs and MFH with special emphasis on the proliferation behavior of the different cell types in these tumors.

In vitro incubation of GCTs and MFH has revealed that in semithin sections nuclei of mononuclear stromal cells are labeled, but with varying density of silver grains (Fig. 10). In contrast, the giant cell nuclei are unlabeled. In some places labeled mononuclear cells are seen closely adjacent to unlabeled giant cells. At higher magnification of semithin sections, macrophages are barely distinguishable from fibroblast-like stromal cells, since lysosomes in macrophage cytoplasm are just visible at the border of light microscopic resolution. When the sections are surveyed by light microscopy, no labeled macrophages will be found. The labeled cells are always identified as stromal cells of the fibroblast-like type.

Electron microscopic autoradiographs showed some labeled nuclei of mononuclear stromal cells. They belonged exclusively to the fibroblast-like cell type (Fig. 11). Silver grains were mostly distributed loosely over the whole nucleus, though sometimes with preference in electron-dense chromatin areas. The cytoplasm of these cells is quite free from silver grains and only a negligible background is observed. Giant cell nuclei, in contrast, are unlabeled and so are the nuclei of macrophages (Fig. 12).

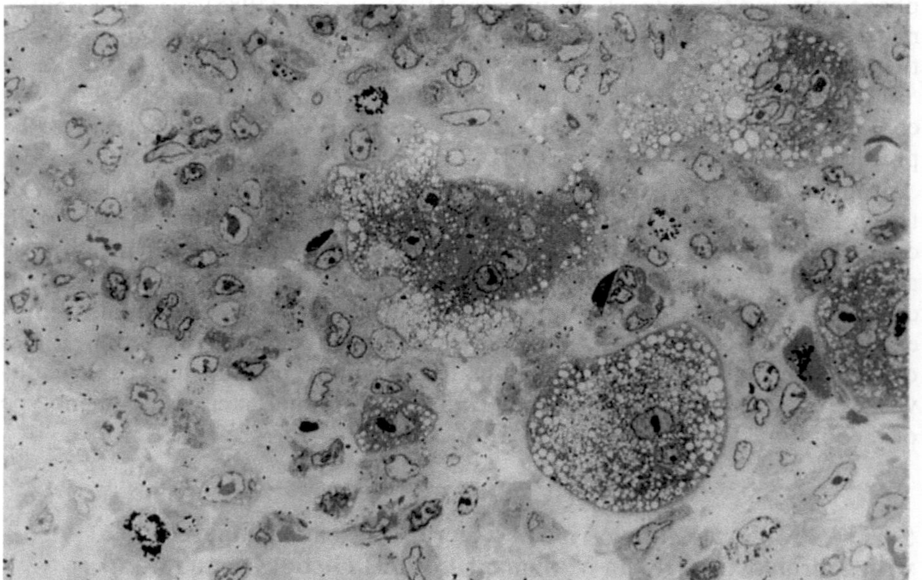

Fig. 10. Autoradiographic-light microscopic preparation of GCT after in vitro incubation with ^{3}H-thymidine. Silver grains can be observed over the nuclei of mononuclear cells. The nuclei of giant cells are always negative. (×330)

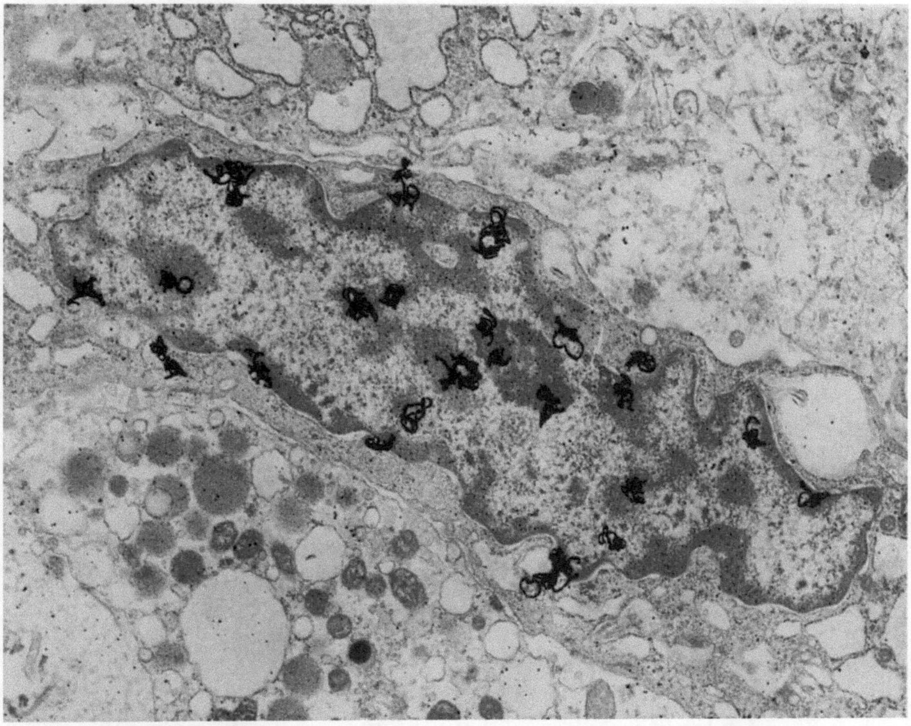

Fig. 11. Autoradiographic-electron microscopic picture of a fibroblastic tumor cell in GCT revealing silver grains over the cell nucleus, pointing to the proliferation of the cell. (× 10 500)

In GCT, the reaction of antibodies against cells of the mononuclear phagocyte system showed that labeling with 25-F-9, an antibody specific against mature tissue macrophages, revealed strong positivity in numerous mononucleated cells, but the majority of mononucleates reacted negatively. The analysis of proliferation rates with the monoclonal antibody Ki-67 demonstrated that some 5% of mononuclear cells in these tumors were actually proliferating. However, by staining with the antibody alone it cannot be decided whether these proliferating cells are of the histiocytic or fibroblast-like type. The nuclei of osteoclast-like giant cells on the other hand always reacted negatively (Fig. 13). These results coincide very well with the autoradiographic results.

To find out which population among the mononuclear cells was indeed proliferating we used simultaneous labeling with Ki-67 and 25-F-9. It became evident that only the 25-F-9 negative mononuclear cells were labeled with the proliferation-associated marker Ki-67; the nuclei of the 25-F-9 positive macrophages showed a negative reaction to Ki-67 (Fig. 14).

In MFH the reaction pattern was very similar to that in GCT. With the antibodies Ki M1 and Ki M2 the cytoplasm of some mononuclear cells showed positive reactions, but the majority were negative. OKM 5 and anti Leu M3

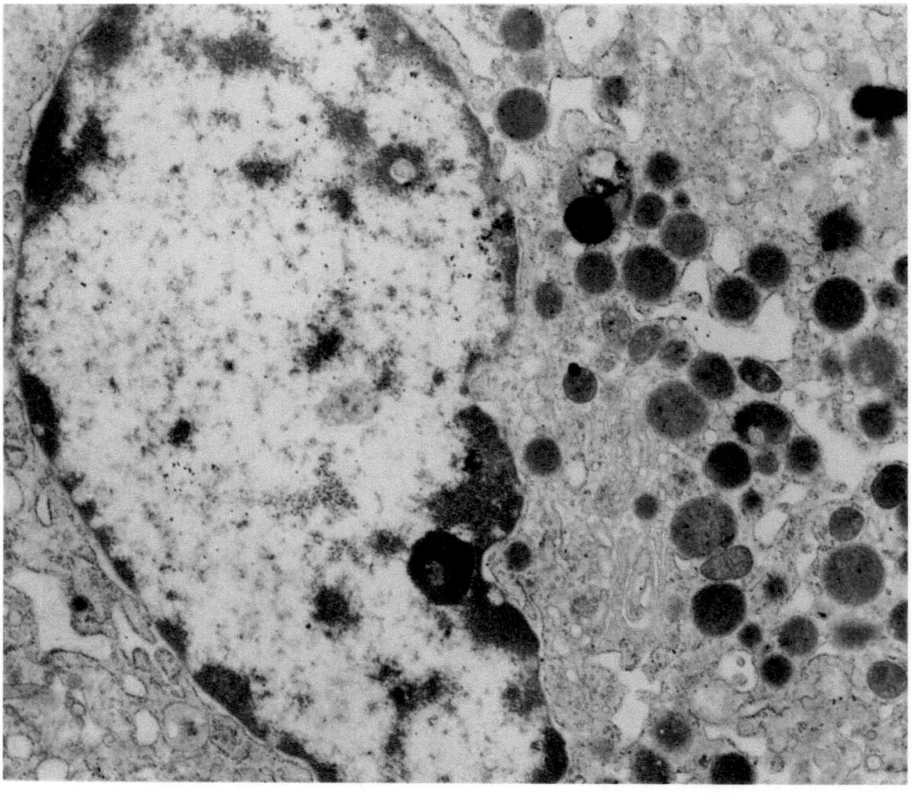

Fig. 12. Autoradiographic-electron microscopic picture of a macrophage without silver grains over the cell nucleus. (×9500)

only revealed a faint reaction in some mononuclear stromal cells. In some of these stromal mononucleates, a strong reaction was observed with the antibody 25-F-9 against mature tissue macrophages.

Double labeling with Ki-67 and 25-F-9 was also performed in MFH in order to verify whether the proliferating cells were indeed of the macrophage type. In accordance with our results in GCTs, it was demonstrated that the nuclei of macrophages with 25-F-9 positive cytoplasm reacted negatively to Ki-67 against a proliferation-associated nuclear antigen. However, the proliferating cells with brown staining nuclei had negatively staining cytoplasm (Fig. 15). Obviously the proliferating tumor cells were not macrophages. When discussing these results it has to be pointed out that previous investigators have attempted to draw some inferences on the histogenesis of MFH from analysis with polyclonal antibodies that were considered to be markers of mononuclear phagocyte system cells, such as α_1-ACT and lysosyme (DU BOULAY 1982; KINDBLOM et al. 1982; NATHRATH and MEISTER 1982). Recent results have confirmed that these markers are not sufficiently specific, as they also

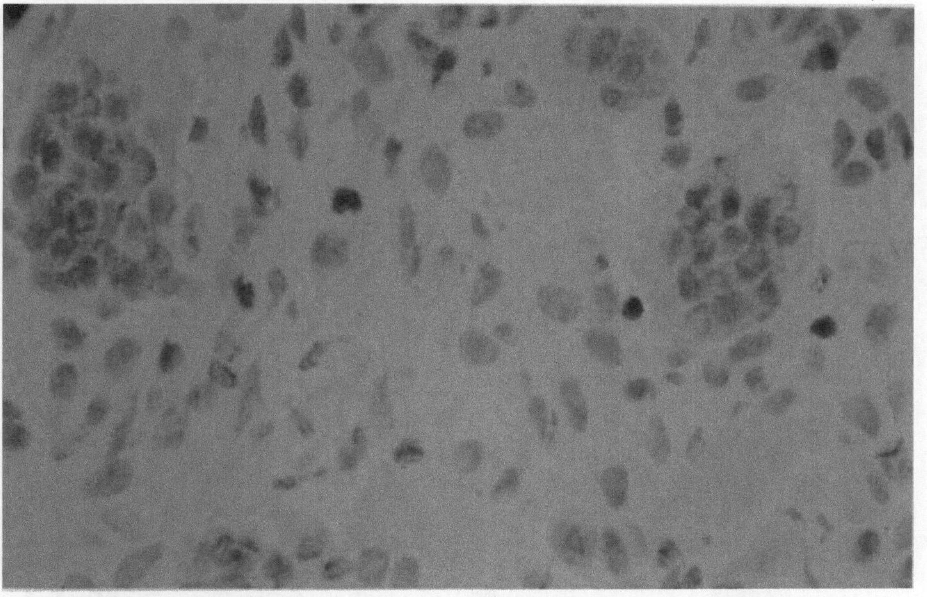

Fig. 13. Frozen section of GCT after staining with the antibody Ki-67 directed against a proliferation-associated nuclear antigen. Only nuclei of mononuclear cells show a reaction. The nuclei of giant cells are negative. (×330)

react with tumor cells from other types of bone neoplasms (ROESSNER et al. 1987). Thus, the results of the above – mentioned studies, apparently pointing to a bimodal differentiation of tumor cells into fibroblastic and histiocytic phenotypes, must be considered unsatisfactory (LAWSON et al. 1987).

Today, monoclonal antibodies are an appropriate tool for identifying subsets of cell populations that were formerly considered as homogeneous (RADZUN and PARWARESCH 1983). This is particularly helpful for recognizing the elements of the mononuclear phagocyte system that were previously identified only by rather nonspecific and unstable markers (ZWADLO et al. 1985). The additional development of proliferation-associated markers made it possible to determine which of the cell populations in the given neoplasms was actually proliferating (GERDES et al. 1984). These markers were useful in assessing the growth rates of bone tumors, together with other methods for the evaluation of cell proliferation such as flow cytometry (HIDDEMANN et al. 1987). Several years ago, electron microscopic investigation of GCTs and MFH revealed two main cell types: fibroblast-like cells and histiocytic cells (STEINER et al. 1982; FU et al. 1975; ROESSNER et al. 1979). In accordance with these findings the application of monoclonal antibodies in the present study has enabled us to identify mature histiocytes as a cell component in MFH, as well as in GCTs. The majority of cells, however, were found to be negative. Similar results were recently described by ROHOLL et al. (1985). According to these authors, MFH tumor

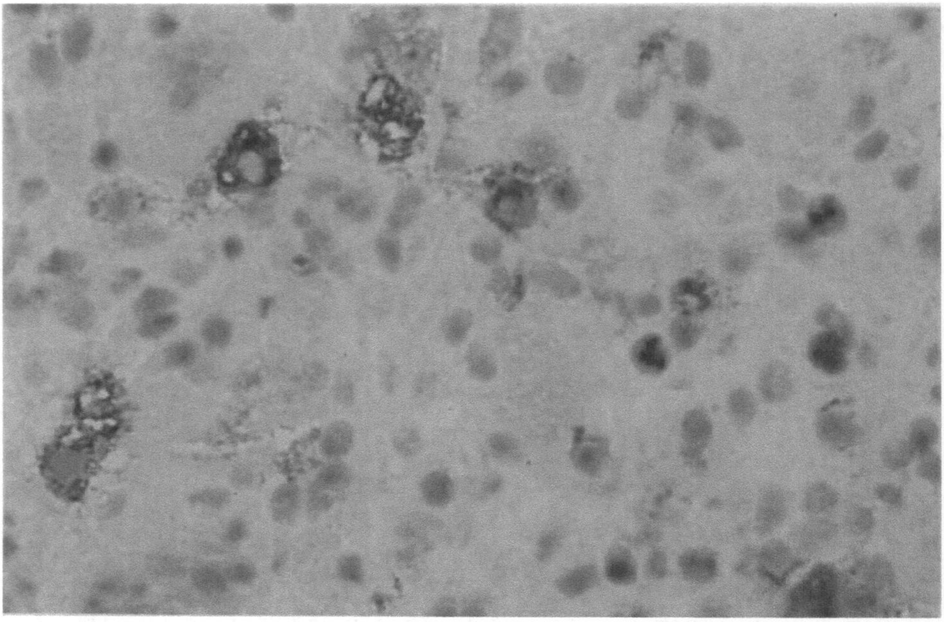

Fig. 14. GCT after double labeling with the monoclonal antibody 25-F-9 directed against mature tissue macrophages (*red*) and the antibody Ki-67 directed against the proliferation-associated nuclear antigen (*brown*). The proliferating cells do not react with the antibody against macrophages. (Frozen section, ×330)

cells show fibroblast-associated determinants with other soft tissue tumor cells, strongly suggesting that MFH is related to fibroblast-like cells. This result is confirmed by our observation that only the fibroblast-like cells negative to these markers against mononuclear phagocyte system cells were found to be positive for the antibody against proliferation-associated nuclear antigens used in an immunohistological double labeling test. Macrophages in these tumors revealed no sign of preference when compared with the fibroblastic cells. A low proliferation rate has been observed in known neoplastic peritoneal macrophages (DAHMS and DE BAKKER 1982). However, the proliferation of tumor cells in MFH and GCT is obviously much greater. Consequently it can be inferred that the histiocyte populations are reactive, infiltrating cells rather than active tumor cells. In contrast to these findings in MFH and GCT, true malignant histiocytosis has been shown to yield different results with strong positivity of its tumor cells to antibodies against MPS (ROHOLL et al. 1985). It remains an open question whether some rare cases of true fibrohistiocytic tumors might exist whose histiocytes could be appraised as active, neoplastic cells. Our study, however, strongly suggests that in true entities belonging to what is called the fibrohistiocytic tumor group (GCT and MFH), the tumor cells are fibroblast-like and not of histiocytic origin. It is probable that on the basis of our present findings the current concept of fibrohistiocytic tumors of bone should be recon-

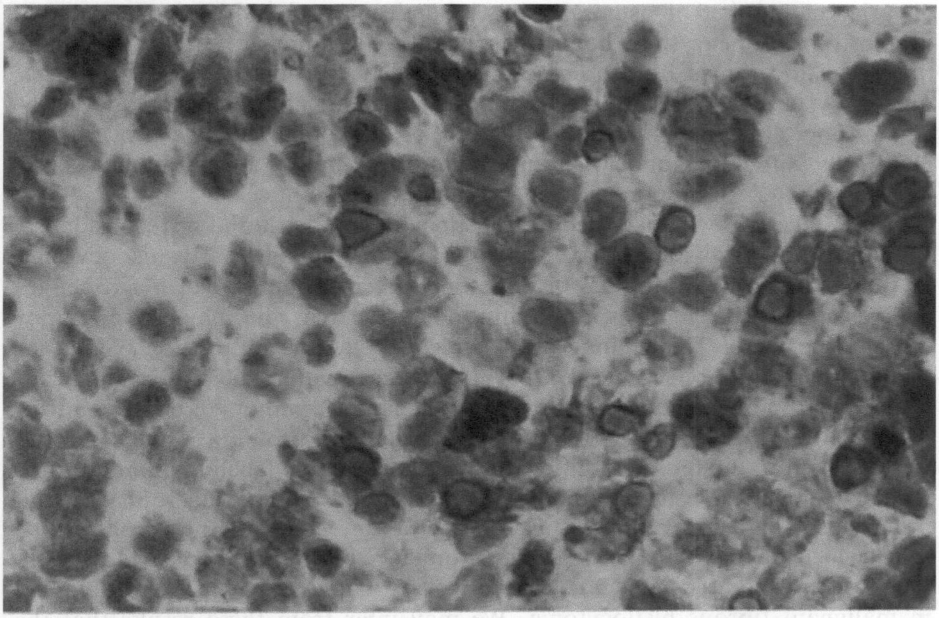

Fig. 15. MFH after double labeling with 25-F-9 against macrophages (*red*) and Ki-67 directed against a proliferation-associated nuclear antigen (*brown*). The nuclei of the macrophages do not react positively with Ki-67. (Frozen section, × 330)

sidered. They are generally not related to true histiocytic tumors derived from MPS cells, but rather neoplastic transformations of local mesenchymal cells (ROHOLL et al. 1985; LAWSON et al. 1987). The histiocytic component should be considered as a reactive infiltrate.

6 Summary

Recent investigations have suggested that osteoclasts and osteoblasts belong to different cell systems: osteoclasts originate from hemopoietic stem cells, most probably via precursors of the mononuclear phagocyte system. Osteoblasts, however, arise from local mesenchyme. The present classification of bone tumors issued by the WHO, however, is still based on the assumption of osteoclasts and osteoblasts being merely different manifestations or differentiations of the same basic cell type. Consequently, histiocytes or macrophages as well as osteoclast-like giant cells are interpreted in most bone tumors as an autochthonous component of the tumor.

In the present study, this theory is contradicted by histological immunohistological, electron microscopic, and autoradiographic-electron microscopic results on a larger number of osteosarcomas, chondromas, chondrosarcomas, chondroblastomas, aneurysmal bone cysts, giant cell tumors of bone, malignant fibrous histiocytomas, fibrosarcomas, desmoplastic fibromas, Ewing's sarcomas, fibrous dysplasias, nonossifying fibromas, and malignant hemangioendotheliomas of bone. In order to elucidate the role of macrophages and osteoclast-like giant cells, different monoclonal antibodies were applied to bone tumor specimens as markers of mononuclear macrophages and giant cells.

The concept of what is called fibrohistiocytic tumors should be reconsidered. Immunohistological studies have shown that in malignant fibrous histiocytoma as well as in giant cell tumors of bone only a certain portion of macrophages will react with the highly specific antibodies, whereas the majority of tumor cells are negative. This finding alone suggests that the infiltration of macrophages is a reactive phenomenon. It is in agreement with earlier autoradiographic and electron microscopic investigations on giant cell tumors of bone, confirming that only the fibroblast-like tumors are actually proliferating. These data were verified in the present study with the aid of double labeling immunohistological techniques, using antibodies against mature tissue macrophages and others against a proliferation-associated nuclear antigen. Only the fibroblast-like cells, which do not react with the macrophage-specific antibody, will express the proliferation-associated nuclear antigen. Analogous results were obtained in malignant fibrous histiocytoma. We may infer from these results that the majority of these tumors must be neoplasms of local mesenchyme, mostly in fibroblastic differentiation, while the considerable number of macrophages is seen as a reactive phenomenon. The role of these reactive macrophages and their possible function in bone tumor biology deserves further study. No significant relationship between the grade of malignancy of a tumor and its macrophage content could be confirmed as yet, possibly due to the comparatively low number of cases in our study. As the majority of macrophage markers can be readily applied to paraffin sections the question should be studied further in a significant number of cases.

The cytogenesis of osteoclasts and osteoclast-like giant cells in bone tumors is still under discussion. There is some agreement that their precursors are not to be found among the local mesenchyme, but rather among hemopoietic cells, probably of the mononuclear phagocyte system. This concept has not been refuted. Some authors advocate the possibility that even mesenchymal cells may be able to differentiate to osteoclasts in the course of bone development. In opposition to this opinion, our immunohistological analysis, conducted in view of the phenotypic characterization of osteoclasts by means of monoclonal antibodies, suggests, in agreement with the results of other authors, that a close relationship exists between these cells and the macrophage system. Antibodies against mature tissue macrophages in particular yield a slightly posisitive reaction with osteoclast-like giant cells, while antibodies against blood monocytes give a negative reaction. Further immunohistological investigations are certainly needed to give a clear definition of the relation of mononuclear osteoclast precursors to the macrophage system.

Acknowledgment. This work was supported by Deutsche Forschungsgemeinschaft grant no. Ro 648 1/2.

References

Alguacil-Garcia A, Unni KK, Goellner JR (1978) Malignant fibrous histiocytoma. An ultrastructural study of six cases. Am J Clin Pathol 69:121–129

Aparisi T, Arborgh B, Ericsson JLF (1977) Giant cell tumor of bone: fine structural analysis of acid phosphatase. Virchows Arch [A] 376:299–308

Ash P, Loutit JF, Townsend KMS (1980) Osteoclasts derive from haematopoietic stem cells. Nature 283:669–670

Athanasou NA, Bliss E, Gatter KC, Heryet A (1985) An immunohistological study of giant cell tumor of bone: evidence for an osteoclast origin of the giant cells. J Pathol 147:153–158

Athanasou NA, Quinn J, McGee JOD (1988) Immunocytochemical analysis of the human osteoclast: phenotypic relationship to other marrow-derived cells. Bone Mineral 3:317–333

Breard J, Reinherz EL, Kung PC, Goldstein C, Schlossmann SF (1980) A monoclonal antibody reactive with human peripheral blood monocytes. J Immunol 124:1943–1948

Brooks JP, Pascal RR (1984) Malignant giant cell tumor of bone: ultrastructural and immunohistologic evidence of histiocytic origin. Hum Pathol 15:1098–1100

Burger EH, van der Meer JWM, Nijweide PJ (1984) Osteoclasts formation from mononuclear phagocytes: role of bone forming cells. J Cell Biol 99:1901–1908

Byers VS, Levin AS, Johnston JO, Hackett AJ (1975) Quantitative immunofluorescence studies of the tumor antigen bearing cells in giant cell tumor of bone and osteogenic sarcoma. Cancer Res 35:2520–2525

Chambers TJ (1978) Multinucleate giant cells. J Pathol 126:125–148

Cordell JL, Fallini B, Erber WN et al. (1984) Immunoenzymatic labelling of monoclonal antibodies using immune complexes of alkaline phosphatase and monoclonal anti-alkaline phosphatases. J Histochem Cytochem 22:219–229

Dehner LP (1988) Malignant fibrous histiocytoma. Nonspecific morphologic pattern, specific pathologic entity, or both? Arch Pathol Lab Med 112:236–237

Dimitriou-Bona A, Burmester GR, Waters SJ, Winchester RJ (1983) Human mononuclear phagocyte differentiation antigens. I. Patterns of antigenic expression on the surfaces of human monocytes and macrophages defined by monoclonal antibodies. J Immunol 130:145–152

Du Boulay A (1982) Demonstration of α_1-antitrypsin and α_1-antichymotrypsin in fibrous histiocytoma using the immunoperoxidase technique. Am J Surg Pathol 6:559–564

Erlandson RA (1984) Diagnostic immunohistochemistry of human tumors. Am J Surg Pathol 8:615–624

Fishman Da, Hay ED (1962) Origin of osteoclasts from mononuclear leukocytes in regenerating new limbs. Anat Rec 143:329–338

Fu SY, Gabbiani G, Kaye G, Lattes R (1975) Malignant soft tissue tumors of probable histiocytic origin (malignant fibrous histiocytomas): general considerations and electron microscopic and tissue culture studies. Cancer 35:176–198

Gerdes J, Lemke H, Baisch H, Wacker HH, Schwab U, Stein H (1984) Cell cycle analysis of a cell proliferation-associated human nuclear antigen defined by the monoclonal antibody Ki-67. J Immunol 133:1710–1715

Göthlin G, Ericsson JLE (1976) The osteoclast. Review of ultrastructure, origin, and structure-function relationship. Clin Orthop Rel Res 120:201–231

Hanaoka HB, Friedman B, Mack RP (1970) Ultrastructure and histogenesis of giant cell tumor of bone. Cancer 25:1408–1423

Hanaoka H, Yabe H (1985) A new concept of the origin and development of the osteoclast (abstract). Dept Orthop Surg School of Med, Keio University 35 Shinanomachi Shinjukuku, Tokyo 160

Hiddemann W, Roessner A, Wörmann B et al. (1987) Tumor heterogeneity in osteosarcoma as identified by flow cytometry. Cancer 59:324–328

Hogg N, Shapiro IM, Jones SJ, Slusarenco M, Bovde A (1980) Lack of Fc-receptors on osteoclasts. Cell Tissue Res 212:509–516

Horton MA, Rimmer EF, Lewis D, Pringle JAS, Fuller K, Chambers TJ (1984) Cell surface chracterization of the human osteoclast: phenotypic relationship to other bone marrow-derived cell types. J Pathol 144:281–294

Huvos A (1979) Bone tumors. Diagnosis, treatment, and prognosis. Saunders, Philadelphia

Isaacson P, Jones DB, Judd MA (1979) α_1-Antitrypsin in human macrophages. Lancet II: 964–965
Iwasaki H, Kikuchi M, Takii M, Enjoji M (1982) Benign and malignant fibrous histiocytomas of the soft tissues. Functional characterization of the cultured cells. Cancer 50: 520–530
Jee WSS, Nolan PD (1963) Origin of the osteoclasts from fusion of phagocytes. Nature 200: 225
Kasahara K, Yamamuto T, Kasahara A (1979) Giant cell tumor of bone: cytological studies. Br. J Cancer 40: 201–209
Katenkamp D, Stiller D (1981) Malignant fibrous histiocytoma of bone. Light microscopic and electron microscopic examination of four cases. Virchows Arch [A] 391: 323–335
Kindblom IG, Jacobsen G, Jacobsen M (1982) Immunohistochemical investigations of tumors of supposed fibroblastic-histiocytic origin. Hum Pathol 13: 834–840
Knowles DM, Iolidijiana B, Marboe C, D'Agati V, Grimes M, Chess L (1984) Monoclonal antihuman monocyte antibodies OKM 1 and OKM 5 possess distinctive tissue distributions including differential reactivity with vascular endothelium. J Immunol 132: 2170–2179
Kölliker A (1873) Die normale Resorption des Knochengewebes und ihre Bedeutung für die Entstehung der typischen Knochenformen. F.C.W. Vogel, Leipzig
Lawson CW, Fischer C, Gatter KC (1987) An immunohistochemical study of differentiation in malignant fibrous histiocytoma. Histopathology 11: 375–383
Loutit JF, Sansom JM (1976) Osteopetrosis of microphthalmic mice – a defect of the hematopoietic stem cell? Calcif Tissue Res 20: 251–262
Loutit JF, Nisbet NW (1982) The origin of the osteoclast. Immunobiol 161: 193 Clin Orthop 153: 92–105
Mason BY, Taylor CR (1975) The distribution of muramidase (lysozyme) in human tissues. J Clin Pathol 28: 124–132
Meister P (1984) Immunhistochemische Methoden bei der Diagnostik von Weichgewebstumoren. Pathologe 5: 90–98
Meister P, Nathrath W (1981) Immunohistochemical characterization of histiocytic tumors. Diagn Histopathol 4: 79–87
Motoi M, Helbron D, Kaiserling E, Lennert K (1980) Eosinophilic granuloma of lymph nodes – a variant of histiocytosis X. Histopathology 4: 585–606
Nash JRG (1982) Macrophages in human tumours: an immunohistochemical study. J Pathol 136: 73–83
Nathrath W, Meister P (1982) Lysozyme (muramidase) and α_1-antichymotrypsin as immunohistochemical tumour markers. Acta Histochem [Suppl] 25: 69–72
Oursler MJ, Bell LV, Clevinger B, Osdoby PH (1985) Identification of osteoclast-specific monoclonal antibodies. J Cell Biol 100: 1592–1600
Permanetter W, Meister P (1984) Distribution of lysozyme (muramidase) and α_1-antichymotrypsin in normal and neoplastic epithelial tissues. A survey. Acta Histochem 74: 173–179
Radzun HJ (1985) Immunhistochemie des menschlichen Mononukleär-Phagozytischen Systems. Immunohistochemical analysis of the human mononuclear phagocyte system. Gustav Fischer, Stuttgart
Radzun HJ, Parwaresch MR (1983) Differential immunohistochemical resolution of the human mononuclear phagocyte system. Cell Immunol 82: 174–183
Radzun HJ, Parwaresch MR, Feller AC, Hansmann ML (1984) Monocyte/macrophage-specific mononuclear antibody Ki-M-1 recognizes interdigitating reticulum cells. Am J Pathol 17: 441–450
Roessner A (1984) Zur Zyto- und Histogenese der malignen und semimalignen Knochentumoren. Gustav Fischer, Stuttgart
Roessner A, Hobik HP, Grundmann E (1979) Malignant fibrous histiocytoma of bone and osteosarcoma. A comparative light and electron microscopy study. Pathol Res Pract 164: 385–401
Roessner A, Zwadlo G, Vollmer E, Sorg C, Grundmann E (1987) Biologic characterization of human bone tumors. IX. Occurrence of macrophages. Pathol Res Pract 182: 336–343
Roholl PJM, Kleijne J, van Basten CFH, van der Putte SCJ, van Unnik JAM (1985) A study to analyze the origin of tumor cells in malignant fibrous histiocytomas. A multiparametric characterization. Cancer 56: 2809–2815
Schajowicz F (1961) Giant cell tumors of bone (osteoclastoma). A pathological and histochemical study. J Bone Joint Surg 43A: 1–7

Shen H, Talle MA, Goldstein G, Chess L (1983) Functional subsets of human macrophages defined by monoclonal antibodies: a distinct subset of monocytes containing the cells capable of inducing the autologous mixed lymphocyte culture. J Immunol 130:698–705

Steiner GC, Ghosh L, Dorfman HD (1972) Ultrastructure of giant cell tumor of bone. Hum Pathol 3:569–586

Talle MA, Allegar N, Makowski M, Rao PE, Mittler RS, Goldstein G (1983) Classification of human lymphocytes and monocytes with the OK series of monoclonal antibodies. Diagn Immunol 1:129–135

Todd RE, Biondi A, Roach JA (1985) Human macrophage antigens. In: van Furth R (ed) The mononuclear phagocytes. Characteristics, physiology and function. Martinus Nijhoff, Dordrecht

Tonna EA, Cronkite EP (1961) Use of tritiated thymidine for the study of the origin of the osteoclasts. Nature 190:459–463

Ugolini V, Nunez G, Smith RG, Stastny P, Capra JD (1980) Initial characterization of monoclonal antibodies against human monocytes. Proc Natl Acad Sci USA 77:6764–6768

Vollmer E, Roessner A, Gerdes J, Mellin W, Stein H, Chong-Schachel S, Grundmann E (1986) Improved grading of bone tumors with the monoclonal antibody Ki-67. J Cancer Res Clin Oncol 112:281–282

Yoshida H, Akeho M, Yumoto T (1982) Giant cell tumor of bone. Enzyme histochemical, biochemical and tissue culture studies. Virchows Arch [A] 395:319–330

Zwadlo G, Feige U, v. Bassewitz DB, Bröcker EB, Sorg C (1983) Monoclonal antibodies against human macrophages: distribution of macrophage subtypes in normal, inflammatory, and tumor tissue (abstract). Immunobiology 165:242

Zwadlo G, Bröcker EB, Bassewitz v. DB, Feige U, Sorg C (1985) A monoclonal antibody to a differentiation antigen present on mature human macrophages and absent from monocytes. J Immunol 134:1487–1492

Zwadlo G, Schlegel T, Sorg C (1986) A monoclonal antibody to a subset of human monocytes found only in the peripheral blood and inflammatory tissues. J Immunol (in press)

Subject Index

The numbers set in *italics* refer to those pages on which the respective catch-word is discussed in detail

AFP = α-fetoprotein 188, 191, 195, 199, 200, 201
APUD-system 14
α_1-AT = α_1-antitrypsin 208
α_1-ACT = α_1-antichymotrypsin 208, 212, 220
α_1-antichymotrypsin (α_1-ACT) 208, 212, 220
α_1-antitrypsin (α_1-AT) 208
α-fetoprotein (AFP) 188, 191, 195, 199, 200, 201
adenoma, pleomorphic 186, 198, 199
aggressive fibromatosis 95, *107*, 108, 110, 156
  osteoblastoma 122, 123, 124, 131, 146, 147
anaplastic osteosarcoma 42, 44, 47, 53, 68, 70, 71, 72, 73, 75, 77, 78, 81, 83, 84, *86*, 96, 97, 110, 123, 126, 129, 130, 132, 208, 209, 216
androgen receptors 159
aneurysmal bone cyst 95, *104*, 106, 110, 210, 212, 214, 224
angiosarcoma 94, 103
annulate lamellae 18, 22
antibodies against bovine osteonectin (bON) 32, 33, 42
    human osteonectin (hON) 32, 33, 42
avidin-biotin-peroxidase technique 2

bON = antibodies against bovine osteonectin 32, 33, 43
BrdU = bromodeoxyuridine 92
bone cyst, aneurysmal 95, *104*, 106, 110, 210, 212, 214, 224
    solitary 95, *104*, 110, 135
  dysplasia 133
  formation, enchondral *56*
    in osteosarcomas *66*
  metastases 94
  sialoprotein 49
  tumors, proliferation behavior *91*
bromodeoxyuridine (BrdU) 92

CEA = carcinoembryonic antigen 177, 188, 191, 194, 199, 200, 201
CK = cytokeratin 176, 177, 178
calcitonin 155
  receptors 155
callus 32, 35, 36, 37
carcinoembryonic antigen (CEA) 177
cartilage 36, 37, 38, 56, 57
  calcification 57, 80
  zones 56
catecholamines 11, 20
central osteosarcoma 95, 109
chondroblastic osteosarcoma 97, 123, 126, 129, 130, 132, 133, 208, 209
chondroblastoma 32, 42, 45, 52, 224
chondroblasts 38
chondroclasts 57
chondrocytes 37, 38, 56, 57
chondroid bone 36, 37
  chordoma *165, 173*
chondroitin sulfate 190, 198
chondroma 95, *107*, 110, *133*, 134, 146, 147, 170, 172, 173, 177, 185, 209, 224
chondromyxoid fibroma 32, 42, 185
chondrosarcoma 32, 42, 45, 52, *91*, 94, 98, 109, *133*, 140, 146, 147, 165, 168, 169, 170, *171*, 174, 176, 178, 179, 185, 198, 199, 201, 209, 224
  clear cell 171
  dedifferentiated 133, *134*, 135, 146, 171
  extraskeletal myxoid 173, 185
  low-grade *165*
  mesenchymal 97, 109, 170, 171
  myxoid 170, 171, 172, 173, 175, 185, 199, 201
  chorda dorsalis 140
chordoid sarcoma 173, 185
  tumor 173
chordoma 14, 94, *98*, 100, 109, *140*, 146, 147, 169, 170, 173, 174, 177, 178, *183*
  anaplastic 183
  chondroid *165*, *173*
  immunohistochemical investigation *183*
  periphericum 185
chromogranin 2, 13, 16
clear cell chondrosarcoma 171
collagen type II 56
columnar cell zone 60
concollagenous bone proteins (NCPs) *49*

cytokeratin (CK) 2, 6, 7, 13, 25, 176, 177, 178, 185, 186, 188, 190, 191, 193, 199, 200, 201

DNA index (DI) 116, 117
ploidy *116*
DOPCs = determined osteoprogenitor cells 52
dedifferentiated chondrosarcoma 133, *134*, 135, 146, 171
dermatan sulfate 190
desmin 23, 188, 191
desmoid 156
desmoplakin 8
desmoplastic fibroma 210, 224
determined osteoprogenitor cells (DOPCs) 52
dysplasia, fibrous 32, 38, 42, 95, *106* 110, 210, 224

EMA = epithelial membrane antigen 177, 188, 191, 195, 199, 200
ecchondrosis physaliphora 171
embryonal rhabdomyosarcoma 1, *20*
enchondral bone formation *56*
calcification 85
ossification 73
enchondroma 107, 133
enchondromas, multiple 133
enchondromatosis 107, 171
endolymphatic stromal myosis 156
ependymoma, myxopapillary 167, 199
epiphyseal growth plate *56*, *58*
epithelial membrane antigen (EMA) 177, 188, 191, 195, 199, 200
estrogen 155, 161
receptors 156, 157, 158, 159, 160, 162
estrophilin 161
Ewing's sarcoma *1*, *3*, 32, 42, 45, 68, 69, 92, 94, *97*, 99, 109, *144*, 146, 147, 210, 213, 224
after chemotherapy 213
atypical 4, 10
large cell 4
extraskeletal myxoid chondrosarcoma 173, 185
osteosarcoma *131*, 146
factor VIII-related antigen 5
fibroplastic osteosarcoma 42, 44, 48, 53, 97, 123, 126, 129, 130, 132, 208, 209
fibroblasts 36, 38
fibroma, chondromyxoid 32, 42, 185
desmoplastic 210, 224
nonossifying 135, 206, 209, 210, 213, 224
fibromatosis, aggressive 95, *107*, 108, 110, 156
fibronectin 197, 198, 199, 200
fibrosarcoma 32, 42, 94, 103, 133, 134, 135, *139*, 146, 210, 214, 224
fibrous dysplasia 32, 38, 42, 95, *106*, 110, 210, 224
histiocytoma, benign 95, 101, *107*, 109
histiocytoma, malignant 94, *99*, 101, 104, 109, 133, 134, 135, *138*, 146, 147, 168, 206, 210, 211, 213, 214, *217*, 224
osteoclasia 135

gAg = glycosaminoglycans 190, 191, 198
gFAP = glial fibrillary filament 16, 188, 191, 198, 199
germinative zone 59, 63
giant cells *205*
in osteosarcomas 209
reparative granuloma 135
tumors 115, *135*, 140, 146, 147
benign 95, 105
of bone *103*, 105, 110, *153*, 206, 209, 210, 212, 213, *214*, 215, *217*, 224
of bone, metastasizing 137
malignant 94, 105, 111
malignant, of soft tissue 138
glial fibrillary acidic filament (gFAP) 16
protein 178
glycogen 4, 5, 8, 13, 17, 19, 23, 25
glycosaminoglycans (gAg) 190, 191, 198
growth plate, epiphyseal *56*, *58*

hON = antibodies against human osteonectin 32, 33, 42
hemangioendothelioma, malignant 210, 224
histiocytoma, benign 95, 101, *107*, 109, 206
malignant 94, *99*, 101, 104, 109, 133, 134, 135, *138*, 146, 147, 168, 206, 210, 211, 213, 214, *217*, 224
classification (subtypes) 138
histiocytosis, malignant 222
Hodgkin's disease (lymphoma) 94, 100, 144, 145, 146
Homer-Wright type of rosettes 4, 12, 20
hyaluronic acid 190, 198
hydroxyapatite 31, 49, 50
hyperparathyroidism 135
hypertrophic zone 56, 61, 64, 65

iuxtacortical osteosarcoma 123, *130*, 132

Ki-67 *91*, 116, 141, 189, 193, 207, 219, 220, 221, 222, 223
keratin 2, 188

LCA 13, 23
leiomyosarcoma 32, 42
liposarcoma 140
myxoid 94, 100
lymphangiomyomatosis 156
lymphoma of bone 1, 25
malignant, of bone *143*, 146, 147
lysozyme 208, 220

MFH = malignant fibrous histiocytoma 94, *99*, 101, 104, 109, 133, 134, 135, *138*, 146, 147, 168, 206, 210, 211, 213, 214, *217*, 224
macrophages *205*
distribution in bone tumors *208*
malignant fibrous histiocytoma 94, *99*, 101, 104, 109, 133, 134, 135, *138*, 146, 147, 168, 206, 210, 211, 213, 214, *217*, 224
classification (subtypes) 138
giant cell tumor of soft tissue 138
hemangioendothelioma 210, 224
histiocytosis 222
lymphoma of bone *143*, 146, 147
osteoblastoma 131, 141
xanthogranuloma 138
medullary osteosarcoma 123, 132, 146
meningeal sarcoma 32
mesenchymal chondrosarcoma 97, 109, 170, 171
monocytes 208, 215, 224
multinucleated giant cells *205*
multiple enchondromas 133, 171
myeloma 94, 100, 109
myoglobin 23
myositis ossificans 32, 36
myxofibrosarcoma 138
myxoid chondrosarcoma 170, 171, 172, 173, 175, 185, 199, 201
extraskeletal 173, 185
liposarcoma 94, 100
myxopapillary ependymoma 167, 199

NCPs = noncollagenous bone proteins *49*
NOF = non-ossifying fibroma 206, 209, 210, 213, 224
NSE = neuron-specific enolase 2, 6, 12, 13, 14, 18, 25, 188, 191, 197, 199
neuroblastoma 4, *10*, 142
peripheral 12
neuroectodermal tumors *1*, *10*
neuroepithelioma 11
neurofibroma 156
neurofilaments 7, 13, 16, 25, 178, 199
neuron-specific enolase (NSE) 2, 6, 12, 13, 14, 18, 25, 188, 191, 197, 199
nidus 122
non-Hodgkin's lymphoma *23*, 143, 146
non-ossifying fibroma (NOF) 135, 206, 209, 210, 213, 224
notochord 166, 169, 170, 171, 177, 183, 185, 198, 199, 200
5′-nucleotidase 178

ossification, enchondral 73
osteoblastic osteosarcoma 42, 44, 46, 67, 68, 70, 71, 72, 73, 74, 77, 78, 79, 82, *85*, 97, 123, 126, 129, 130, 131, 132, 208, 209
osteoblastoma *122*, 131, 146, 147
aggressive 122, 123, 124, 131, 146, 147
malignant 131, 147
osteoblasts 32, 35, *38*, 46, *51*, 56, 57, 58, 73, 74, 77, 78, 205, 223
osteocalcin 49
osteochondroma 133
osteoclasia, fibrous 135
osteoclastoma (giant cell tumor) 146
osteoclasts 56, 57, 58, 74, 77, 78, 104, *124*, 205, 214, 216, 217, 223, 224
osteoclastlike giant cells in bone tumors *205*
osteocytes 58, 67, 68, 74, 77, 78
osteoid 32, 36, *38*, 45, 50, 67, 68, 79, 81, 84, 86, 87, 100, 123, 133, 140
osteoma 32, 42, 43, 122
osteonectin *31*
osteopontin 49
osteosarcoma 32, 34, 42, 44, 51, *55*, 94, *95*, 100, 104, 108, 111, 120, 122, *123*, 134, 135, 140, 142, 146, 172, 208, 210, 213, *214*, 224
anaplastic 42, 44, 47, 53, 68, 70, 71, 72, 73, 75, 77, 78, 81, 83, 84, *86*, 96, 97, 110, 123, 126, 129, 130, 132, 208, 209, 216
bone formation *66*
central 95, 109
chondroblastic 97, 123, 126, 129, 130, 132, 133, 208, 209
enzymatic activities *72*
extraskeletal *131*, 146
fibroblastic 42, 44, 48, 53, 97, 123, 126, 129, 130, 132, 208, 209
intramedullary 95, 109, 123, 132, 146
iuxtacortical 123, *130*, 132
medullary 95, 109, 123, 132, 146
osteoblastic 42, 44, 46, 67, 68, 70, 71, 72, 73, 74, 77, 78, 79, 82, *85*, 97, 123, 126, 129, 130, 131, 132, 208, 209
parosteal 68, 69, 70, 71, 72, 73, 74, 77, 78, 80, 81, 83, *86*, 94, 95, 97, 108, 109, 115, 121, 123, 130, 132, 146
periosteal 123, 130, 132, 146
small cell sclerosing 67, 69, 70, 71, 72, 73, 74, 77, 78, 79, 80, 81, 82, *86*
superficial 123, 130, 132, 146
teleangiectatic 97, 110, 123, 126, 129, 130, 132, 209
after chemotherapy *127*, 146

PNET = primitve neuroectodermal tumors *1*, *10*
parachordoma 173, 185
parathyroid hormone 155
parosteal osteosarcoma 68, 69, 70, 71, 72, 73, 74, 77, 78, 80, 81, 83, *86*, 94, 95, 97, 108, 109, 115, 121, 123, 130, 132, 146
pepsin digestion 2

periosteal osteosarcoma 123, 130, 132, 146
peripheral neuroblastoma 12
  primitive neuroectodermal tumors (PNET) *1*, *10*
pheochromocytoma, malignant 94, 102, 110
plasma cell myeloma 94, 100, 109
plasmacytoma 94, 100, 109
pleomorphic adenoma 186, 198, 199
preoperative chemotherapy 127, 128, 146
primitive neuroectodermal tumors, peripheral (PNET) *1*, *10*
progesterone receptors 156, 157, 159, 160, 162
proliferation behavior of bone tumors *91*
proliferative zone 56, 60, 61, 63
protease digestion 2
protein blot 32, *33*, 52
proteoglycans 49
pseudorosettes 4, 14

von Recklinghausen's disease 156
remodeling zone 58, 61
reparative granuloma, giant cell 135
resting zone 56, 61
rhabdomyosarcoma 14, 23, 24, 25, 32, 42, 94, 100, 134
  embryonal 1, *20*
rosette formation 12, 16, 17, 19
  like formations 4, 9
rosettes, Homer-Wright type 4

SC = secretory component 188, 191, 196, 199, 200

S 100 protein 2, 13, 15, 177, 188, 191, 196, 198, 199, 200
Schwann cell tumors 15
secretory component (sc) 188, 191, 196, 199, 200
small cell sclerosing osteosarcoma 67, 69, 70, 71, 72, 73, 74, 77, 78, 79, 80, 81, 82, *86*
solitary bone cyst 95, *104*, 110, 135
spindle cell sarcoma 168
steroid receptors *153*
stromal myosis, endolymphatic 156
superficial osteosarcoma 123, 130, 132, 146
synaptophysin 25
synovial sarcoma 94, *102*

teleangiectatic osteosarcoma 97, 110, 123, 126, 129, 130, 132, 209
tonofilaments 6, 8, 10
type-I collagen 31, 45, 49, 52
type III collagen 51

vimentin 2, 4, 5, 13, 15, 20, 24, 177, 186, 188, 191, 194, 199, 200, 201

Xanthogranuloma, malignant 138
xanthosarcoma 138
zone, columnar cell 60
  germinative 59, 63
  proliferative 56, 60, 61, 63
  remodeling 58, 61
  resting 56, 61
  of hypertrophy 56, 61, 64, 65
  of palisades 56

Index of Volumes 75–79 Current Topics in Pathology

Volume 75: The Human Thymus. Edited by H.K. MÜLLER-HERMELINK

B. VON GAUDECKER, The Development of the Human Thymus Microenvironment
G.G. STEINMANN, Changes in the Human Thymus During Aging
G. JANOSSY, M. BOFILL, L.K. TREJDOSIEWICZ, H.N.A. WILLCOX, M. CHILOSI, Cellular Differentiation of Lymphoid Subpopulations and Their Microenvironments in the Human Thymus
N. DOUROV, Thymic Atrophy and Immune Deficiency in Malnutrition
CH. NEZELOF, Pathology of the Thymus in Immunodeficiency States
H. WEKERLE, H.K. MÜLLER-HERMELINK, The Thymus in Myasthenia Gravis
H.K. MÜLLER-HERMELINK, M. MARINO, G. PALESTRO, Pathology of Thymic Epithelial Tumors

Volume 76: Neuropathology. Edited by C.L. BERRY

J.H. ADAMS, The Autopsy in Fatal Non-Missile Head Injuries
J.R. ANDERSON, Viral Encephalitis and Its Pathology
R.O. WELLER, A General Approach to Neuropathological Problems
C.L. SCHOLTZ, Dementia in Middle and Late Life

Volume 77: Morphological Tumor Markers. Edited by G. SEIFERT

G.L. WRIGHT JR., A.D. COX, Monoclonal Antibodies to Human Tumor Antigens
T.M. CHU, Immunohistochemical Markers for Human Cancer
H. DENK, Immunohistochemical Methods for the Demonstration of Tumor Markers
R. MOLL, Epithelial Tumor Markers: Cytokeratins and Tissue Polypeptide Antigen (TPA)
G. KLÖPPEL, J. CASELITZ, Epithelial Tumor Markers: Oncofetal Antigens (Carcinoembryonic Antigen, Alpha Fetoprotein) and Epithelial Membrane Antigen
T.O. ROGNUM, P.S. THRANE, F.R. KORSRUD, P. BRANDTZAEG, Epithelial Tumor Markers: Special Markers of Glandular Differentiation
W. ALTMANNSBERGER, M. OSBORN, Mesenchymal Tumor Markers: Intermediate Filaments

H.F. OTTO, R. BERNDT, K. SCHWECHHEIMER, P. MÖLLER, Mesenchymal Tumor Markers: Special Proteins and Enzymes
R.V. IOZZO, Proteoglycans and the Intercellular Tumor Matrix
J. CASELITZ, Basal Membrane Antigen as Tumor Markers
J. CASELITZ, Lectins and Blood Group Substances as "Tumor Markers"
PH.U. HEITZ, Neuroendocrine Tumor Markers
P. KLEIHUES, M. KIESSLING, R.C. JANZER, Morphological Markers in Neuro-Oncology
TH. LÖNING, K. MILDE, Viral Tumor Markers
I. DAMJANOV, Cell, Tissue and Organ Specific Tumor Markers: An Overview

Volume 78: Ovarian Pathology. Edited by F. NOGALES

I. DAMJANOV, Ovarian Tumours in Laboratory and Domestic Animals
H.-E. STEGNER, Hormonally Related Non-Neoplastic Conditions of the Ovary
L.L. ADCOCK, L.P. DEHNER, Surgical Staging of Ovarian Tumours: The Individual and Integrative Roles of the Oncologist and Pathologist
C. NUÑEZ, Cytopathology and Fine-Needle Aspiration in Ovarian Tumours: Its Utility in Diagnosis and Management
S.G. SILVERBERG, Prognostic Significance of Pathologic Features of Ovarian Carcinoma
H. FOX, The Concept of Borderline Malignancy in Ovarian Tumours: A Reappraisal
E. SAKSELA, Advances in Immunohistochemistry of Ovarian Tumours

Volume 79: Cell Kinetics of the Inflammatory Reaction. Edited by O.H. IVERSEN

O.H. IVERSEN, The Cell Kinetics of the Inflammatory Reaction. Introduction and Overview
H.B. BENESTAD, O.D. LAERUM, The Neutrophilic Granulocyte
I.C.M. MACLENNAN, S. OLDFIELD, Y.-J. LIU, P.J.L. LANE, Regulation of B-Cell Populations
G. JANOSSY, D. CAMPANA, A. AKBAR, Kinetics of T Lymphocyte Development
S. FOSSUM, The Life History of Dendritic Leucocytes (DL)
R. VAN FURTH, Origin and Turnover of Monocytes and Macrophages
D.O. ADAMS, T.A. HAMILTON, The Activated Macrophage and Granulomatous Inflammation
L. ENERBÄCK, K. NORRBY, The Mast Cells
J.L. VAN LANCKER, Molecular Events in Liver Regeneration and Repair

MIX
Papier aus verantwortungsvollen Quellen
Paper from responsible sources
FSC® C105338
FSC
www.fsc.org

If you have any concerns about our products,
you can contact us on
ProductSafety@springernature.com

In case Publisher is established outside the EU,
the EU authorized representative is:
Springer Nature Customer Service Center GmbH
Europaplatz 3, 69115 Heidelberg, Germany

Printed by Libri Plureos GmbH
in Hamburg, Germany